Alan Close has been in love, and had sex. He lives in and around Sydney.

Other books by Alan Close

The Romance of the Season (1989)

The Australian Love Letters of Raymond Chandler (1995)

Men Love Sex

Edited by Alan Close

VINTAGE

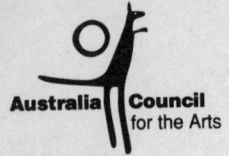

This project has been assisted by the Commonwealth Government through the Australia Council, its arts funding and advisory body.

A Vintage Book
published by
Random House Australia Pty Ltd
20 Alfred Street, Milsons Point, NSW 2061

Sydney   New York   Toronto
London   Auckland   Johannesburg
and agencies throughout the world

First published in 1995

Copyright © in this collection Alan Close 1995

Copyright © in individual stories remains with the authors

All rights reserved. No part of this publication may be reproduced, stored in a retrieval system, or transmitted in any form or by any means, electronic, mechanical, photocopying, recording or otherwise, without the prior written permission of the Publisher.

National Library of Australia
Cataloguing-in-Publication Data

Men, love, sex.

ISBN 0 09 183101 6.

1. Men - Attitudes. 2. Interpersonal relations. 3. Love.
4. Sex. I. Close, Alan, 1955- . II. Title.

305.31

Typeset by Midland Typesetters, Maryborough
Printed by Griffin Paperbacks, Adelaide
Production by Vantage Graphics, Sydney

10 9 8 7 6 5 4 3 2

For my father
John Frederic Campbell Close
born Sydney 1916
suburban hero, backyard warrior
big man of the seventeenth hole

CONTENTS

Introduction
Alan Close

This Is Our Secret 1
Steven Lang

When That Shark Bites 7
Mike Johnson

The Ten Dollar Ticket 27
Damien Lovelock

His Eternal Boy 39
Peter Wells

In Praise of Eva 51
Julian Davies

Dream Lovers 67
Archie Weller

Three Ways 79
Gerard Lee

Black Mud and Braille 95
James Cockington

Lovelawn: A Fantasy 103
David Owen

Japan 131
William Yang

My Feminine Side 147
Mark Mordue

Green Eyes 155
Angus Strachan

I Asked the Angels For Inspiration 161
Venero Armanno

Surrender 179
Roger McDonald

When a Man Realises He's Bad 189
John Birmingham

Running Hot and Cold 199
Chad Taylor

Baby Oil 209
Robert Drewe

Still 217
Christopher Cyrill

Natural Healing 225
Alan Close

Matchbooks 239
Matthew Condon

Ngomo Manza 265
Tom Carment

The Dark Stars 273
Clinton Walker

Whisper It 293
Jonathan Griffiths

Neighbours 297
Tim Winton

And Then a Funny Thing Happened 303
John Stapleton

Where the Mine Was 329
John Dale

Room 311 349
Lex Marinos

Ex-Wife Re-Wed 359
Frank Moorhouse

Upstream 383
Ian Beck

He Found Her In Late Summer 389
Peter Carey

The Ultimate Act of Living 405
Eric Rolls

Acknowledgements 421

List of Contributors 423

Introduction

A few years ago I was driving out of town with one of my good men friends, another writer, when one of the many small, incremental episodes of confusion took place which were, for me, the genesis of this book. We were heading north up the Pacific Highway, I was driving and we were talking easily. Around the Bulahdelah bends, a winding and heavily wooded section of the highway, I tried to turn the conversation to some particularly anatomical aspects of our sex lives and my friend went silent.

This is a man I have known for many years, as close a friend as I have got, another touchy, huggy 70s sort of guy, a funny and articulate man who I thought I could talk with about anything. I tried to understand what had happened. He had clammed up completely.

'What's wrong? What's the matter?' I flourished the wheel through the bends and looked across at him, trying to make eye contact. But he avoided my eyes—and I knew I had crossed The Line.

'Go on,' I pestered. 'What's wrong?'
'Nothing's wrong,' he said. 'Just ...'
'Yeah? Just what?'
'When you talk like that you sound like a woman.'
'Um ... Yeah?'
'Well ... it makes me feel uncomfortable.'
End of conversation.

Later we were making camp and because I'd organised the trip I was giving instructions—what I would have called offering information—about what we had to eat, how to erect the tent, where the wind would come from, that sort of thing. And again my friend went silent.

'What now?'

'When you talk like that,' he said, 'you make me feel like a woman.'

Since that day I think I have had this conversation—or lack of it—circled in my mind. 'Yes, must get back to that some time, must see what was really going on there.' Well, the time came. I found the opportunity to get my friend talking, to cross the line of male silence. He was one of the first men I asked to contribute to this book.

Like most books, this one started with questions, with a desire to sort a few things out. I was swimming one day (during another incremental bout of confusion), puzzling over some trouble I was having with my girlfriend, trying not to let my discomfort become panic, when I started wondering how other men dealt with such periods of emotional uncertainty in their relationships. Or—panic now!—if they even experienced them at all. My mind started turning over. How different, or how similar, are we? When it comes to love, to sex, to relationships, what, as men, do we share?

And I had the idea. Ask around. Gather some stories. Find out.

That's how this book came about. At first I was simply curious, voyeuristic. I wanted to find out how other men dealt with the issues of love and sex and gender which I feel so present in my life. I wanted to see if I was different from other men. I wanted to see what we had in common. I wanted, I suppose, to feel less alone.

It was only later, as I proceeded down the track, negotiating with publishers, enlisting contributors, talking to people, that I started to see where this book fitted in a wider context. I realised, for a start, that such a book—a collection of stories about love and sex, all by men, straight and gay—has never been done before, and that there was immense interest in reading the result.

(I should like to say here that because I am heterosexual I feel hesitant speaking about 'men' as a single gender when my experience only refers to relationships with women. But the gay men I have spoken to indicate that the issues they face with their partners often aren't that different from those that heterosexual men face with women. Our commonality is that we are men, our sexual leaning comes second.)

Every person I talked to thought this book was a good idea. It touched a nerve with both sexes. Repeatedly I was told by individual men that they felt neglected, overlooked and undervalued by the attention and opportunities available to women over the past decades. They felt silenced—just as women did before feminism. More than once men told me they had had the idea for such a book themselves. I had tapped into a wide vein of male frustration that I only suspected was there.

Women were interested for perhaps the opposite reason. Anything to get men talking seemed a good idea with them, anything to enter the hollow caverns of the great male silence, to start filling the huge empty space of knowledge.

The hunger was great to find out what men really do think about the whole business of love, sex, relationships. Women told me again and again *'Men don't talk'*.

Like air into a vacuum, the empty space is ready to be filled. A huge thing has happened—is happening—between men and women and this book is both timely and necessary. I wouldn't say it is long overdue—probably even five years ago the engine of change did not have up enough steam to carry such a book—but I would say now that this was a book waiting to happen.

'Men can't talk about their feelings.' 'Men aren't in touch with their emotions.' We hear this all the time—mostly from women. I would like to bounce back and defend my gender. 'Yeah, of course we talk. We just do it different to you.' But unfortunately I think it is true. I have a dozen women friends I can ring any time and chat with easily about the emotional goings-on in our lives, but with even my close men friends such conversation feels uncomfortable, if not out of bounds completely. Most men—and I include myself in this—simply aren't comfortable talking with other men about their inner feelings, their desires, their hopes, their fears—their business. I believe we need to.

I have realised, in retrospect, that what I was actually trying to do with this book was to get men *talking*.

From infanthood everyone develops systems of survival and adapts these to suit the challenges of growing up. We accumulate responses to our environment based on our biological makeup, our conditioning, and our experience—until, without our knowledge, these systems become our identity. But eventually this catches up with us, and most people reach a time in their lives when they realise that the fundamental way they have been used to thinking about themselves doesn't work anymore. The survival systems stop functioning. It is at this time that one confronts—often with great discomfort—how the blueprint from the past has created one's identity. Often, because many of us are still childless, this happens to the men of my generation in our thirties. We have what used to be called our mid-life crisis.

This, at least, is what happened to me. My systems started breaking down in my mid-thirties. My relationships weren't working. For several years I was non-specifically unhappy and didn't know why. Eventually, when things got bad enough, I started making enquiries, saw people, attended programs, and gradually pieced together the stories I had been telling myself of my life—who I was, why I did things, who I thought I was supposed to be.

For me a large part of this was circling around the business of what it meant to be a man, how this affected my relationships (with both men and women), and what were my attitudes to love and sex. I tried to understand where these attitudes had come from, and how I would change them if I could.

I came to the conclusion that I was anything but alone, that although of course I had my own particular circumstances, I fitted right into the great male predicament. I wasn't that different. I was, in fact, depressingly bloody typical. And I realised that the business of *being a man*, of *acting like a man*, of *manhood* was a straightjacket which I would have to somehow untangle myself from before it strangled me.

And I was lucky. I was born in 1955, I came of age in the 1970s, I was a member of the first feminist generation. The women of that generation have offered men the example that it is possible to examine and reassess and try to change what doesn't suit about being brought up with a certain gender conditioning. Men, I think, have a lot to thank feminism for. Feminism has given us our future.

Feminism has changed everything for men and women. Since those years there are no fixed landmarks in the landscape of sexual and emotional identity. What it means to be a man, what it means to be a woman at the end of the twentieth century—in this country at least—is becoming a matter of individual choice. The bastard offspring of choice is confusion, and there is no doubt (just look around) that we are a population cast adrift in gender confusion—but from confusion comes possibility. It is a necessary state to pass through on the way to change.

Men, I believe, are trapped in isolation. It is the bottom line, the essence, the poison of the male predicament and I am convinced that the only way out of it is to start talking, to ease ourselves into the understanding that we are not alone. This is the only way we will not remain trapped in our past.

The model of female friendships is sitting across a table, face to face, sharing. Men have friendships, of course, but our intimacy is shoulder to shoulder, side by side, not face to face. We *do* things together, but we find it difficult to simply *be* together. We remain trapped inside our skin bags, strapped into our straightjackets.

Women complain that they don't know where they stand with their men because men won't talk about their feelings. This isn't some kind of brute stubbornness, it is because most of us don't have the language. We don't know how to articulate our emotions. Men, on the surface, might not *want* to talk about these things, but most often we don't want to because we don't know how to. We're not taught to. In fact, we're taught *not* to. It is an integral part of our training as young boys to become grown men, especially old style Anglo-Celtic men. 'Don't display emotion,' we are told. 'It reveals weakness.'

Most men are familiar with only a narrow, masculine

sliver of themselves. We are comfortable with the expressions of masculinity, the 'hard' emotions, but an essential part of being a man is not letting our guard down on our soft, feminine side. Because of this we don't get to *know* these feelings, and they scare us. Men love facts and figures, we thrive on them. They order our lives. But feelings are unempirical and contradictory. They are hard to grasp, to enumerate and, often, to understand. They are, therefore, *unmanly*. And our feelings present us with uncertainty and vulnerability, and these are not socially prescribed masculine qualities. So we run from our feelings. We find some place to hide until the unpleasant sensations pass, and then go back into our habits. We go to the pub, we 'drink away our sorrows'.

Wittgenstein theorised that what you can't talk about doesn't exist. Because, as men, we can't speak of our feelings they don't exist for us. So, until we learn to talk, we remain excluded from ourselves. Language is the first, crucial stage of empowerment.

The conditioning and social construction of the feminine identity has been 'outed' conclusively over the past three decades, and men are merely at the start of the process which women put themselves through in the early years of feminism. Of hard self-examination, of addressing our own desires and needs and choices. Scratch through the layers of defensiveness, complacency and fear and I think many men—younger men especially—would agree that the way men are supposed to be does not work. And quietly, at their own pace, in their own lives, they are asking their own questions, trying to find what does.

The next twenty or thirty years will, I believe, see a great transition in male identity. And language is the key to this. We will find our own empowering language. Not necessarily the feeling-speak of women, and certainly not the impoverished grunting of our fathers, but a new hybrid which gives us our future, allows us to be comfortable with ourselves, to change.

Not that I said any of this to the men I asked to contribute to this book. Most of them probably would have told me to go pack it. I didn't want to set an agenda, to frame a picture—although perhaps I am doing that now. I wanted, simply, to hear some stories, to present a snapshot of where men are at now.

Love and sex. It's a broad canvas, a big ask. My brief to contributors was deliberately vague. I asked them to address issues which were relevant to them, for their stories to be personal and honest and heartfelt. I hoped each story would be a torch shining into the darkness, lighting its small corner of the big picture, illuminating the experience of being a man in love. Or out of love, or trying to love, or avoiding love. Or searching for love. Or loving too much. In some way dealing with the business.

Sex comes into it, of course. Scratch away at sex, I suggested, and pretty soon you get to all the other stuff: love, family, responsibility, women, kids—even jobs, money and mortgage. It's all there. Sex is the engine, love is the journey, death is the peace at the end.

As Raymond Carver might have said, 'We've all seen some things.' These were the things I wanted to get in this book.

The book isn't composed only of 'writers'. I asked actors, musicians, and artists. One of the stories comes from a bloke I ran into one night at a party. Another time I was in a taxi and I noticed the book the driver had on his dashboard. (It was—how could I not notice?—*Once Were Warriors*.) I looked across at his glasses and desk-dwelling pallor and knew he was one of us. We got talking, I told him about the book, he sent me some stories, and one of them is in here too.

I got on the phone to a man who reviews books in New Zealand. He gave me a list of names. I sent off letters and three of those stories which dropped in my mailbox in due course are here. I went back to writers I admired, to favourite stories from favourite books and some of them are here too.

The word got around and stories started arriving from people I'd never heard of. One batch arrived and I went through them but they didn't read true. The voice was off, as if the writer was writing the way he thought he should, rather than how he wanted to. I sent them back. Later, by letter, the writer revealed herself to be a woman. I felt vindicated, but wouldn't have minded being fooled. Perhaps it would have proved some sort of point. She would, at any rate, have had an interesting time at the launch.

One day a story arrived from Tasmania. I read the first paragraphs and my heart sank. It was science fiction. I hate science fiction. And how could anyone pull off a sci-fi story, complete with weird jargon and wacky names, about matters of the heart? But this writer did. It is an astute and funny story. And sci-fi, after all, is one of the established male playgrounds. Men love gadgets. That story is in the book.

What we have ended up with is, I think, an extraordinary collection, an amazing range of voice, style and content. Young men, old men, family men, single men, straight men, gay men. In the end the makeup of a book like this comes down to personal taste and I would like to acknowledge all those writers who offered contributions which did not, in the final selection, make it in. Ain't no party without guests—thank you all for coming.

A hundred people make a book, and for the support and attention they have given this book, and for the good humour which was always present, I would like to extend special thanks to Jane Palfreyman and Julia Stiles, and to everyone else in the back rooms at Random House.

But most importantly, of course, there would be no book without those men whose stories you are about to read. This is their book, their voices, their achievement. Thanks guys. Good talking to you. It's been a hoot.

Alan Close
Maianbar
July, 1995

This Is Our Secret
Steven Lang

I am alone, without even the dog. I climb the back fence and cut across the new-mown field to the farmyard, between the white-washed buildings, over the muck-covered cobbles, past the stinking byre and the lowing cattle. A little gravel road leads down to the railway line, dipping under it at a bridge made of red bricks. Brambles grow up the side of the embankment there, but the fruit is not as good as those further along near the station. Even though I am expressly forbidden, I once walked all the way along the track. For the last half-mile the line is in a cutting carved out of the rock and there is hardly room to get out of the way of trains.

After the bridge the road divides into two. One way, towards town, leads to the sewage works with its smells and odd trapeze-like structures that turn, slowly dribbling water onto large round circles of gravel. The other way leads to a field and then peters out. It is shady between the high railway embankment and the trees on the other side of the road. I go down to the field and walk along the edge of the wood until I come to the water. There used to be a bridge at that point and its metal girders are still stretched across the top of the water like lengths of railway line. It's possible to cross the river there, if you're brave and if the metal is not too slippery. On the other side the pine forest starts.

Even the river is quiet here, forming a long clear pool under the bridge. Trout hang motionless in the stream. My father knows how to guddle trout. He says they like places where the bank overhangs the water. You find somewhere like this and crawl over to it on your belly (because they can see your shadow even from under the surface) then very slowly you put a hand into the water and wait and watch. If you are very still the fish will come to you, and if you're patient you can grab them behind the gills. I tried it but couldn't keep still for long enough. I like to sit on the metal girders and watch the fish, hanging in the water in threes or fours or fives, dark fish, brown trout. The water is clear and the bank, covered in pine needles, comes neatly to its edge.

Further into the forest an old canal leads to a small loch. There is a lock gate on the canal and lily pads on the loch. No-one goes to these places except me and my father's dog. The little loch with its overhanging trees has been forgotten, but someone must have made it because it has a dam wall and a sluice gate which lets the water run back into the river again. The sluice gate is rusted shut. The loch would be no good to fish because of the lily pads. It is round and still and there is something unappealing about the water. I do not swim in it.

Mostly I come here by myself, although very occasionally I come with friends. It is possible to come in from the other side on bicycles and we have done this, playing games in the rhododendrons which line the driveway. It is all part of The Estate.

There is a man in the forest today. He is dressed in an

old coal worker's coat and thick baggy trousers, black leather boots and a dirty white shirt. He is unshaven and mysterious. He strikes up a conversation with me, walking along between the trees with his hands in his pockets, the flaps of his jacket held back by his arms.

'I work on the Council,' he says, but does not specify further.

He talks about women. He wants to know if I've had a woman yet and tells me about the women he's been with. I am shocked and intrigued, drawn by his candour. The women in his stories seem to want to do it with men whereas up until this time everything I have heard has seemed to suggest that women don't like this sexual business, that they only consent to do it with men reluctantly, or out of love.

I am excited by his talk and affect a knowledge of these matters I do not have concerned to appear a man of the world.

After a time he says,
'Here, d'you want to know what I've got in my pocket?'
'Okay,' I say.
'Guess,' he says.
'I don't know, cigarettes?'
'No, they're up here.'
He pats the breast pocket of his jacket with his free hand.
'What do you think I've got in this one here?'
'Money,' I say.
'No.'
'Sweets.'
'No.'
'I give up.'
'You wanta feel for yourself?'

I do not know about this, but at the same time I do not want to say no to this man. He talks to me like I am an equal, not a child, telling me his stories about women. So I come up beside him and he takes his hand out of the pocket of his dark blue trousers which have a thin white pinstripe to them. I put my hand in. His penis is right there, hard and soft and silky skinned all at the same time. I pull my hand out and jump away. The touch of his intimate skin is electric, frightening, fascinating, weird.

He laughs.

'That fooled you,' he says, but it is not true. I realise I had been expecting this.

He leans back against a tree.

'D'you want to see it?' He doesn't wait for an answer. He undoes the buttons on his fly and exposes himself to me. He has a big penis, a great thick uncircumcised thing which he strokes with his right fist, pulling the foreskin back off its head and then letting it slip forward again. I have seen lots of penises at school but nothing like this. It is enormous, a broad stump, a man's equipment.

He is pleased with my awe and becomes very coarse in his language. He says he can't get a frenchie to fit him, he is so big. He says he had a woman last week who was too tight and she'd split open while he was giving it to her. He laughs again.

I laugh too, but this sort of talk scares me. That such things are possible, or even desirable, seems horrific, terrifying. I have never seen a vagina, except my sister's, when we were small, but I imagine them to be extremely sensitive things. My mind often wanders into the realms of torture; I think of the soldiers in the war who were tortured and I wonder how I would bear it. I lie in my bed in the dormitory at school and shudder at the idea of things being pushed under my fingernails, of endless drops of water falling on my forehead and feeling as though they were boring into me, worst of all, of being strapped down over fast-growing bamboo so that its points push slowly up through my flesh.

But I can never bear to imagine the injuries which people might inflict on each other in the place between their legs, of the things men might do to this frail part of other men, or of the things they might choose to use to fill with pain this mysterious vacancy of women. Surely these are left alone, surely there are some safe places.

But I do not want to seem ignorant in front of this man, so I laugh. During the summer I had seen a boy wank himself until he ejaculated. I tell him this.

'Show us yours then,' he says.

I need no further invitation. I open my trousers and pull out my penis, a thin slender thing beside this man's stout trunk. It is almost hard and I pump it to make it appear as big as possible.

The man stays leaning against the tree milking himself.

'D'you want to touch it then?' he says.

I go over to him and reach out tentatively to hold it, fascinated but also slightly revolted. His voice has become very strange.

'Move it a bit then,' he says, and I do, holding it gingerly between thumb and forefinger. But I cannot keep going. I step away again and he takes over in my stead, wanking himself until he comes, his semen spilling on the pine needles, thick and white.

I want him to know that I can do the same so I rub myself vigorously, but cannot come. When at last it happens nothing comes out of the end.

'Don't you worry about it,' he says. 'It'll happen soon enough.'

But quite suddenly it is not my failure to produce semen which disturbs me. I am possessed of a profound shame. This shabby man with his unshaven face and undone fly fills me with disgust. The whole business disgusts me. I am ashamed. I want to escape.

He is telling me some other story but I interrupt and tell him I have to go, that my mother is expecting me.

'Here,' he says, 'don't go telling anyone about this now. This is our secret.'

'Of course not,' I say, horrified at the prospect of my mother or father discovering what has happened, and my complicity in it.

'Good-bye,' I say and walk away until I have put a little distance between us, then I start to run. I cross the metal bridge, glad that he will be unable to follow.

I am sorry it happened in my pine forest, which was mine alone, no-one else's, a pure place, now sullied.

When That Shark Bites
Mike Johnson

It was seeing Shona Blake that gave Parker the idea.

We kids had been sent off up the beach away from the adult party to chase each other around playing tag; mostly it was Parker and I chasing the screaming Tessa Hinds so we could touch her somewhere with Rebecca Langdon getting red in the face trying to trip her up for us, and Jumbo Jim lumbering around as an afterthought. Parker and I wanted to get Tessa down on the sand so we could tickle her, but she had long flying legs she was always showing off and could run almost as fast as a boy.

We'd just got her down when a girl I'd never seen before came wandering over from the adult group. She stood a little way off and watched us shyly. I got the impression of an oval face and long, shiny hair blowing in the sun. Parker and I both jumped off Tessa.

'Shona!' Rebecca shrieked, and ran over to her.

Tessa Hinds got to her feet, giggling and smoothing down her frock. Rebecca Langdon had already taken her friend in tow and was talking close to her ear the way girls do.

I looked at the new girl and she looked at me. Then I looked somewhere else, maybe at Jim who was eyeing the surf or maybe at Tessa Hinds' legs, and when I looked back she was still looking at me. Her brown eyes had these long dark lashes she somehow held absolutely steady. Her skin was creamy and lightly freckled.

'This is Shona Blake,' Rebecca said in a possessive voice. 'Her parents have just arrived for the wedding.'

'Hello,' said Parker in a very friendly voice.

She said something and I said something at the same time; she had a throaty, scratchy voice, like an adult. There was an awkward pause as we listened to the braying of our parents out in the water.

'Didja want t' play tag?' Parker asked the new girl.

But Rebecca put her bossy arm through Shona's and took her off up the beach; after a quick look at Parker and me, Tessa followed them.

'She's hot,' Parker said, watching the girls. There was a hard, narrow look on his face. I agreed with him but didn't feel like saying so. Being the bridegroom's son by a former wife, while I was only a visitor for a week or so, Parker had the kingpin position; he knew the run of the house, where the biscuits were stored, where his father kept his condoms and live .22 shells and where his mother-to-be kept her black lacy knickers. He'd even promised to steal the .22, go up the beach and shoot some seagulls.

Then Jim, Parker and I hit the water and rolled around in the surf. The cool, fizzy water made my body tingle.

'Hey,' Parker said, coming up out of a wave, his pale body sleek and fish-like. 'Let's get the girls to play spin-the-bottle. We can take them to the sandhills down the end of the beach.' He gave me a big wide grin, more like a grimace.

'I don't want to take my clothes off,' Jim said. He was like a ponderous whale in the water.

'You will, though,' Parker said. 'It's as easy as feeling up Tessa Hinds.' Jim wallowed away, pretending to go for a wave.

'He's chicken,' I said, seeing the girls coming back along the beach. Parker saw them too.

'He's a goose,' Parker said. 'But you're not chicken, are you?'

'No,' I said. Even from a distance I could see that Shona was looking out towards us. Parker gleefully knifed his hand through the water as if it was the fin of a shark.

Rebecca and Shona were sitting on the sand when we came out of the water, Rebecca talking frantically behind her hand. I thought she was talking about me and was bothered about that because Rebecca hardly knew me at all. Tessa was sitting a little way off, busy pouring sand over her legs.

We were just about to join them when I got shy and sheered away; Parker wasn't bothered though and went right up and sat beside Shona whose pleated yellow skirt made a pattern like a shell on the sand around her. I felt pretty stupid standing there with nothing to do so I pretended to talk to Jim. Parker was going for it, throwing his body around, talking and laughing and making himself generally entertaining; Shona was listening and nodding and sometimes laughing but her eyes were on me the whole time. No matter which way I turned I could feel them. I thought about spin-the-bottle and felt naked with just my bathing costume on. Jim said something stupid, and I said something stupid back.

The adults started packing up and Uncle Owl shambled over to us. He was already half-pissed with a silly grin on his face which he was unsuccessfully trying to wipe off on the back of his hand. Even on the beach he was wearing the same dowdy brown suitcoat that he wore on the farm. He had this lopsided walk, as if one leg was shorter than the other.

'You kids git yourselves on t' the ute,' he said. Then he leered across at the girls. 'What's all these secrets then?'

'I'm going t' be a bridesmaid,' Rebecca said.

Uncle Owl snorted, 'You'll be lucky.'

Parker and I scrambled onto the ute together, him going to one side and me the other. Shona came up and sat beside me, pushing in close to make room for the hefty Rebecca. I took this as a good sign, and tried to think of something to say to her.

Dad was already powering up the ute while the other adults piled into cars. Betty, Parker's mother-to-be, went past still in her bathing costume. Dad leaned out the window and whistled. 'You keep your eyes on the road, Tom,' she said. I looked at Parker and he rolled his eyes. Through the window I could see the back of Mum's head locked in disapproval mode. At the same time I heard her laugh.

On the other side of me, Jumbo Jim sat upright and solemn like some kind of totem. When we went around corners the totem just stayed upright and Shona was pushed against me or me against her. My head kept swivelling around to look at her, and I could feel the softness of her against my thigh and hip as if it were the most important thing my body could feel. She looked at me just as often. Her eyes were big and clear and brown; a full face and a mouth shaped like a heart. I could only face her for a few seconds at a time. I asked her where she was staying.

'At the Langdons',' she said in her throaty voice. I didn't know where to put my awkward legs except keep them away from Tessa's.

Dad took a pretty sudden turn, Shona's head banged against me and her thick, light-coloured brown hair spread all over my shoulder. I caught a scent, something deep and sweet. She stayed that way, briefly, head on my shoulder, even when the ute had righted itself. When she did pull away a couple of shiny strands were left on my shirt. Then it occurred to me that she was short, much shorter than she'd seemed on the beach. I furtively looked to see if she was sitting lower than me but she wasn't; I couldn't understand it and I got confused and couldn't think of anything more to say. Also I was getting distracted by Tessa's cynical looks and the way Parker was eyeing Shona up and down.

Back at Parker's house there were more adults and little kids running around everywhere. Some of the men were digging a pit in the back garden where the meat and potatoes would be cooked the next day. Jumbo Jim went home and the girls went next door to the Langdons'. A little later Parker took me aside, all business.

'Tomorrow night, at the sandhills.' He gave me a knowing look.

'Have you asked the girls?' I could see them over the fence going through the Langdons' front door. Before she went through Shona looked over at us and I'm sure she was looking at me; there was a question in her face.

'I've talked to Tessa. She's going to talk to the rest of them.'

'Rebecca will talk them into it.'

'She thinks Jim's good-looking,' Parker said with disgust, adding 'I hope that new girl comes. Did you see those boobs of hers?'

Quickly I said, 'When will we go?'

'After the wedding, when the oldies are all pissed.'

It looked like that wouldn't be long. There were mattresses all over the floors in the house and crates of beer stacked everywhere. Just outside the kitchen Parker's father George was loudly bragging about something to Dad, who was going red in the cheeks and squinty around the eyes from drinking. In the kitchen Mum and Betty were at the bench making club sandwiches. Mum was cutting the crust off the bread with quick ruthless movements. I kept moving in case I was given a job.

Back in the boys' room, Parker kept talking about Shona all the time, about how big her tits were, saying her name often, getting his foul mouth used to it. While he wasn't looking I took the strands of hair off my shirt and put them under my pillow.

Later that night while the adults were partying on, Parker and I got dressed and made it out the back window to the street.

'Did you really feel Tessa up?' I asked him.

'I told y', didn't I?'

'Will she go further?'

He tapped his index finger against his teeth. 'She might,' he said distractedly. 'I can't wait to get my hands on Shona's big tits.' He gave me a sudden, fierce look.

I got away from him, went to the beach and waded in the sand around the rocks and watched the black waves surging between them. They made a sucking, frothing sound. I wanted to write Shona a note or something, maybe a poem. It was a thrill to imagine her opening up a piece of paper and reading something I'd written. I sat on the beach and tried to think of a poem but the words were harder to get than the feeling.

The adults played jazz, Louis Armstrong, all night, especially 'Mack the Knife', Dad's favourite song; it had to be him putting it back on all the time ...

You know when that shark bites
with his teeth dear

scarlet billows start to spread ...

The next morning I got up before Parker and wrote the poem I'd tried to write the night before. It didn't come out much better except for one line I liked. *My fingers play among your shining skin.* I knew *among* was wrong and I didn't properly understand what I meant, but it sounded quite sleek.

All I needed was an opportunity to give it to her, but once Parker was up he stuck to me like glue. To complicate matters the adults were all in a fluster getting ready for the wedding and every now and again a bunch of instructions would be floated our way; we were supposed to be finding clean shirts and looking after the little kids and all sorts of things. I saw Dad talking earnestly to George, who was looking morose and drinking already; apparently the bride and groom were not on speaking terms this morning.

I got my chance when Betty came over and started giving orders to Parker. She had dark hair with a small, pale face and spoke in a hard, flat voice; I'd often heard Mum say how pretty she was. All the while she spoke Parker didn't look at her but stared straight ahead with a bored expression; she'd been living in for three years and he'd heard it all before. After he'd gone I asked Mum if I could take something over to the Langdons'. She was cutting things up again, the knife flashing down on the cutting board so close to her fingers I thought she was going to chop them up too. She gave me a pile of stuff to take over for the girls and I was lucky enough to see Shona as soon as I walked in the door.

'I'm going to be a bridesmaid too and wear a white dress,' she said, excited. She had a trick of being able to pull back her eyebrows and make her eyes bigger. When she did that and laughed at the same time her whole pretty face came out at you. I didn't know what to say, so I gave her the poem on a piece of paper folded up lots of times.

'I wrote it last night,' I said, feeling stupid, 'when I was on the beach.' She opened it up right then and there, and, as she read it, the blood crept up her neck and face. The freckles on her arms came up like gold flecks. I wondered if she'd got to the good line. Then she hugged the poem to her chest, gave me a quick, wide-eyed look, turned and ran off.

Back at Parker's, we watched the adults put the hot stones in the pit and the foil-wrapped food on top.

Parker was brooding. 'You might have to help with Jim,' he said. 'We can't let him chicken out.'

'Sure,' I said.

'I can hold him down while you get his underpants off.'

'Sure,' I said.

We watched the adults shovel earth back over the food until there was nothing left of the pit but a warm patch of ground.

The wedding was pretty boring. I just waited for time to pass. All the adults had these cheesy grins on their faces and there was a lot of moaning and droning and standing around. It didn't do much for Parker either; getting a new mum didn't seem to be impressing him greatly. In the bridal procession Shona walked right past me in her white dress, her eyes shining as if she were the bride. I worked out that she looked tall because of the upright way she carried herself. She gave me a quick, shy look.

After the wedding things soon went back to normal. The adults got into drinking and shouting and laughing as if they'd been holding it all in for hours. They dug up the steaming food which smelled of clay and stood around the pit stuffing their faces and making speeches. Betty and George were standing together all lovey-dovey.

I found Parker twisting Jim's arm halfway up his back.

Jim looked so scared I thought his eyes were going to fall out. Later we slipped away to the beach. Parker was carrying a knapsack but wouldn't let us see what was in it.

'Are you ready to get your gear off for the girls?' Parker said to Jim.

'I told you I didn't want to,' Jim said in a weak voice. His face turned white and blobby. 'I'll tell my father.'

'He'll tell his father,' Parker said to me as if I couldn't hear. He turned back to Jim. 'Don't worry, Jim, you won't be the only one, we'll all be getting our clothes off.'

'Will we?' I said, sickened by the queasy look on Jim's face.

'Of course we will,' Parker said.

'I thought we were playing for kisses,' I said, thinking of Shona's small, plump mouth.

Parker just curled his lip.

The girls didn't arrive until near dark. We didn't say much when we met up. Shona and I could hardly look at each other but could hardly look anywhere else either. I kept thinking of her quick fingers unfolding my poem. Parker led us along the top of the sandhills; we moved in single file and I was right behind Shona, admiring the way her small, neat body bobbed up and down. Once, from the top of a dune, she stopped and looked back at me, smiling, which made me smile too. After that we could look at each other and every time we did we smiled to make it easier.

Parker stopped and pointed dramatically out to sea. We all saw it, a shark's fin moving with fastidious calm through the swells not far from the beach. The swells were dark and the shark moved through them the way things can move in twilight, smooth and silent and only half in the world. 'Shit,' said Parker. 'And we went swimming today.'

Shona looked at me with big round eyes. I thought of Parker's hand sliding through the water.

'Hey,' Jim said, looking back. There was someone coming up the beach. I could tell from the lopsided walk it was Uncle Owl.

'D'you think he's following us?' I said to Parker.

'Fuckin' old pervert,' Parker said.

Tessa giggled, shook her blonde curls and put her hand to her mouth. Shona moved closer to me, her bare arm brushing mine. The fair, delicate hairs on her arm were standing up.

When we looked back out to sea, the shark was gone.

After that we ran, flying up and down the sandhills until we got right away from where the houses ended. Parker took us to a deep shady hollow hidden by dense marram grass. I sat down on the cool sand and Shona sat down beside me. Wisps of long hair floated over my shoulders. When I looked at her she gave me a big cheeky grin that changed her face and made her look like a tomboy. Parker plonked himself down on the other side of Shona, opened his knapsack and took out two small boards and two bottles, one empty and one full. We all watched while he solemnly flipped the lid of the full one.

'We're going to play spin-the-bottle,' he announced grandly as if none of us knew, smoothing down a mound of sand for the two boards. He sounded like the minister at the wedding.

'What do we have to do, if it points to us?' Rebecca asked, watching the empty bottle spin happily on the boards.

'Take off a piece of clothing,' Parker said, adopting the tones of a teacher explaining something to the class.

'What about going off with somebody to the next hollow?'

'That comes afterwards,' Parker said.

There was a silence during which the moment of consent

passed by without notice. I figured since none of us was wearing much it was going to be a short game.

Assuming the right to first go, Parker leaned forward, his jaw working tensely and, with a triumphant flourish, spun the bottle. Everybody watched the turn of their fate and thought about their underpants. Parker drank. The bottle did several full turns and ended up pointing back at himself. He looked at it, frowning.

'That means *you* have to take something off,' Rebecca said. Parker took off his T-shirt and I saw he was wearing a singlet he hadn't been wearing before.

It was Shona's turn; she took a swig of beer and gave the bottle a quick flick. Jim moaned when he saw it settle on him. 'Just get on with it,' Parker said in his teacher tones.

'He means get off with it,' Rebecca said and everybody giggled. Jim took off his shirt; his chest was white and flabby in the half-light.

It was my turn and I came up with Tessa. Calmly she took off her blouse; she had nothing underneath and everybody looked at her breasts, which were small and pale and high on her chest. She didn't mind leaning back on her hands and giving us a good look. Shona tried to catch my eye but I avoided her gaze. Tessa gave me a mocking look.

'She hardly has any,' Rebecca said in an undertone.

'It's not fair, I didn't have a bra,' Tessa said when Shona's turn came to take off her blouse. She was pale and soft-shouldered and there were gentle curves at the back of her neck. Her bra carried a visibly full load.

Poor Jim was the first to get down to his underpants. Parker had to twist his arm to get his shorts off. He sat with his legs crossed and his body bent forward. He was so scared it made everybody tense. The next turn brought Rebecca to her knickers. She had large, bouncy breasts which pointed off in different directions.

'Like a cow,' Tessa said.

My T-shirt came off, and I was aware of how my brownish skin glowed dark in the fading light, and how Shona kept sneaking glances at me. The turn after that saw Shona's bra come off. She had full, dipping breasts with large dark nipples. She let us have a look then covered them with her arm.

So Parker got his eyeful. When his turn came he grabbed the bottle and spun it with a fixed, feverish quality. When Jim copped it he immediately started bleating, accusing Parker of doing it deliberately. Parker ordered him to shut up, grabbed hold of his arm and twisted it. Jim started to struggle and Parker ordered me to come and pull down his underpants. I didn't like the tone in his voice so I didn't move. When I failed to jump Parker looked across from me to Shona and back again with a bleak look; when he looked at me he could see the betrayal in my face and when he looked at Shona she looked right back, her head held high in her 'tall' look, daring him to say something.

An ugly look came over his face. He turned to Jim and gave his arm a couple of vicious twists. Jim screamed in falsetto. 'I surrender,' he said.

'I'll do it,' Rebecca said, getting up.

'No,' Jim wailed, and, shaking, took down his briefs; he nearly fell over when he had to stand on one foot. His balls were already quite dark with hair and his cock, although shrivelled up in fear, was still big. It all hung at awkward angles. He quickly tried to cover himself up, but Parker knocked his hands away.

'Keep playing,' he commanded, keeping one hand on Jim's arm.

When Shona was knocked down to her knickers she didn't stand up to take down her skirt but wriggled out of it on the sand. Although she was deep-breasted, her hips were small and pert, her legs neatly shaped and her ankles slim.

'Perhaps I can help you?' Parker said.

'I can do it, thanks,' she said, not looking at him.

Rebecca was the first girl to go. The rest of us were holding out in our briefs. When the moment came, the bossy Rebecca was suddenly shy. She turned her back to take down her last bit; she had a solid body with big buttocks and thighs, and the light, curly hair she was growing didn't hide the swelling between her legs. She stared back aggressively at anyone who looked too hard at her, especially Tessa, but she didn't try to hide herself.

Tessa was next and she didn't make any fuss but crossed her legs when she sat down. Then Parker got his and he made a show out of it, standing up and facing us, dropping his briefs and pushing forward his hips so we could all see his cock standing out rigid from between his legs like some tense little animal. Tessa made the kind of sound girls make when they're trying not to laugh. I tried to catch Shona's eye but she wouldn't respond. Parker gave her a superior look. 'Let's play pairs now,' he said.

'It's not fair,' Rebecca said. She gestured to Shona and me. 'They're not naked yet.'

'It doesn't matter,' Parker said. His voice had gone hoarse. With a savage movement he bent over and spun the bottle. When it stopped at Jim everybody laughed. 'I get another turn,' Parker said, and spun again. This time he came up with Rebecca.

'Come on then,' she said, getting up. Parker looked desperate.

'Let's just all feel each other up,' he said.

'We've got to play properly,' Rebecca said.

'It takes too long,' Parker said, his eyes sliding around all the time towards Shona.

'It's my turn,' Shona said, taking the bottle firmly, closing her eyes and spinning it. When she opened them again the bottle was pointing at me. Tessa Hinds let out a long hiss. Parker picked up the bottle and looked at it as if it were the bottle's fault. He took a long drink from the full one.

Shona stood up, 'Michael and I get to pair,' she said to Parker. It was the first time she'd used my name and in her mouth it sounded like somebody different.

'And so do we,' Rebecca said to Parker.

'We're not playing properly,' Tessa said, not looking at the pathetic Jim.

We left them arguing. Shona took my hand and we slipped through a cleft in the dunes to the next hollow. She quickly took off her briefs and I did the same. We tucked up under a big lupin and she took my hands in hers. Shy and solemn, we sat that way for a moment, very naked.

'That was a wonderful poem,' she said, a tremor in her voice. 'No-one's ever written me a poem.' She put her hand around my neck and rubbed her arm against my cheek. Her freckles had gone dark, making her skin look mysterious. There was a humid odour coming off her body.

I touched her breasts which were the softest things I'd ever touched. I cupped them in my palm and stroked the upper slopes with my thumb. Her nipples swelled up when I played with them. She ran her hands over my face and chest, her fingers feeling everywhere, took my hand, placed it between her legs, and I touched something even softer; warm and swollen and as slippery as the flesh of a shellfish. I remembered the line I'd written, *My fingers play among you shining skin*, and realised that *among* wasn't wrong at all, but exactly right. Then she rubbed my cock so gently I seemed to feel the slide of it on the inside of my skin. At the same time she put her head on my shoulder and sucked at the soft flesh on my neck, making my body tingle the way it had in the water.

'You'll write another poem, won't you,' she said. 'Promise?' I promised, and we lay quietly touching each other and kissing with our tongues. Her mouth tasted the way she smelt. When I slipped my fingers up into her silky moistness she gasped and wriggled her hips around and bit hard into my neck. We both stopped when we heard something. It was like the cry of a child or a seagull; although it sounded far away it had a piercing, lonely quality. 'That's Tessa,' Shona whispered, gripping my arm, but I wasn't sure.

The shadow, when it fell, slid right across the sand in front of us. 'There's someone there,' I whispered.

We grabbed our briefs and scuttled back to the other hollow. Jim was lying on the sand with Rebecca bent over him sucking at his cock which stood out thickly from his body as if it had been transplanted there from another creature. His face was all putty.

Tessa was on her back too, her legs splayed at awkward angles, while Parker jerked around on top of her, holding her arms above her head. As soon as he saw us he jumped off her and made straight for Shona. Planting himself in front of her, he reached out and started fingering her breasts. She waited for a moment as if she were going to let him, then slapped his face. He stood his ground as if he might slap her back, then turned away.

Tessa was sobbing. 'I didn't want to,' she said, pulling in her breath as if she were hiccupping. 'I didn't want to go all the way.'

'There's someone here,' I said to Parker. 'An adult.'

It took a moment to register. Then he swung around, his eyes on the now moonlit sandhills; his cock swung around ferret-like after him as if it too were joining the search.

There were significant shadows everywhere. 'Scatter,' he barked.

There was a mad scramble for clothes and we all scattered. Only Jim didn't move fast. He just lay there after Rebecca jumped off him, his cock hanging at a sad, bloated angle. I stayed with Shona, and near home we caught up with Tessa who was walking along the street alone. When she saw us she started crying all over again. 'I didn't want to. They held me down like it was tickling. Look.' She stopped and lifted up her dress and there was a trickle of blood on her thighs.

'Who's they?' I said.

'Rebecca helped him.'

'There'll be trouble over this,' Shona said, taking my hand. She walked along beside me with firm, determined strides, not letting go my hand. When we got to the Langdon house she wrapped her arms around me and put her head on my chest and kissed my neck on the place she'd bit me. She was trembling.

'Tomorrow,' I whispered. I didn't know what to say to Tessa.

The adult party was still in full swing when I got in, and I managed to slip past everyone unnoticed. I didn't feel tired and hunted out some lemonade. I couldn't see Uncle Owl anywhere. Parker came in soon after, but he wasn't as lucky as me; his father saw him and got a nasty look on his face. 'Where have you bloody kids been?' he yelled. Parker turned stubborn. His father took a swipe at him as he went past.

'Hold on there, George,' someone said.

'Sneaky little bastard,' George said.

I sneaked to the bathroom and had a pee. In the mirror I saw the mark her teeth had left where they had broken the skin; when I touched it there was a tender soreness.

Back in the bunkroom Parker hardly looked at me except to give me the kind of nasty look his father had given him a few moments before.

There was no hope of sleeping. They must have played 'Mack the Knife' a thousand times. And 'When the Saints'. I thought of Shona and put my fingers up to my nose and dozed with her dark slippery odour in my head.

I came to with the sound of shouting in the next room. Parker was already sitting up. The adults were having a row. George was shouting at someone. I heard Uncle Owl's carping voice. Then I heard Dad playing his peacemaker role by telling the other guy he'd push his face in if he kept causing trouble. He said he'd been in the bloody army and wouldn't have any problems. Someone else was also trying to help, telling Dad he was full of crap. A moment later there was the sound of tumbling bodies and breaking glass. The women started screeching. Parker gave me a significant look.

My mother came through the door. 'Get dressed,' she said to me. 'We're leaving.' There was a grim, tight look on her face.

'We can't go now,' I said.

'Right now. And don't bloody argue.'

I turned away from the gin on her breath. She hustled me through the front room, which looked a mess. Betty and George were in the kitchen screaming at each other and clawing at each other's faces. There was a wet red wine stain down the front of her wedding dress and food all over the floor; Uncle Owl was lying in the middle of it, making weak attempts to get up. Betty screamed something about Parker being a big problem.

'Problem! Problem!' George bellowed. 'You're my fuckin' problem!'

As we went past the front of the house someone came

backwards through the bay window in a great shower of glass. A bottle came spinning out after him, smashing on the verandah post, and I heard George shouting that he'd get his .22 and kill the bugger. I could hear Betty screaming that she was going to divorce George and George screaming back that he'd be better off without her and all her fucking old boyfriends. All the lights had come on next door at the Langdons'. Dad and Mum piled me between them in the ute.

'Do you think we should go?' Dad said at the last minute. 'It's a long way to drive at night.' I held my breath.

'Of course we should,' Mum said in a voice that was made of wire. Dad knew better than to argue.

I caught a glimpse of a cluster of faces at the window of the girls' room at the Langdons' as we took off, and touched the tender wound on my neck.

Dad drove home drumming his fingers on the steering wheel and I could hear the song in the rhythm, *You know when that shark bites, with his teeth dear ...* At least they chose to be silent rather than fight all the way home.

I realised I hadn't brought the strands of hair I'd put under my pillow.

After that my parents crossed Betty and George off their list and I never saw any of the kids again. Nobody so much as mentioned the subject of the wedding. For a while the bruise turned dark and interesting looking. I wrote Shona a poem about it, but had nowhere to send it. I went into the post office and looked up Parker's number. When I rang a voice I didn't know said the Parkers had moved out. I didn't have a copy of the first poem and forgot it all but for the one line. After that the bruise faded and got less interesting, and when it disappeared I threw the second poem away.

Once, in my twenties, I drove back that way and found the sandhills turned into a housing development where bulldozed sections sprouted houses, lawns, shrubs and dry goldfish ponds. I drove around for a while. There were just houses and subdivisions and staring kids on bikes. It took me some driving around until I realised that I was looking for Shona Blake, some clue or sign. I saw a woman who looked a bit like her pushing a pram. Then another, and another. Shonas everywhere pushing prams, but no Shona. In a forgotten but familiar gesture, I rubbed my fingers against my nose as if I could provoke that secret, delirious smell and that night in the sandhills, but there was nothing, maybe the deceptive, sweet smell of nicotine.

And if it turned out that one of these young mums pushing prams was really Shona, would I know her? I doubted it. She'd become too mixed with other Shonas. I'd probably drive right past her blank-eyed looking for someone else, someone whose face had crossed that border from memory into myth. The curve of a neck, the ripeness of a breast; a tomboy smile and a couple of lost strands of hair; a wound and a scent.

I wouldn't know her.

I smoked and drove around a while longer drumming an old song on the steering wheel, but there was nothing there.

The Ten Dollar Ticket
Damien Lovelock

When I was a kid I went to a Catholic school. I believed all the stuff they told us, prayed in church and thought that God was everywhere. Thought that was a cool idea. But I was about eight years old then and thought most things were cool. We used to study from a book called *The Christian Gentleman* and most of us believed all that was in it. I was always suspicious of the kids who didn't believe it. I thought, 'What's wrong with them, don't they *get* it?'

Things went along OK until I was fourteen and I changed schools. Then I wasn't too sure about a lot of the Catholic stuff. Especially morality.

The new state school was non-denominational and much freer and I joined it at the age when we were starting to go to parties. All the guys used to hang in the schoolyard in groups, into which I was readily accepted. Two or three key figures always led the discussion, mostly about the weekend's activities. They were like Telecom. Everything that was going on went through them. Party Marty was one of them. He was the under-sixteen version of Izzy Dye. Always happening, always knew at least three parties that were on and whether they were worth going to.

The party scene was full of us; young guys trying to get across the room and talk to the girls, remaining cool at all costs. It was never difficult being cool in front of the girls, but always difficult in front of the other guys: striking a pose, slow dancing with a girl when the lights were low, pashing off, doing the tongue thing (before the parents arrived). That was good. I really liked that. It was great fun.

Back at school on Monday and it was all 'Yeah, I did OK,' and 'She nearly did it, if they'd only not come around the corner at that minute ...' But I always thought it was kinda weird because I really liked these girls. Most of them. A lot of them were people that we had all grown up with and knew well. But the whole thing was changed by the new social stage that this stuff was played out on—the Saturday night inevitable. I guess it was a rite of passage.

Pretty soon I began to get the impression that I was the only guy in town who wasn't scoring heavily with the girls. Everyone else seemed to be doing really well. There were different groups in the schoolyard—the surfies, the sharpies—but the rave was pretty much the same. There was also all the bus stop stuff; who was sitting next to whom on the bus. I always found this difficult because at fourteen I was walking around with a virtually permanent erection. Trying to get down the aisle of the bus with a suitcase carefully placed in front of you and still look cool and nonchalant was not so easy.

I was unimpressed by the language and the discussion that accompanied this stuff. The act itself was great; the kissing, the slow dancing and the excitement and nervousness were really cool, edgy, but the Monday note-swapping I felt was tacky. I liked girls. I didn't want to talk about them the way most of the other guys did. I got the impression too that, individually, most of them were like me but the group dynamic seemed to toughen up the language and the people with it.

So my disinterest grew. It was helped by drugs coming into the scene. Smoking dope at these parties made it much harder finding the energy to spend three hours trying to sit next to some girl and go through all the right moves at the right time to eventually ease an arm around her. The music always sounded so much better when you were stoned ...

There was the fashion too. I was really into Brian Jones, the guitarist from the Rolling Stones and on one of their albums he was pictured wearing a pink corduroy suit. It looked great on him (I still think it does, even though my son is disgusted when I point this out to him). One day I was in town with Mum to get a new pair of pants. In Surf, Dive and Ski there were the regular Levis and one pair of pink corduroy flares. And I knew I had to have them. They were actually nothing like Brian Jones', more like Bozo the Clown's, but they were pink and they were mine. My mates, quietly and individually, thought they were pretty cool. But as a collective, they put heaps of shit on me, which made me even more determined to wear them.

The next thing, of course, I was called a poof. Because I was not trying to screw the girls at the parties, and I was wearing pink pants, I must be a poof. I felt sort of betrayed by my mates giving me all this bad PR.

But now I was in a real dilemma because the Catholic ethic was still in the back of my mind. I knew that if I was going to sleep with a girl at the age of fourteen, I had to love her and want to marry her and have kids with her. Taking someone's virginity was the biggest responsibility in the world. It was special and had to be cherished but I couldn't see how I was going to be able to do this with the girls I knew especially now that I had my pink pants and I was a poof. So on one hand I was confused and defeated but inside, the erection machine was on non-stop and getting bigger all the time.

I didn't know about masturbation. I was an only child, from a single-parent family, so I hadn't figured it out yet. Kids didn't talk about wanking at school, they talked about wankers. I thought it was some kind of disease, a loser trip. I assumed most of the other guys had it together because they were really obsessed by girls. I was into my sport, football and athletics and surfing, and music and other stuff that these guys didn't seem to take much interest in.

The crowning thing for me was the fact that the guys who tended to do best with the girls at the parties were generally guys whom other guys at school wouldn't piss on. They were phony, bullshit artists and wimps who weren't well thought of, merely tolerated. I couldn't believe that most of these girls couldn't see through this shit because everyone else could. *We* could.

I lived about ten minutes from the Cross and used to go up there on the way to the footy. I knew what all the 'workers' up there were about. My Mum had told me about who they were and what they were for but I'd never really thought much about them, having been into that Catholic morality thing of trying to be non-judgmental and forgiving. I knew about Mary Magdalen and was always prepared to turn the other cheek ...

It was the sixties. The Vietnam war was on and the R&R guys were coming to Sydney in droves; the prostitution scene had really exploded. There were workers everywhere, on the streets twenty-four hours a day. They were different then. Most workers were engaged in a 'profession' rather than a means of survival. It was definitely a different scene to the junkie thing that is so predominant today.

One day after footy I was walking through the Cross with my constant companion, a three-quarter erection, and suddenly it hit me. The girls were there and I thought: Man, *this* is what I can do. I really wanted to know about sex. I really had to do this or I knew I'd go crazy.

I figured it all out. I knew I had to get hold of ten dollars. (I had walked past many times before and had been asked 'D'you wanna girl, love? Ten bucks a go.') This was a lot of money then. I had no idea how I was going to get it. But it still seemed easy, logical. OK, I thought, they want ten bucks and they're prepared to do it. And I want to do it, and all I need is ten bucks. I assume I don't have to lie, to bullshit, in fact to say anything at all.

I brewed on it for a couple of weeks. I couldn't stop thinking about it. Every time I went to the Cross I was staring out the window of the bus and salivating all over my shirt front and thinking about this but I was aware that it was a big moral step. I just knew it was wrong. It couldn't be right because it was too much fun, too easy. There had to be rules against it. The parameters of the fun factor at age fourteen weren't wide enough to include something as cool as this. I knew that. But fuck it.

I finally psyched myself up. My stepfather was out selling houses in the far western suburbs and came home each night and drank half a bottle of Scotch. Not so that he was really pissed, but so that he was not quite fully aware of what might have been going on around him. I decided Friday night was the night. I hung in until he'd had his Scotches, his dinner, watched a bit of TV and then crashed at around 10.30. I gave it about ten minutes then I crept into my parents' room and there was the wallet. There was about $70 in there so I snipped a tenner. I was sweating, freaking out, I couldn't believe I'd done it, but I was driven; I knew that this was the night that I was going to find out about all this stuff, all this sex stuff.

I was totally convinced that I was only ever going to do this once, then I'd wait until I got married.

I wanted to look kind of cool, rather than fourteen and on the case, so I got my old school suit, minus the tie, and I thought, yeah, now I look older. I put some grease in my hair, ran out and jumped on the bus. Once I'd got there, I looked around and there had to be fifteeen girls lined up at the bus stop, facing me. But it was so public. I knew that the minute I spoke to one of them a bus would pull up on the other side of the road with all the teachers from my school, and most of my relatives and they would all look out the window at the same time and see me. And there was the Big Guy ... He was gonna know too. But I figured I could deal with the Big Guy 'cause it was a personal thing. I could figure that out. The relatives and the teachers, though, I couldn't deal with them at all.

So I walked. Because it was my first time, I really wanted to get it right. I looked at the girls and wandered around in a loose figure eight through the Cross. Most of this Kings Cross doesn't exist any more. It was much more rambling, Dickensian, than it is now. Every time I saw a girl I tried to avoid eye contact. If they succeeded in catching my eye, I turned red, sweated even more and walked even faster. My heart was beating until I thought it was gonna pop out of my chest. I would see a girl I thought could have been the one, then would stand psyching myself up, thirty-five deep breaths, then come back and of course she'd be gone. This went on for about four hours, maybe five. It was about two in the morning and I was starting to get leg cramps. I was soaked through with perspiration and almost at the point of giving up because I was so fucking exhausted from power-walking around the Cross, my brain going at 300 miles an hour and this pogo stick poking through the front of my pants. Maybe it's just not worth it, I thought.

One last lap. By now I was getting hip to my own shortcomings. I figured that if I walked into a less populated area, where there were fewer buses and less likelihood of public apprehension. (A vision flashed through my head: front page of the Sunday Mirror—SCHOOLBOY CAUGHT IN BROTHEL INCIDENT. Yuck. Life would be over. I'd be sent to St Joseph's or something. No, I couldn't even imagine the punishment for such a crime.)

Down the hill, just outside Joe Bardetta's barber shop, opposite the United Nations Club, I saw her. She was probably in about her mid-thirties, had an eighteen-inch peroxide blonde beehive and was big in all the parts that you'd want to be big in in that profession. She wore skin-tight leopard-skin pants, which came about four inches above her ankles, and an amazing pair of stiletto heels. She had a smoke hanging out of her mouth. I though she looked great. She just looked like *sex*. I had to fight with every ounce of strength and self-control in my body to not walk past her. I was just dying there, about to have a coronary. I had cramps in both legs, and the fourteen kilos I'd sweated from my body had soaked into my shirt and my pants.

I walked up to her.

She said: 'D'you wanna girl, love?'

'Yeah,' I replied in as deep a voice as I could muster.

'Ten bucks.'

'Yeah.'

So that's it.

The next thing we were walking around into an alley and up some stairs. I was shaking so much even my dandruff was trembling. She tried to put the key in the door but it wouldn't go in properly. At that moment I knew God was watching. I knew He was doing this, He was trying to save me because I could no longer save myself. But I didn't want to be saved. That was the problem. I appreciated the gesture, in fact I was profoundly grateful to know that God was there watching, but not at that very moment please, and not in such a direct manner. I could think of many other occasions in my life when I had wanted some direct intervention and didn't get it. Why now? So I stood there wanting to do nothing but jump off that balcony and run home screaming. I just didn't think I could go through with it.

But she spoke: 'It's because I always slam the door with the key in it, and I've bent it. Just give me a minute, love,' and she worked away. It took two or three minutes but felt like four weeks.

Finally the door opened and we went in. She stood there and casually removed her clothes. I couldn't believe it. The next thing everything was off and her body was there. Other than my mother's I'd never seen one up that close. I was in shock. She looked at me and I figured she must have known I was so young.

She said, 'Come over here, love, I just have to make sure you're clean.'

I walked towards her, no idea what 'clean' might mean. Was she going to inspect my fingernails, check to make sure my shoes were shined? She unzipped my fly and this thing emerged, which was so hard by now and had been in this position for so long it was practically petrified. She got a bowl of warm soapy water and gave it a little wash and then stroked it a couple of times. My whole body just about came through the end of it. Forget the semen, it was the rest of my body I was worried about.

She gave me the OK.

I didn't really know what was going on. I thought maybe that was it. Had we already done it?

THE TEN DOLLAR TICKET

Then she just lay back on the bed and told me to take my clothes off. I took my jacket off, leaving everything else on, including my shoes. She was lying there with her legs spread wide apart and motioned me on top of her. I wanted to look but I couldn't so I just fixed my gaze around the neck, earlobe, shoulder vicinity so I didn't make eye contact and start crying or something. I got on, the next thing I'm in there, and bang. I took to it like a duck to water, as they say.

It's done. All of a sudden it's over.

Now I was just amazed. The act itself was pretty good and had impressed me; I thought I did everything that I was supposed to do and I felt it went pretty well, but more than that, I was really proud of myself. I couldn't believe I'd actually done it.

I put my clothes back on and I felt fantastic, light and loose and really great. She gave me a little pat on the back as we walked out. I think she thought it was kind of cool to have such a young client, it was probably a change for her. So off I went with that really weird smell of sex and sweat and six-hour-old Old Spice running down the back of my neck and pooled up in my shorts somewhere.

I was at the bus stop with an idiot grin and dazed look on my face. I probably looked more stoned than when I was stoned; glassy eyed. On the way home I was thinking two things. One, I did it. Not 'I can't wait to do it again,' just 'I did it. I did it.' And two, all those guys at school are bullshitting. Now I knew for sure. Just the way they talked about it. None of them had done this. I felt on one hand a sense of one-upmanship but on the other hand I realised that the main reason I had wanted to do it was that I thought that everyone else had done this thing and I hadn't, and I rolled this notion over in my mind: they were all *bullshitting*.

The next day I was still pretty happy but the guilt thing

was huge. Fuck, I was thinking, I can't tell anyone, imagine if someone finds out, and I wondered if they could tell just by looking at me. I went out to visit a couple of my mates down the street and hung out for a while to let them have a good look at me, but they didn't say anything so I breathed a sigh of relief. Things were cool. Funnily enough the permanent erection subsided.

But about Wednesday I started to get the urge again. And I started thinking about it and remembering how good it was. The same old rave was going on at school. 'What are you doing this weekend?' Party Marty had a party happening at Bondi, no parents, all these girls from Dover Heights. But I couldn't get excited about it.

So Friday night came, I couldn't even wait until Saturday night. Stepfather came home, had his half-dozen whiskies and I was into his wallet before he even went to sleep. I snipped the tenner, and I was outta there by nine o'clock. I was back by one. Same girl, same place and now I was really killing it. The second time was completely different to the first time but it was still really good. Now I really couldn't believe it. I've never been one of those guys who was into something nobody else was into at school. So this was a whole new thing. It went on for a few weeks.

Finally I had to tell someone. What was the point of having something like that, getting into all this stuff if nobody knew? Not that I wanted to boast to the world, that was the last thing I wanted to do, but I wanted to share with a couple of my mates this amazing find I'd made: if you have this money, you can do this thing and it's really good. I was sort of sure they were all going to hate me and think I was a devo, but I had to tell them. Just one or two of them.

My best mate lived in my street, and one day on the bus

after school when we were looking at the girls as usual and figuring out who we'd sit next to if we weren't so petrified, I said: 'Guess what I did last Friday?'

'Dunno. What?'

'I went to a brothel.'

He just looked at me and burst out laughing. But he wasn't laughing at me, he just couldn't fucking believe it.

'What?'

'Yeah, I did it. I went to a brothel.'

'What was it like?'

'It was unreal.'

'Take me,' he says.

'Yeah, sure. Yeah, that'll be great. We'll go together, it'll be more fun.'

Friday night came, six-thirty. My mate was down there with his ten bucks, his best clothes, ready to rock. Off we went. It was a tremendous success. By the next weekend word had spread and now there were about five guys who showed up at my place. Over the next couple of months it built up to this thing where I felt like a tour guide on a Butlins holiday camp. Up to a dozen guys. But we couldn't meet at my place any more because there were too many of us. I didn't want the publicity. My Mum wondered about this new-found popularity but I explained it away. I think I told her we were going to the wrestling or the roller game or something.

We'd get on the bus and hit the Cross and we'd all do a huge circuit and everyone'd find the girl they liked and then we'd break up into groups of two and three, depending on the area that we were going to go back to. I was loosely the leader of this but there wasn't a whole lot to lead.

Every week there seemed to be at least one new guy who hadn't done it before and it was fantastic. It was a wild time. And then it just stopped. The numbers dwindled and I stopped wanting to go every week, the novelty had worn off.

For about six months though, that was the scene, the ten dollar ticket to Paradise.

His Eternal Boy
Peter Wells

I went late to my appointment, as I saw it, on Tuesday. Deliberately I left it until a few minutes before the shop officially shut. I knew this could make my appearance at home irregular, if I stayed any time with Mr Kernow, but I decided that I would risk whatever problems this created.

I felt dread, oddly, as I went towards the door. The Open sign was still there, and inside I saw the figure of my lover, as I liked to think of him, head lowered, inspecting, I saw, when I stood by the door, hand frozen as I reached towards the doorhandle, an embroidery which had been mended. He was inspecting this with such minute attention—he was famously particular as a dealer, refusing shoddy or second-rate work, a real epicure—that when I turned the handle it was he who started and laid aside the piece of embroidery slowly, his hand falling as if it had suddenly lost all power. But his eyes were looking into mine intently and there was something almost pleading in them.

'You came,' he said, and I knew he was grateful. We

stood there uncertain how to go on. I sensed this meeting was the most important one we had yet had. Somehow we both knew more about each other, or at least I had begun, I felt, to get an insight into him. He did not move. He stood there looking at me as if it was the first time he had ever seen me totally, and his gaze moved over my body slowly, until our eyes once again, yet shyly almost, met.

He smiled. He *smiled*.

My power over him felt complete. Without saying another word I turned to the door and with a brazen casualness which I felt would be completely convincing to any passers-by outside, I flipped the Closed sign over and walked, as if I worked out the back, behind the curtain.

Behind the curtain.

Once in the shadowy dark, lit only by a single high window. I felt breathless with my daring. I leant against a high-backed chair. My fingers felt nerveless. I did not undress.

He came in after several minutes. The length of this time seemed deliberately calculated to make me pass through a number of transitions or emotions. I felt certain he would not leave me there alone, even though this was, apparently, what he seemed to be doing: I longed to touch him, and to bury my tongue in his mouth, possessing him, or pulling him towards me so that we could merge again as we had done before. But his absence, his silence, seemed to point to the intensity of the decision-making process he was going through.

He pulled the brocade curtain across. It seemed he had been standing there all the time, almost in the room, feeling for me, listening. He turned away from me and, carefully, with that nicety I recognised in him, rearranged the curtain so that there was not so much as a splinter of light entering the room. The traffic, the world outside, was muffled. The room was pleasurably dark.

He came and stood beside me. Again, we looked at each other, and I found myself smiling. He began to undress.

His undressing, like everything about him, was deliberate. I watched his fingertips calculate the undoing of the buttons. The small ivory disk as it slipped sideways through the carefully stitched hole. The sharp susurration of his singlet. The sound, slithering, of his shirt falling on to the arm of the chair. He slid his singlet over his head. It was like a theatrical curtain rising up, revealing for me the vulnerability of his chest with its valley and river of hair running down in a furrow, towards that juncture: his leather belt. He stood for the slightest moment without his shirt, so that I could see him. His eyes, dark, they looked, grazed against mine. I was aware of the sound of my own breath.

When he was certain I was captured, as it were, by my own glance, he leant towards the curtain. He twitched a dim wattage of light into the room, and stood deliberately within it, showering in its fusillade. I looked at his body, which I had never seen. My eyes felt like starving thieves, full of hunger.

Yet he stood there showing his body to me in a prosaic, unerotic light. It was as if he was saying: look, this is the body of a man aged forty-two, this is what you are making all this romance around. Look at it, see the way the chest muscles are starting to slip, read these lines, running in sharp scars, down under the arms. See the slight swell of a belly, and the jellied tensity of the body of an aging man. Look at the hair, and the way it is tufting all over my body: see my flesh and feel how it has been carried round, year after year, through any number of encounters and sagas, sadnesses and ecstasies.

He stood there, defiant, mute, in front of me: allowing me to inspect him.

'I knew a boy once,' he began to speak. His voice was thick. 'Somewhere else. Another town. I was working in an auction house then. He ... he *thought* he loved me. He was like you.' His grey eyes mockingly saluted me. 'Sweet, nice. Naive.' I blinked. 'This boy was just about your age ... and I ... was ... unlucky enough, or ... lucky enough ... to be ... his starting point.'

He drew in a long breath. I sensed this telling was painful to him—and more possibly, would be painful to me. 'At first it was just sex. Good sex. Then ... he fell in love with me. I could tell. I could read it in his eyes. His face. I was ... frightened, at first, to love him back. What is the point?' A pause. I fought my inclination to speak. 'But what sense is there in living like that? So we loved each other. And we planned to leave the small town where we had met. Where I was living.'

There was silence a moment and outside, like a soft rain falling, I could hear the sound of cars passing and people walking. I listened to this for one moment then it fell out of focus.

'... it was ridiculous,' he continued, undressing now, as if he were not thinking. His thick fingers unlatched his belt. 'I had grown too casual with ownership, you might say. One afternoon, in the municipal park. Surrounded by ferns. I lowered my head on to his shoulder. He leant his head back and I buried my tongue in his mouth. We thought we were alone ... It was intoxicating, that brief moment.

'There was a cicada down by my foot, I remember that. His tongue. I remember. His tongue was like a river I wanted to follow forever, to its source.' His voice was deliberately cool, as banal in its telling as possible, as if he desired, above all, to strip the facts of their emotion and thus to protect himself.

'Someone saw us. They took a photo. I was blackmailed. I had to leave town. Leave my job. Even him. His parents were told. His parents ... who had left him in a boys' home. I left that town. He was to follow.' He let out a short laugh here. 'We promised each other,' he said. 'We swore.'

He now began to unbuckle his belt. I was silent. His belt slid slowly through cloth loops. He reached down and pulled the zip of his fly open. Released, his pants began to slide down his legs revealing his stocky, densely black-haired thighs. Briefly I lost a sense of what I should do—to look, to touch, to speak.

'What happened?' I tried to make my voice sound casual. He was silent a moment, as if he had not heard. Then he shrugged, but it was as if he were shrugging something off. 'Nothing,' he murmured, his voice reduced to its essence, stripped to a tonal darkness which seemed to me, at that moment, the essence of masculinity, of manhood, even in its shyness and unwillingness to express emotion. He leant down and casually stepped out of his underpants, so he stood in front of me, almost accidentally it seemed, naked.

'He killed himself,' he said to me, avoiding my glance, looking down at the floor in silence. He made that same, futile shrugging motion. Then he looked at me. 'I killed him,' he said softly, so softly I had to lean forward to hear him. Perhaps this was his aim. For one almost terrifying moment, he leant towards me and raised his eyes to look into mine. But before this had happened, my own mouth had betrayed me. My youth.

'What do you mean?' I cried out. 'You didn't kill him. You couldn't have.' He looked at me for one second of coruscating intensity: there was a bitter irony, even cynicism, in his glance as he looked into my face. I had the hallucination that he wasn't seeing me at that moment. He was seeing this other boy.

'He held the razor.' His voice was again deliberately banal. 'He bled to death. On his own. In that park ... where we were photographed.' Again that shrug. 'Sure ...'

I took my clothes off, unconscious almost of what I was doing. It happened so quickly, he seemed caught off guard. And when I was naked, there was the briefest pause in which we both rested in the rarity of the moment.

It was such a novel sensation to be naked with him. I felt a whole, almost impersonal, quality of discovery overcome me as the palms of my hands investigated the contours of his body. In my excitement I began to kiss him, almost frantically. Pulling my head away, we stopped there.

We looked at each other in one of those series of looks which seemed the most significant moments or stations in our friendship: they were like glances which grew fractionally closer each time, with a remorseless momentum inwards, a form of surgery almost, exploratory, removing barriers. Yet as I leant in towards him, preparing my face to receive his kiss—or to kiss him, if he so much as hesitated—his hands rose up and held my arms in a brace. He pulled me away from him.

I felt his eyes move over my face, almost cautiously. When he spoke there was a kind of carefulness in his words and I felt a distance grow and widen between us, even as we stayed there, not moving, silent.

'You know what we do together ... doesn't mean anything ...' he said to me carefully, '... anything more than what we're doing now.'

My answer was to move towards him, to try and bury that questioning face, to blind it. However he pulled my face away from his, holding me by my face quite painfully. I felt

HIS ETERNAL BOY

the pressure of his hands on the sides of my face and for one moment, as the pressure increased, the thought crossed my mind that I did not actually know him at all and that he might actually be violent: if that were the only way to make me understand—comprehend the little, or in fact, how much, I meant to him.

'You don't get it, do you,' he said to me. His voice was thick. '*You really don't get it at all.*' He said this so quietly it was barely a whisper.

'Yes—' I said to him, in a low voice. 'Yes ... I do get it.'

When he went on looking at me, in silence—in disbelief—I repeated my words—'I do'—in a lower voice then murmured the words again, and again, a prayer, a purr, my supplication, 'I do, John ... I do ... I do.'

He seemed as if he was on the point, not of being convinced, but at least persuaded out of the darkest recesses of the mood which had overtaken him.

'I ... love you,' I whispered.

This was the worst thing I could have said.

He let out a short, derisory laugh. He hit me sharply, on my backside.

Our faces were very close together—he could see the tears start out in my eyes and he hit me again, harder. I looked at him. Into his grey eyes. He seemed to be staring right into me. He hit me harder still, but with a slow processional rhythm which allowed me to see he was not so much out of control as leasing out his power, suggesting what might await me if I continued on with this lunacy—the lunacy of love. He paused, drawing his hand back. '*You—don't—love—me,*' he whispered in my ear, and his voice was curved and carved with whatever had happened to him during his life.

I cannot explain this. I felt an incredible and wonderful

safety at that moment. I did not fear danger. I felt he was expressing, on the contrary, the depth and intensity of his love. No matter how he might try to hide it, or choose to express it.

'What you *love*—' he whispered to me, as if what he was saying was so essential only I should hear it, 'is—' he pulled me towards him, so there was only a fraction of space between us, but a space nonetheless. His fingers were digging into my flesh. He pulled me into him, violently.

The pain was sharp, and I heard myself crying out. I heard my own voice, as if it were a stranger's, because my own voice was not saying any words at all, but making these small noises which sounded as if I was enjoying whatever power he had over me as much as being hurt by it. I felt this person, whoever it was, had to be expressed—it was as if some part of me was being born—and his power was his recognition of this in me, and his mastery over this transformation of self.

'This is what you like doing.'

And his finger, dry, slid into my pucker.

Gradually, his full, dry finger was inside me and I felt the pores on his skin, the irradiating pattern of them, and more distantly, the pull and lull and throb, like a tide, of his heart, and the blood in his body pumping through, and then back through his finger and into me.

His face filled my entire vision; I saw an angry eye, an animal's eye, like a fish on a hook, an eye which accuses you when the body, or heart, is dead. Yet if his eye had looked into me, my eye, in equal part, had looked back, into him. And I too had seen.

He lowered his hands then, slowly.

'Don't love me,' he said in a flat voice, as if to prove, simply by saying it, that it was an obvious, proved point.

'No—' my own voice surprised me with its disembodied

strength. I felt for the first time in my life—so this is what it is to be adult. 'No. I do not love you.' And yet it was as if, by saying these words, I had proved the exact opposite.

An almost overpowering feeling of sadness ran through me: a quake. Perhaps he felt it too. He went over to the basin and he simply stood with his back to me. He turned the tap on; the water seemed an expression of his feelings. I went and stood behind him. In the mirror, a small elegant mirror with a flaw in it where a piece of mould was caught, like a trapped moth in glass, I saw his face: and for the first time I saw Mr Kernow—John—as another human being. Not an adult. Not as someone older who could teach me essential things about myself. But someone human like myself: confused, uncertain, torn.

Perhaps this should have been disillusioning, the moment in which I turned and left him. Instead I wanted perversely to stay. I could not stand that face in the mirror, the way his face, always so intact and firm—chiselled and elegant was how I saw it—was now distended, eyes red, pockets of flesh dragging under them, his mouth half-open with pain. I forced him round to face me and slowly, very slowly and silently, so that the sound of my tongue on his skin was the only sound, I found my tongue moving all over his face.

I held his face between my hands. His eyes were lowered. Taking the initiative in a way which surprised and even shocked me, yet I felt only an exhilaration at the discovery of this new self within me, I placed my lips against his and pressed against them, so that, at first inert, almost stilled with shock, he began to respond and soon I was pushing him against the handbasin as my mouth and tongue searched him out.

I did not want to talk. I did not want words. I only wanted whatever it was we could work out together, eliminating the space between our two bodies. He cried out as my teeth, amateurishly, grated against his skin. But I kept on going until I felt the strain, and fight, and stiffness ebb out of his body, and he began, just lightly, to moan.

Now we began to struggle, like two humans within a sack, struggling to be made free.

It was an almost unspeakable relief to have entered that zone in which the only question is the arrangement of limb to limb, and of answering symmetry, and then the remorseless drive towards convergence. For me, at that age, still half-animal as it seemed, it was as if I were being made human, as if in reverting to that most basic of all instincts and motions, I was reaching out towards a realisation of my self, that inchoate form located inside my flesh. I wanted him in me, inside me; I possessed him as much as he took me and I felt he gave me some quality of humanness simply by making me realise the animal which I was.

The pleasuring he gave me was long, intense, and with many gradations in pitch, motion, intensity, depth and even feeling. I felt he was both angry with me and protective of me. I felt at moments he hated me even while he was making love to me, and I felt he was loving me even while he was hardly even mentally, it seemed, beside me. It was an endurance test and it was as if he wanted to make sure, at its end, after he had come and I finally came, that there was almost nothing of my old self left. Or as if my old self was simply that spurt of liquid, now growing cold, which he was leisurely smearing, back and forth, forth and back, slowly, abstractly, on my chest.

He cradled me for a while, and breathed in my ear. We held still like this. I could smell him. I could smell me. In the zone of our smells lay a minute arena: seconds ticking away the hour.

Suddenly, as if he were swallowing back a hiccough too enormous to be suppressed, he burst into tears. This was profoundly shocking to me. He turned his face away from me, as if ashamed. His weeping was hot and deep and passionate. I lifted his arms which were like deadweights and placed them around me. I crawled into his body, straddled my own arms around him and sticky from tears and visceral juices, I stuck myself to him.

I held his face between my hands. I kissed his tears away. That moment when he looked up at me. That moment.

Warrior of tears, geisha boy of fear, alone in our lake, drifting.

In Praise of Eva
Julian Davies

Yes, she was a tall woman, but one whose sense of purpose made her body seem more powerful than it really was, that gave her a physical presence that demanded to be taken seriously. Right now I can see her standing in front of me in the doorway of her bedroom, her arms raised to the sides of my face where they press my cheeks. I can feel the force of those hands, the heat from her palms, the pressure from her fingertips, all these things containing the urgent impatience of her mood, a mood of love for me. She slaps me suddenly, slaps my cheeks with both her hands and tells me I am nothing but her 'gorgeous little toyboy'.

   She, Eva, was what is called a *mature-age student*. These older students have quite some reputation for achievement. They've gained experience of life, discovered what interests them and learnt to concentrate on it, and have outgrown the distractions of youth. At that time I was only twenty and easily distracted, so easily distracted that I didn't really notice Eva until I'd already shared classes with her for almost two years. Then, one day, arriving late to a lecture, I sat down next to her by chance and began a passing conversation with her as we left the room an hour later. As though accidentally, we continued to walk together under a calm, blue spring sky out of which floated the drifting downy fluff from the flowers of an avenue of tall eucalypts. I noticed the down as it floated past Eva's face and sometimes landed in her hair, but it wasn't a romantic thing to me then as it is now—romantic, and sexual just to think of. We had coffee together, seated at an outside table where we could see our fellow students passing by, and I became aware that I enjoyed Eva's conversation—but not with the overwhelming pleasure that even the faded sound of her voice moves in my memory now.

Right now I see the slow drifting strands of gum blossoms, I hear Eva's voice, and I remember the startled joy with which I took her nipples into my mouth. Each time I felt freshly the disbelief that I was allowed to take her nipples between my lips. But that came later.

Still, something began to happen that day beneath the trees and at the cafe table even though I didn't know it and, if challenged, would have considered it totally impossible that anything could. I like to remind myself how impossible so many things have seemed to me before I've gone on to succumb to them. Ever since only its consummation made imaginable my affair with Eva I've tended to question my own judgment in most things, especially my ability to understand my own responses. You see, with Eva I didn't for a long time know what was happening to me.

I remember my first visit to Eva's house, a substantial suburban building where she'd lived for over twenty years and which wasn't unlike the house my parents owned, the house where I'd grown up. This parallel may have occurred to me unconsciously even as I followed Eva through the front door because I recall a feeling akin to queasiness as we came out of the light of a summer's day and into the cool shade of her domestic life. Both her daughters were there. They were standing together in the kitchen making themselves toast and coffee. Eva greeted the girls and—her self-possession was always quite stunning—betrayed no hint of awkwardness as she introduced me to them. Certainly, there was no reason for her to behave in any other way. Eva and I weren't lovers, indeed we'd never touched. I was only a friend from university. But in that situation I suddenly felt the implication of something more than that. I tried to talk to the girls, Emelia and Kitty. And from some bizarre need to win their favour, and a confused desire to please Eva, I made a supreme effort, was charming, but also somehow knew to resist any excess of unctuousness. And yet it became clear that by accompanying their mother I had set myself aside. I saw a glance, a flicker of communication, which passed between the girls, and a look their grey-blue eyes shared as they spoke to me, a look of ironic complicity.

I think of what soon became the taut, shrewd, unforgiving judgment of those daughters and, yes, I remember the startled joy with which I took Eva's nipples into my avid mouth. Each and every time I felt such disbelief that I was allowed to take her this way. I think of that, and then of women young and older. Everywhere back in my youth I recall forbidden fruit. In an age which believed in its own liberality I remember dogmatic precepts enforcing constraint and denial. You see, in the days when I met Eva it was, even among the young men I knew, unfashionable to pay much attention to a woman's breasts. To do so was to disclose a *tit fixation* and also, most likely, an ineptitude with women. Yes, it was as though the least sign of interest in breasts betrayed an unresolved juvenile obsession with the memory of a mother's milky nipples, with those fleshy baubles of dependency. In those days, you also carefully avoided any mention of your own cock. To talk about cocks among the undergraduates of my era was truly *retrograde*. When you talked about sex you tried to make the point, but in as subtle and off-hand a way as possible, that you knew how to make a woman come, that your fingers and your tongue had unequalled talents. Oh Lord, how we thought we lived in sophisticated times. When I fell in love with Eva I also fell in love with her breasts. Perhaps the passion I felt for them was a reaction to denial—in any case, I adored them, both of them equally. And the most wonderful thing was that she loved me to love them.

In the first awkward, sticky sexual contacts of my late teens I recall how I attempted to keep my hands away from the breasts of girls. I recall how desperate I was to show that I knew what I was doing, desperate to display skill, to give pleasure and disguise what pleasure I took. Not that it was difficult when in fact I took so little. I certainly wasn't unique. There was such desperation in the love we young men felt for young and desirable women, a desperation of utter lustfulness controlled by the fear of disapproval and failure. There was the fear of some naive or awkward act, fear of what could be said in the void after sex, fear of commitment, fear of disclosing that we feared commitment—or, in fact, that we might really yearn for it. And, always lurking most devastatingly, there was the fear of rejection.

At first I wanted nothing from Eva and therefore feared nothing too. I carelessly enjoyed the times we met without anticipating them. Then, one day when Eva and I had just finished lunch together, again at a table outdoors on campus—it was probably about a month after our first walk through the falling fluff of gums, and not long before my first visit to her house—something happened. We stood up to part and, as Eva turned and walked away, a friend of mine, another student, stopped to speak to me. He gestured towards Eva's retreating back with a nod of his head.

—So, who's the old woman? he asked.

It was the anger I felt at his question that surprised me. Why should I react so strongly? Oh, I should have already known. I should have understood a quality in her presence there beside me in our lectures, a quality that caused the lecturer's voice, a man whose classes had not seemed boring previously, to begin to dissolve into irrelevance. Now, in anger, I was unnerved by an unwanted glimmer of understanding. But, no, it was true—wasn't it?—she was quite old, and the mother of two grown daughters. The moment passed, and perhaps I explained away my anger as just arising from a basic sense of human empathy. Perhaps I reassured myself and felt protected by her age without even bothering to consciously define for myself the certainty that nothing, surely, other than friendship could happen between us. It must have seemed self-evident.

When we sat together, talking, close across a table, there was another discrepancy between us caused by age. We knew, and sometimes even enjoyed, a teasing battle of wills, a contest between my confident undergraduate opinions and Eva's gently amused impatience with them. I see her opposite me, her elbow on the table top, her chin cupped in one hand, the tip of her little finger resting at the corner of her mouth, touching the delicate edge of her smile. She would listen as I—well, in those days, like most of my contemporaries, I was so in the thrall of a fashionable form of relativism that I might well have argued that gravity was a cultural construct foisted upon us by western science. So, in a case like that, Eva would listen and then ask why it was, in this world of foisted gravity, that she and I and the cafe table didn't float away together high above the campus. I sometimes wonder why she continued to meet me. Throughout what were for me, self-protectively, the unconscious stages of our 'courtship', she remained patient. I am amazed by this now when I consider how much her life contained: a part-time job, her studies, an array of friends, her daughters, and then a boy like me as well, accommodated too without being made to feel a mere adjunct. Later she explained that she was physically attracted to me and not much interested in my opinions—something I could never have understood at a time when I believed one's existence was validated by the views one held. She told me she saw a sweetness in my nature that was all the sweeter for my being unaware of it.

I still do not remember myself as being sweet but rather as suddenly desperate. Perhaps it was in reaction to what was happening unconsciously with Eva, but I began to chase girls in a predatory way that had never been mine before. I calculatingly pursued several women my own age. To be fair to myself, the girls often participated too in those subtle and not-so-subtle verbal ploys and manoeuvres when our minds tried to help position ourselves and our bodies for contact. And then there were also one or two preposterously blatant and yet strangely inconsequential seductions, seductions as much of myself as of anyone else. It was at just this time that I propositioned a woman at the checkout of a supermarket.

I can still hear that woman's voice.

I have arrived at the cash register with a jar of caviar. I am buying the caviar because I plan to take a friend, another woman who attracts me, on a picnic to celebrate her birthday.

—Fish eggs, the woman on the till comments as she takes the jar from my hand. She surprises me by speaking to me in this way, but, then again, she is young and full of it, full of the fresh, rich profligacy of her own youth. I can see that clearly. She projects it, almost wantonly. But there is also a tautness to her abundant sense of self.

—Fish eggs, she says. It is as though she teases me a little with my purchase of this luxury. She taunts me, but lightly. It is as though she says: *Are you such a rich boy that you can afford this stuff?* Fish eggs.

—Yes, I say, but I doubt they'll hatch.

She too is startled now and looks at my face. Although it is she who has mentioned fish eggs, her expression holds measures both of distaste and amused surprise as though it has never occurred to her that fish might have been born from caviar. Suddenly she smiles.

—You can forget it. She taps the metal top of the jar with a red polished nail. I'd prefer the champagne any day. What about you?

—Yes, perhaps I would. So, when you finish here would you like to share a bottle with me? Of champagne? This is what I say to her. And I say it unselfconsciously, without a doubt, without cringing inwardly. I'm capable of this, of being so glib in the certainty of lust.

—OK. I finish at six.

I can hear her voice now, replying so easily too. But—do you know?—although we screwed later, these first glib phrases were, in the end, about all we had to say to each other. It seems quite strange to me, now, the liberties, the physical intimacies, we will allow ourselves with people with whom we can't even conduct an enjoyable conversation. It can be so easy to come to terms with the attraction of strangers—if you aren't afraid. Or if you are confused and hiding from the fact that you are in love with a woman older than you by almost thirty years.

How can I continue to describe Eva for you? It is perhaps true that she wasn't a particularly distinguished woman to look at. But how am I to know anything about these things when at one time she seemed to me to be middle-aged and matronly, and then, not so much later, to be quite exquisitely beautiful.

The first time Eva asked me out at night—and it was she who asked—I was increasingly overcome by anxiety. The invitation, made nonchalantly while we sat together waiting for a lecture to begin, unnerved me not immediately but as the day slipped away. By the time I saw her sitting in the driver's seat of her car, by the time I reached out a hand towards the handle of the passenger's door, I was overcome by fear.

I was living in university accommodation at that time and she picked me up there before we drove downtown. That night as she drove me into the city my fear became complicated, in the shifting semi-darkness of the car's interior, by the now familiar pleasure of her company. Although we were unusually silent my uneasiness began to dissolve in the company of Eva as we moved together through the shifting pattern of light cast from outside the car. I heard the regular pattern of her breathing there beside me in that light, light which slid across the tiny dimples of the dashboard vinyl, across the upholstery of the seats, and on in limpid sections, in little trapezoids and triangles, formed from streetlight that slanted in on us out of the random geometry of an urban landscape. I started to relax in this sway of motion and unnatural light and the intimate rhythm of Eva's breathing. She sat forward in her seat, her limbs in line with mine, in parallel existence, except that her hands were raised to grip the wheel. I saw slivers of light pass luminous over my legs, clad in white light cotton trousers, and travel on to define the roundness of Eva's knees, to slide across the fine grain of her stockings.

She took me to a nightclub, a low-lit place where a kind

of showmanship held sway, where the bartender wore black, the waiters wore black, the piano player and the saxophone player wore black and the performer—a woman who was doing a cabaret act on a small black stage—wore black too, but also bright red knee-high boots. She sang a selection of Kurt Weill songs—until Eva told me about him that night I'd never heard of Kurt Weill—while the saxophone, staccato and lushly flatulent by turn, punctuated her phrasing of the words and heightened the rich but anxious qualities of her voice. Eva sat close beside me at a table near the stage, and at one point in the evening she, in the extent of her enjoyment, reached out a hand to grasp one of mine where it lay in my lap. I glanced around at her just as she looked at me, and I thought I saw, quite clearly, how perfectly unencumbered her face was by anything other than her pleasure in that music and her delight in being able to share it. Then, as I looked at her and believed that her expression was free from any implication or insinuation, I knew I'd begun to love her.

Later, yet not so much later, I wondered how naive I'd been and how much her pleasure was, in fact, enhanced by wanting me and having me right there. I also wondered how carefully she'd performed for me, how restrained she'd been. Was the look of entrancement on her face as she listened to Kurt Weill contrived, or if not contrived then actually born from the extent of her intent concentration on me? Later she told me how much she'd wanted me even before that night and how she'd carried the embarrassment of her foolish desire for this boy about with her for several weeks. So, at the moment that I suddenly found Eva inescapably loveable for her apparent lack of artifice, she was fighting to disguise and control her lust. Later, with Eva, I discovered so many of the complexities of love, and the complexities to be met in a worldly, older woman. Among many other things, I saw just how much her face could insinuate. She was, I learnt, capable of the full range of moods and teasing ploys that thrive in any one of us.

In the car, parked somewhere on the way back after the cabaret, Eva kissed me—and it was she who gave the kiss and I who received it. There, at the edge of the road, a hand of hers slipped inside the cotton of my trousers, slipped beneath white cotton made grey in the half-light of a distant street lamp, and touched my cock. In my room, a little later—the room we returned to because her daughters would be there at her house—we undressed to an orchestration from beyond the door, an orchestration made up of the sounds of people talking as they passed, of a ringing telephone, of the opening and closing of other doors. Yes, in that little room, which now seemed to be a flimsy thing at every moment endangered by careless and encroaching, if not malignant, public forces, Eva began to undress.

You've noticed, of course, that my reactions, my patterns of thought, tend to seem rather deliberate. I have been accused of holding back, of being aloof, lazy or even slow-witted, and while there is some truth in all these things, with Eva I was truly, deeply in awe of the full weight and measure of her existence, of her separate existence. Even now I remain aghast at the memory of Eva undressing. In my room, to the sound of passing laughing students, Eva took off her clothes quickly, as though she'd decided to avoid any attempt to show me herself in seductive incre-ments. Rather, she made me see quite clearly what she was. The first aspect of her body that I noticed—I'd knelt down naked right in front of her—was the skin of her stomach. Unimagined marks spread a loose and pale tracery there, stretched wide from the carrying of babies, one of them before I was even born. I can't deny that I was overpow-eringly dismayed, but also so fascinated that my hand went

IN PRAISE OF EVA

up to touch that skin and, lower, her pubic hair, curving downwards hypnotically, a triangle already greying. Lower still there were some veins grown proud and delicately blue on the side of one of her legs. Unnerved I looked up at her face. I saw her eyes look down at me quite patiently. Penitent and suddenly emotional I bent to kiss her thighs, a luscious breadth of them that seemed at first incongruously strong when all I'd until then known had been their unobtrusive movement under cloth. I raised my head again to the glorious revelation of her breasts, breasts not so much large as ungrudgingly, abundantly available to me and still nobly resilient against half a century's persistent drag of gravity. I put my lips upon them, each in turn, in the first of many such soft embraces.

But I was still shocked, yes, shocked and dazed, as though the signs of Eva's age might somehow contaminate my youth and drag me through my life, might take me too quickly closer to the edge of death. And so, confused this way, I looked up again, my chin now against her stomach, my head tipped back to gaze upward along the foreshortened splendour of her torso. Her smile was broad and so indulgent from so far above that in the influence of its sweet beneficence I reached my hands with ardour what seemed a mile aloft to take both nipples each between two fingertips to squeeze them there. In the lifting of those limbs of mine, which suddenly seemed twice their normal weight—while the skin of my inner arms grazed Eva's stomach and the palms of my hands glancingly met the fullness of her breasts—I saw how she was waiting there for me, waiting, almost with amusement, to see what I would do. And—how can I describe what happened then inside me? Perhaps at that moment I began to understand, almost as the promise of some greater, blinding revelation, how much might be given by one person to another if given willingly and without conscious procedure or any fear at all. In that blissful anticipatory state I stayed upon my knees, stayed to press her nipples still between the tips of my trembling fingers, my being as though poised there between my fingers too, exquisitely pinched in the first discovery of love.

I remained stunned and elated for several days—in retrospect comically so—and, if I became slightly less stunned over the weeks and months that followed, my elation did continue. If you are a man, you, like me, have probably had someone at some stage repeat to you that old saw that before marrying a woman you should look at her mother to see what she will become. Well, at the time of my passion I would have retorted that one of the advantages of taking an older woman for a lover is that you already know what she has become. It was absurd of me, perhaps, but I felt as though I'd been allowed a rare discovery: the discovery of a mature woman's love. I increasingly felt as though I had entered what I can only call a *state of grace* from which my own sexual past, and the continued activities of my contemporaries, would have seemed pathetic were they not too petty to achieve pathos. Had I been a more zealous boy I might have told them this, but I said nothing. I felt altogether far too blessed to carp. I moved about more intently, outwardly focused, continuing the various aspects of my life, and actually a little less self-obsessed than in the past. I moved and did these things, but inwardly it was as though I was perfectly still. Perhaps you've known this too, the complete, if fleeting, stillness of euphoria? I would certainly have married Eva had she allowed it.

Such a hope was hardly consistent with conventional wisdom. There came an evening at Eva's house, an evening when she spoke to me while she washed her hair. She was in the bathroom leaning over the bath, kneeling on a mat, clothed only in her underwear. She spoke to me while lathering the shampoo into her hair.

—Allan, your mother phoned me this morning, Eva said, not facing me but the bottom of the bath, the quality of her voice strangely distant.

—My mother? Really?

—She was angry.

—What did she say? I stood motionless in the doorway, leaning forward slightly, my hands gripping the architraves, my gaze fixed on the motion of her hands, on the shampoo foaming white between her fingers. I watched the shampoo in her hair and wondered how she, my mother, had got Eva's number.

—She asked me why I have no sense of seemliness.

—Seemliness? You're joking?

—She asked me why I have to ruin the life of a young man. She told me I've had my chance and should let you have yours. She asked me how I can be so selfish.

—Jesus, she said that?

Eva did not answer me immediately but continued to lather her hair. And I continued to watch her, spellbound by this situation and, not least, by her beauty there, on her knees, almost naked, her hands and arms in fluent motion, her head adorned with foam, her eyes shut, her face somehow naked too in its blind concentration above the white enamel of the bath.

—She told me I have corrupted an innocent boy, Eva continued and seemed to smile slightly. She accused me of cradle-snatching and of not being able to grow old gracefully.

—I hope you hung up on her.

—No, I listened. I thought I owed that to her. Eva half-turned her face towards me. Her eyes were still shut but it seemed she was sharing her expression with me, an expression which suggested, incredibly to me, the acceptance of blame.

I was furious. My equanimity was gone. I could hear my mother's voice, full of concern for me, it was true, but also intolerably self-righteous. Oh yes, my parents believed I was a victim of a lascivious experienced woman. Jesus. *What a joke!* I shouted. And I could hear a contained prurience implicit in their criticisms. I could hear them telling me about the way I was wasting my life. There was a tone in their voices that suggested they'd been there, peering around the door of Eva's bedroom or my college room while we lay together, disapproving but also somehow titillated.

But for Eva the accusations could not be completely dismissed. Guilt does have such mysterious and irrational powers. When I remember the way I was sometimes daunted and shamed in the presence of her daughters I think I begin to understand how she must have felt. Then I knew the full weight of accusation. Theirs was the contempt of contemporaries—in fact Emelia was over two years older than I was—and they increasingly saw me, I am sure, as some sort of vile opportunist who had been rejected by the girls of his own generation. Even her former husband, another of those men who have walked out on their families for the company of a younger woman, was unmistakeably snide to me when we met a few times in passing.

Now when I think of Eva on her knees, her head white with shampoo, I feel the inevitability of loss. Even then I began to sense it, to breathe it in with her kisses. Eva became increasingly tender with me, more lingering in her love. It was as though she knew something I didn't, as though I had faced judgment, been found guilty, and that I was the only one yet to be informed of the sentence.

There came another evening, an evening when I was

overwhelmed by the intensity of Eva's mood, a mood which I felt sure presaged my own impending banishment. It was an evening when everything seemed deliriously off-balance, an evening through which Eva flirted with me recklessly in front of Emelia and Kitty. She called me her 'toyboy', her 'luscious toyboy', and took me to her room. I went with her although we usually tried to protect her disapproving, jealous daughters from any obvious brandishing of our love. We undressed to an accompaniment from the kitchen of someone, one of the girls, banging utensils together and slamming cupboard doors. And as Eva straddled me on the bed, her thighs and shoulders gleaming in subdued light from the bedside lamp, there was whispering from somewhere close outside our door and an unidentifiable thumping noise. Eva made love to me that night, despite the sound of continued disruption, of laughter and loud music elsewhere in the house, and was completely unperturbed, her torso upright in its fluent and exquisite movements on my cock, as though this was not merely her passion but also her vocation. I reached my hands to touch her face, the beloved details of her face, and fought to resist the tears as they pushed up behind my eyes. I was overcome by her determination to give me pleasure and the desperation I felt about everything I would lose with the loss of Eva. She was my ally, my support, my family when my own family could only criticise the choice I'd made instead of accepting it graciously. I believed they'd betrayed me and thereby forfeited any right to loyalty or love. So, alone in my bliss and accompanied by fear, I clung to Eva. She attended to me tenderly and, as ecstasy approached, leant forward so her hair and breasts hung down together near my eyes and near my mouth, and, as I came, I lifted my head and, no longer able to restrain myself, began to cry. I sobbed and kissed those breasts and that hair made wet with tears, and through blurred eyes saw her looking down at me with great amazement.

Even now, a decade later, I sometimes think only of the loss of Eva. I think of how persistent was the opposition of my parents and, particularly, of her daughters. But now I can't blame them as easily as I used to do. There is no doubt that Eva becomes not less wonderful to me but much more so, yes—but would we have lasted together even without interference?

When Eva broke with me not long after that night of tears, I fought desperately to convince her to change her mind. I argued and, when that didn't work, I cried again like a child. Whether it was only the opposition of our families which decided her I can't say. Perhaps, if I'm honest, I must allow that my youth may itself have been a daunting handicap as well, a problem only too much time could help.

My parents were delighted by what they thought was my escape and so relieved that they bought me an air ticket to Europe. They told me a holiday, a break from study, would do me good. Over the next few years they often said they hoped I would meet a nice girl my own age.

Dream Lovers
Archie Weller

One of my memories is of going to the drive-in in Kojonup, when I was about eight or nine. Because we had no television on the farm this was always a treat for us. We would travel the sixty kilometres or so in the back of the ute or in the back of the car and it would be a pleasant family outing.

The movie we saw this night was called *The Island of the Blue Dolphins* and was about a native American girl who survived the massacre of her tribe. She bore a resemblance to a young Elizabeth Taylor and spent the entire movie in a short buck-skin skirt. I cannot remember her name but I fell in love with her. My as-yet-untainted mind began to wonder what that dress barely hid and, for weeks afterwards, I had curious, exciting but purely innocent dreams about her on that magical island. She was my first girlfriend.

Thus it has been throughout my life. I seem to fall in love with the image of a woman rather than her earthly essence. It is safer for me to plant the seeds of love in my mind and watch them grow under the stormy tumult of my thoughts, which I can control, than it is for me to grasp the reality of another human coming into my close personal life and unleashing something that I cannot control.

I believe love is something special and I do not give it easily. Indeed, I cannot give it easily. And I think this comes from the life I lived as a child. I was raised in the country where I spent much time in my own company playing with friends I had created in my mind. It was a solitary life but I enjoyed it thoroughly. Then, when I was seven, I went to a school in the hills of Perth and there came into contact with that intriguing species known as girls. Just as I was finally getting interested in them (specifically one Jenny Jones who was a little bit older than me, a tomboy, and the niece of one of the two boss-ladies—and who probably never even noticed I existed), I moved to an exclusive all-boys school. So all my adolescence was spent in the company of boys; the only time I saw girls was during the holidays or at the terrible debacle of organised school dances. I am convinced that this lack of communication when I was a young man clumsily experimenting with equally curious and interested young woman was the cause of my eventual shyness with the opposite sex. That and the fact that I was a writer. I knew at the age of twelve that I was—and always would be—a writer. I am never happier than when inventing and creating adventures and characters to go with them. And perhaps I will always be more comfortable with people I create in my imagination than I am with the real people I meet.

I met my first flesh-and-blood girlfriend at a holiday camp run by the YMCA. Her father was Protestant and her mother was Catholic. We held hands and I went to visit her at her parents' house when the camp was over. I wrote to her from school—my first correspondence with a girl—but I was shy of her parents and, foolishly, never visited her again. After about a year of writing to each other she said she'd met another fellah on the school bus. My first kick in the guts by love. I was all of thirteen years old.

A little later, at the only school dance I ever enjoyed, I met a beautiful Aboriginal girl. The effect of the disco lights shining on her face was electrifying. At supper, which we had outside, the shadows curved around her delectable ... unreachable body. I was always a good dancer, letting my dancing do my talking for me in fact, but it took me all of that night just to ask her for a dance. When I did I was so excited. Later she walked with me out to the bus and I asked her whether she would like to go to the Royal Show the following Saturday. But I twisted my ankle, can you believe my luck, and couldn't meet her. I saw her again some years later in Broome where, once more, my shyness destroyed any hopes I might have had of taking up the relationship that was clearly being offered to me.

In the last year of my school life I went to an experimental community school that specialised in the development of the individual and had little time for rules. There, along with the rest of the class, I fell in love with a truly gorgeous girl. Vivienne drifted through the school in an ethereal cloud of beauty. Her hair was long, reaching almost to her knees, and red, being coloured with henna. Her serene eyes were a deep, dark, almost violet, blue. She made her own clothes which seemed to swirl around her or cling to her inviting body. She had a perfect nose and a perfect chin, and a peaceful disposition. She enjoyed smoking dope and listening to Kris Kristofferson.

She was an incarnation of the image of the ideal lover I had always held in my mind. And because of this she was the first girl I ever wrote to expressing my true feelings, and she wrote me a beautiful letter in return. She is also the first girl I wrote poetry—and a short story—for. I poured out my heart to her. I visited her once and dreamed of her often. But, alas, to no avail. The second time I went to her house I saw her getting into an elegant car with someone I didn't recognise. After that I never saw her again. My dream-scape had been crushed. Just as the Navaho Indians will destroy an intricate sand painting so no-one save the person for whom it is intended may see it, so then was the image of Vivienne rubbed out and destroyed. Yet the sand did not blow away entirely and the residue of that painting will always be with me.

Now that my ideal had been shattered, I thrust myself into the real world with youthful enthusiasm. But love still eluded me. It was still an unknown thing, the true touch of a woman's body—a woman, that is, who loved me and I loved in return, not a piece of flesh underneath my gyrating loins.

In the old days before Christianity came slashing and repealing all the old laws, galloping with pious righteousness over the horizon, some of the tribes of Aboriginal Australia believed this about the birth of a baby. A man would sleep beside a sacred water-hole and a baby spirit would creep into his hair or beard. When he slept with his woman she would have a dream and the baby spirit would crawl up her leg just as a kangaroo embryo does. She would kick her feet like a kangaroo and lo! the baby would be conceived.

So the birth of a baby was not connected with the act of raw sex but rather with the spirits all around this spiritual land and with dreams. The actual copulation was only for enjoyment and this is how it came to be for me. Rushed, drunken outings with predominantly drunken partners. Love had little to do with it, although I was always kind to my companions. But there was very little poetry in these adventures. The names of the women are not forgotten, of course, but the incidents hold no true memories for me. Some I feel ashamed to recall.

It was at this time that I went to work in the wheat bins where I encountered a boss with lustful intentions. I was young and still very shy, with long, curly, brown hair and dreamy eyes and he fancied me. The experience of that hot, balmy, summer night is one that will stay with me forever and it took a tood ten years for me to get used to men touching me in the old camaraderie of 'mateship'. A hand on my knee in intense conversation or an arm flung round my shoulder in drunken friendship would make me freeze. Nyoongahs are sociable people, coming from a culture that shares everything from cigarettes to troubles. My aloofness and discomfort at these friendly, innocent overtures caused a lot of unwelcome, unnecessary friction with my peers and mates. The touch of a woman would have healed me, comforted my confused soul. A woman's gentle voice and warm soft touch would have turned my nightmares into dreams again. But there was no-one around.

Well ... there had been one, up in Broome, where I had wandered in my erratic way, happy not to be too close to anyone. She had blonde hair and greenish-blue eyes and several children from other men. She was pregnant again and drank a lot and was untidy and fat. But she was somehow different. There was something about her. And she was real!

I took her to the movies one night in the open air cinema and we saw *Leadbelly*, a movie about the blues musician Huddie Ledbetter and ... *The Island of the Blue Dolphins*. Except now I was all of twenty-two years of age and I could see the flaws in this old relic. Parts that had once scared me now just left me bemused. I was more interested in how they had turned a studio into an island and the other false ways they had of making fantasy appear real. I still found the actress, whose name I can't remember, attractive, but I was sitting with a woman of real flesh and blood, her warm leg touching mine, her hand in mine and her scent in my nostrils. This was the woman I longed for now. After the movies we walked hand in hand back to her home on Kennedy's Hill Reserve—the place where the better girls about town, such as the girl I had met long ago at that school dance, did not live or venture. Just before the police station we stopped and we kissed. I believe that is the first kiss I really remember. The moon cartwheeled through the sky and the starlight shone down turning her into a Princess of Beauty. It was then I knew I loved her.

Our courtship was slow, hindered perhaps by the fact that she was having a baby and liked having a drink and I could never have the first and was trying to leave the other alone. But I loved her and my crazy mind made pictures of her that probably were not true and could never have been. As for sex, that never occurred.

I was one of the first and few people to visit her in hospital when her baby was born. I found a full packet of Drum on the seat outside the TAB and this was my present to her.

Then I left Broome and wandered in my lonely, restless way up to Derby just to see what that town was like. I obtained work there and fell half in love with another girl. But I was to meet my Broome Belle in Perth about a year later and we started our friendship again. It was a shaky affair like all my other trysts, but we had some special times together, not necessarily only sexual. If love is all they say it is in the books and poems of the classical writers and the music of the bards, then I can truly say she was the first woman I held in my arms and loved. She was not an image from some book or movie screen. I had felt her hair blowing against my face and her fingers grasping mine in possessive love. I had smelt on her breath the wine she had drunk and she was oh so alive and, to me, glorious.

Her beautiful life was flicked out one murky, unforgettable night, when she was picked up for drunkenness and found next morning hanging from her own sweater in the Midland lock-up.

I could not fall in love with a woman's body for a long time after that. Her eyes, yes. And the shape of her neck and the slant of her head and the fall of her hair. Women's eyes captivated me, staring down at me like stars in the unreachable heavens. But I had touched a real woman and pulled her out of my dreams, only to watch her flutter lifeless to earth.

From then on I fell in love with other things. Beer and wine, Cinzano, Brandovino and Coruba rum—and the flimsy friendship of false mates. Slow horses and fast women and dry barren patches were the norm now. For five long years fame visited me, but I wallowed in my own company and the bottle was my only true friend. Sexual gratification eluded me—not for lack of trying—and I wrapped my dreams around me like tattered cloth keeping the cold from a poor, scrawny, diseased beggar.

I preferred a good book or a nice bottle of wine or the image of a woman to the actual act of humping and bumping and panting and saying and listening to a lot of lies. I was too withdrawn and unprepared for the reality of sexual relations but not only that, I was also too lazy to perform the rituals humankind demands. I was, in fact, a hopeless bower bird. I could not stamp or whistle out a love song or preen my feathers for the benefit of a female or present little gifts in my bower for my lady-love to inspect. I preferred to act the clown and hide my tears behind the glassy face of my friend the bottle.

But I also had my skill as a writer. Why bother with someone I had to talk to, take out to dinner or the movies, buy things for, when I could create a woman out of all the women I knew? I am sure I would rather have held that woman in my arms and kissed her breasts and run my hands and tongue over her body, but I had to settle for painting her into words. After all that is what I am best at, a song-man of words.

In the old days a song-man was important. He was the one who made up songs for the coming of the rain, the fertility of a fishing expedition, the success of a kangaroo hunt. A *mabarn* man could sing a man to death or a woman into love. There were song-women too and women had their own sacred ceremonies that it was death for a man to see. It is an anthropologist's misconception that Aboriginal women were treated with brutality and disdain by the men. In fact they were treated with respect and often with awe.

In the southwest of West Australia, in the land of the Nyoongah peoples, there were few arranged marriages, unlike the nor'west where the lifestyle and lay of the land decreed it best for an old man to have a young wife to look after him.

If a young Nyoongah girl fell in love with a young man, or vice versa, the lovers would let this be known at a council meeting. First of all, though, the young man, painted in red wilgie, would dance for the girl. He would rub against her and the red ochre would become smeared over her body. If she did not remove it, it was a sign that she liked him as well. If, at the council meeting, no other man made a claim, the woman was protected against other men until the next meeting when, if the couple still felt the same, protection was given against all men, women and tribes. A simple ceremony would then take place and the man would claim his wife in front of the whole family. Gifts would be exchanged, usually a new skin boaka for her and new weapons for him. He would take several strands of hair from her head and entwine them in his fur armband, thus making the marriage whole. Then they would leave on a journey that might take up to a year to complete and would probably result in the birth of their first child. This journey was meant to establish their ties and bring them closer together. A Nyoongah girl, now as then, is very jealous of her man, her *coort-maart*, and won't give him up easily, even though nowadays he may beat her and she may be a slave to his whims. It was the girl's responsibility to uphold the moral code of the tribe. If she came under another's bewitching spell and, literally, screwed up, then her punishment could be mutilation, beatings from other women, or death by starvation.

But white man's laws and white man's alcohol have cut like a scythe into our beliefs and morality and changed love into a shambling sad dance of the damned. The ethics of a proud, strictly moral people have been shattered and destroyed.

Ours is a shadowed secret world embellished with too much drink and too much violence. But there is a lot of love within it if you look for it in a smile, a caress, a gentle mumbled word or a shared laugh. And out of the ashes of the old laws and ethnics is arising a new morality, a new set of standards and beliefs.

Now it is the women who are the powerful ones. In the end it was their magic more than the men's that prevailed. It is the women who look after the children and try to protect their husbands from the tremors of this new world. The men who once were gifted hunters and trackers and bush men are now lost in this land where their skills are no longer valued and there is no solitude to meditate upon the glory of Nature and the intricacies of life. We will always be warriors, although battle was never really our way of solving problems, unlike our more bloodthirsty neighbours. But fighting against such great odds is wearing us down and taking from us all that we desire—our pride and self-worth. It is true we have ideas but nowadays it is the women who usually get those ideas to work.

The main difference between Nyoongahs and *wadgulas* is knowing that together we will survive in this new life before us. Nyoongah women don't leave their men except as a last resort and Nyoongah men might shout a lot but they haven't got the macho Aussie Anzac outlook which so many *wadgulas* carry with them. This relationship between Nyoongah man and woman has nothing to do with prestige or power or money. They are both outcasts in their own land and so really only have each other. And it is pure love, as pure as the flowers upon the wattle tree, or the water that flows from the back of the dancing, prancing blue dolphins.

I am living with a woman now. We have spent three years together with all its ups and downs. Reality, I now realise, is another human not only sharing your bed but your whole life and everything you do and think. For a solitary man, a wandering cloud, this can be hard to accept. But her long black hair that shines a burgundy red in the cheerful hands of the sun fascinates me. Her large black eyes swamp over me and her laughter can lift me to the skies. She is not a Nyoongah and she does not really love me I know, although I think she sometimes comes near to it. But if ever she reads this I hope she knows that I love her with a love which is pure because it comes straight from my heart. And my heart is all that I truly possess. My mind has been trodden upon and dug up for gold, diamonds or opals and, even though it is my sacred site, other people have seen glimpses of its darkened caves and amazing wonders. But my heart is my own, chipped and cracked though it may be, and any who touch it are protected from all men, all women and all tribes—forever.

Three Ways
Gerard Lee

I climb the steps of the Greyhound and arrive self-consciously at the front of the bus. A dozen elderly people watch as I struggle to manoeuvre my pack along the aisle. There's only one seat left, or more correctly, part of it's left. The woman sitting beside it has spilled over into a good portion. Spilled over into what is necessarily my half.

'Is anyone sitting here?' I ask and in answer to the question, she somehow triggers the internal muscles of her buttocks and pulls herself back over the halfway line, at the same time passing a hand through her red Rod Stewart hair. I unload the backpack and sit down, readying myself for 1500 kilometres of pure hell across the top end of Australia from The Isa to The Darwin.

'Hot, isn't it?' I say.

'I'm melting away, boxed in like this.' She shuffles uncomfortably in her crimpelenes, gives me an uncertain smile.

We sit for ten minutes, the bus engine rumbling, waiting,

sweating like pigs. No-one speaks. Her rump is beginning to subside back into my territory. The strain of holding it up must be colossal. Soon we'll have contact. When we do touch, it's more comforting than inconvenient.

Perhaps noticing my enjoyment, she hauls herself back against the window.

I offer her a piece of bubblegum. She refuses. 'I've got to stop eating. I only have one meal a day now.' I nod disinterestedly, like I don't even notice she needs to cut down. 'But I'm smoking again,' she adds, glumly. 'Instead of a meal, I puff on a cigarette. Can't win, can you? If it's not cardiac arrest, it'll be lung cancer.'

She takes out a packet of Benson and Hedges, handles them in her small hands like one unused to smoking and lights up.

'When only the best will do ...' She laughs and looks out the window. I follow her line of sight. There on the footpath, in front of the shops is a haggard, grey-haired man with two boys swinging off the ends of his arms. They're watching her and she's looking back through the tinted glass as if they're a boring program on TV. The boys are smiling at her and pointing.

'That your father and kids?'

'My husband,' she says.

I'm embarrassed but she doesn't seem to mind. She keeps looking out, expressionless. She must think they can't see her face.

As the bus pulls out there's no goodbye. Maybe she's too shy to wave, but he looks back as if he'll never see her again.

'He was a rough rider,' she says, almost to herself.

We're passing beneath the slag heaps of the Isa Smelting Works, heading out into open country. The sun's beginning to set. The earth itself now has a glow to it—outback reds and oranges. There's a breeze coming through the windows.

The driver introduces himself. His name's Dave. He'll be taking us to Three Ways, the crossroads of the north-west. From there, it's east to the Queensland border and across the top to Darwin. He also explains that the toilet's blocked, then adds: 'One more thing, ladies and gentlemen. The rules of the bus are that alcoholic beverages and obscene language are forbidden. They're a no-no, all right? So, if you don't want to find yourself out in the middle of the Never Never with nothing but your luggage ... don't get caught.' My companion giggles. 'Over to the left, you'll see the north-west telegraph line.' All heads turn. Out over the dry grass, about fifty metres off a wire droops between slanting telegraph poles, leading off behind and ahead of us. 'And over to the right ...'—all heads turn—'you'll see absolutely nothing.' A short chuckle from the passengers but behind us a raspy voice pipes up: 'That's not nothing, mate,' and continues with a drunken slur, 'that's some of the best bloody grassland in the Southern Hemisphere.' I turn around to see the speaker. He's about four seats back, wearing a moth-eaten twenty-gallon hat and trying very hard to get me in focus.

'Yeah, I'm still here,' he says to me. 'Haven't gotten off yet.'

I turned back to the front again embarrassed. My companion's looking at me.

'He's a real bushie, been down at the rodeo.'

From behind, more quietly, '... the best grassland any-fucken-where.'

'He'll end up like all the rest. They're all the same in the end. Once they give up the rodeo they don't care. He'll be like my old man ... burnt out. Won't go anywhere, won't do anything. All they want to do is ride. I like to move around a bit. Sometimes I just have to get up and leave a place. I can't stand another minute of it. And my husband's good, he says OK ... couldn't do anything else, I suppose. But if it was up to him we'd still be rotting away in Camooweal.'

'Where are you going this trip?'

'All the way to Katherine. I'm worried though. I've never left him alone before, with the kids.'

'He'll manage.'

'Tonight he'll be all right. I've left them steak and eggs, an easy tea. But it's not right. Him having to come home and cook a meal. It's not man's work.'

'Haven't you heard of Germaine Greer, or didn't feminism get out this far?'

She laughs. 'That's what they said about dollars and cents. But they got out here. We've even got the wireless and the motorcar. Wonderful, isn't it?'

'How old are you?'

'None of your business.' She waves the question away, looks out the window and then back, assessing me. She's facing me directly for the first time. It's a pretty face, slightly angry and bright. The drunk rider from behind is staggering around trying to force his way into the toilet. He finally pulls the door open and a stinking whiff races down the bus. The bus driver announces again over the speaker that the toilet is blocked. In a moment he pulls over and offers the rough rider a chance to relieve himself outside.

While he's gone, Dave says, unofficially, not through the mike: 'This bloke's got no shame. The rest of you will have to wait till it's dark.'

Cackles.

'Where are you from?' she asks.

'Brisbane.'

'Yeah, thought so. Me too. I ran away when I was sixteen.'

THREE WAYS

'How long ago was that?'

'Not saying ... Do you remember in the paper, about a bloke who used to rob check-out girls?'

'No.'

'He'd always escape on a motorbike. They called him the Armed Bikie.'

'Aww yeah, I remember him.'

Her eyes light up: 'I was his girlfriend.'

'Really.'

'Ooh, yeah. He got caught on a Friday afternoon at Morningside Fair. It was going to be his last job. I left Brisbane the same night. Haven't been back since. The only thing I miss is the movies.'

'That means you're my age.'

'What does?'

'If you were sixteen when you ran away from Brisbane. That bikie thing was about ten years ago.'

'Could be.'

'What do you mean, could be? That's when it was. You're sixteen plus ten.'

Her brow wrinkles. 'Don't say it like that ... caught myself out there, didn't I?' She stubs out her cigarette and looks at me carefully. 'We don't look the same age though, do we?'

'I've had a sheltered life,' I say.

She smiles and looks away.

'Have you seen *Close Encounters of the Third Kind?*'

'Yeah, I have,' I say. 'Didn't think it'd get out this far.'

She smiles.

'It arrived here about a light year after everyone else saw it. I really loved that picture. I believe it too. There's always sightings up here in the out-of-the-way places ... there's been too many of them not to be true.'

'Yeah, it could be.'

'The fellas that make those pictures must be real characters—we get that out here too.' She's indicating the *Playboy* I tried to conceal in the seat pocket. 'Good articles in there, mate.' She gives me a nudge. I try to act nonchalant.

Her thigh is resting easily against mine now. 'Talking about movies, you should stop at Camooweal for the night ... for the flicks. Everyone'll be there. The blacks with their kids and all the dogs, fighting in the aisles. They laugh at all the wrong places: like when someone gets shot in the guts, they crack up. And they love John Wayne. One of them even calls himself John Wayne. You should go.' Her eyes are twinkling with the good advice.

I see us both sitting back in the canvas chairs like a couple of kids. She's got three packets of Smith's and I've got one. We're having a great time, her large form rollicking in the light coming off the screen.

We're in open country now. Over to the right, the red sun is disappearing. The earth seems to be breathing again, rolling over, recovering from another day under the heat. You can hear it sighing with relief. I reach for the *Playboy* and open it casually hoping it's not going to be the centrefold. I miss the centrefold but hit something equally shameful—a sweet-faced blonde sitting astride a motorbike. No clothes. Only black stilettos. My companion leans across to take it in.

'What a lovely face.'

'Mmm.'

'I didn't think they had girls like that in these stick books.'

'Stick books! Who calls them that? What's it mean?'

'Not saying.' She's holding her mouth tight against a smirk. She's being naughty.

THREE WAYS

It's not quite dusk. The sun has disappeared below the horizon but streaks of yellow light are still coming across from the west. The ground is already in shadow; just above it, grass and small bushes are high enough to be caught in the last rays. Inside the coach a golden light is being reflected off the panels. In front of us the heads of an elderly couple are bobbing together, bathed in light.

She's playing around with the gadgets above our seat. Her reading light comes on.

'How do you get on with the blacks?' I ask.

'Shoot 'em.' She's watching me to see if I believe her. I smile.

'No, I get on well enough with them. Some stations round here though, they give you a gun as soon as you arrive. One place, they wouldn't hire anyone with Aboriginal blood. I'm glad they didn't ask me because I don't know what's in me. All I know is it was some American after the war.' She looks out the window.

'You mean your father's American?'

She nods, sneaks a look at me. In the light from her reading lamp I see her eyes are reddening. She realises I've noticed and casually reaches up and switches the lamp off.

'I'd like to know who he was ... I still write to my mother.'

She's facing out the window. I pat her on the arm not sure how far I should go. Still facing away, she reaches up and wipes one eye. I glance idly about the bus. Two women in the seat opposite are discussing butter and cheese and how to keep them fresh.

'My fridge has a built-in sealed compartment for butter and cheese.'

'So's mine,' says my companion, turning to me, smiling.

In Camooweal, where she used to live, there's nothing of

note except the General Store. She points it out as we drive past—a corrugated iron shed with a Coke ad along one side.

'Worked in that damn place for two years and then it closed down.'

'What, rude to the customers?'

She grins and threatens me and we're already out of town.

'Some good swimming holes out that way.' She's pointing at arid, thirsty landscape, a pile of empty forty-four gallon drums near a dirt track. 'Kimmy and I went in nude one afternoon and we saw this old fella spying on us. We tried to run for our clothes but we couldn't get up the bank. Kept slipping in the mud.'

'I'd like to have seen that myself,' I said.

'Yeah, you would.'

Ten kilometres out of Camooweal she says: 'It's only now I'm beginning to enjoy the country. I've seen all around Camooweal before ... this is new.'

What we're looking at now is what we were looking at before—dried grass with here and there, a spastic eucalypt or two.

Driver: 'Our next stop is Barry Caves. We'll be there for half an hour, arriving at Three Ways about eleven p.m. for an hour stop.'

'An hour stop!' she says. 'I just want to get on to Katherine to see Kimmy. What can you do for an hour in the middle of the night?'

'Plenty.'

She laughs and takes a drag. 'I could say somethin' but I won't.'

We travelled on. At two she was adopted out, at twelve she found out, at fourteen she left home, at fifteen she met her boyfriend, at sixteen she was in court, at seventeen she was in Camooweal.

'And that was like being in jail,' she says, summing it all up. 'Silly things you do sometimes ... and keep doing.'

I nod.

'I've been yakking on, haven't I?'

'No.'

'I have. Now you tell me what you've done. You've been keeping that very quiet.'

'I'm doing Arts at uni.'

'I thought so. Something like that. You look like an artist.'

At about eight we stop at Barry Caves. The place is a non-event except for a cockatoo chained to a verandah railing, trying to sleep. When she strokes the back of its head, it wakes up and starts to yell at the top of its voice something that sounds like, 'June! June!'

'Aww shut up,' she says quietly, and turning to me, 'it's a mental case.'

The bus snails along comfortably, lights dim, passengers dozing. Outside, the Australian night is slipping away. We read. Carol's is Leon Uris, mine is *The Idiot*.

'That a book about you,' she says, noticing the cover. I nod. She shifts in the seat, trying to make herself more comfortable. Suddenly she crumples up in pain.

'O God, O God Almighty.' Her face is screwed up. She's holding her stomach. 'It's my knee ... O God, it hurts like crazy.' She's breathing hard, her eyes watering. She takes a quick glance at me and looks away, humiliated. I rub her uselessly on the back.

'I'm supposed to be in bed for six weeks. My doctor would kill me if he knew I was on this bus. My knee keeps collapsing under me. All this weight doesn't help either. He'd just kill me. He told me this would happen.'

She seems to be in less pain now. She rubs her eyes with her sleeve.

'But it's no good me staying home, the kids're all over me.'

'What about your husband, can't he look after them?'

'He's not too good himself.' She's looking down at the back of the seat. There's an almost imperceptible sob. She reaches up and switches off the reading lamp again. 'He had a buster off a bull he was riding on one of the stations. We didn't know whether he was going to live or not ... God, I'm telling you everything now.'

She puts her hand up, but it's too small. Beyond it, her face is screwing up. Her whole body begins to shake.

She's asleep, resting against the window. I want to lay my head on her shoulder but fear a rejection. She's no angel, sleeping away there with a piggy snore, but I want to cuddle up to her anyway. I look around to the rough rider. He seems to be asleep but he opens one eye.

'Bad manners to watch a man sleep.'

I glance back at her again, studying her face, the flabby cheeks and there, something I haven't noticed before; her ear, sweet, neat, completely fat-free. I look away. It's probably rude to watch a sleeping woman, too.

I take out the *Playboy* and flick through. Those girls look very thin. They're so thin. I put it away and look back at the sleeping woman.

The bus is tearing along now, pushing smoothly through the black night, passengers wrapped in sleep like sandwiches in tissue paper.

THREE WAYS

At Three Ways there's the atmosphere of an Arab marketplace. The depot is nothing more than an acre of concrete set down in the middle of nowhere with a few buildings on it. There are buses here from everywhere, going everywhere—Sydney, Perth, Alice Springs, Darwin, Townsville. You can almost hear the bleating of camels in the background. People zombied by lack of sleep wander around beneath the harsh neons.

An effort has been made to help you feel at home as you travel through these nether regions. In the cafeteria you can buy all the products:—Coke, Cadbury's, takeaway coffee, Cherry Ripes, even cotton buds. Carol and I are waiting at the counter among the sleepy customers. She's brushed her hair but her face is still crinkled.

'See, she's fat too.' She nods discreetly to the girl serving. 'Out here there's nothing else to do but eat.'

'I could say something but I won't,' I say.

'Get outta here.' She tries to stand on my foot.

She orders a ham sandwich and then looks across at other normal-sized people tucking into plates of steak, coleslaw and chips.

'Love a carton of chips.'

I buy a salad sandwich and a Cherry Ripe and stroll outside amongst the buses, thinking about Carol. I'm standing around eating when I see the rough rider and another man sitting together on two plastic chairs. I tune in to the conversation. The other fellow is English and he's just come back from the highlands of New Guinea.

'They run around with axes and spears up there, nothing on.'

'Mmm, mmm,' the rough rider says.

'No. I'm not kidden you, mate.'

'Mmm, mmm.'

'They do! I saw it myself.'

'Mmm, what else did you see up there?'

I turn and head back to some benches I've noticed.

There she is, sittting alone against a brick wall in her pant suit. She's eating a carton of chips unhappily. I sit down beside her. She offers me the carton, I shake my head and offer her the clean end of my Cherry Ripe. She shakes her head and throws the carton under the seat. She's holding her greasy fingers out to dry, her hands so small and dainty.

'Want to come for a walk?'

'Where?' She's dubious.

'Out there, through the grass, under the stars.' She looks at me with that little bright face.

'The grass, the stars, eh?'

'Yeah, the grass and the stars.'

She looks away, then back. I can't figure out what she's thinking. 'That grass you're talking about is spinifex. It's all spikes, pricks ya.'

'We could take a blanket.'

She studies me a long moment.

'You don't want me.' Then barely mumbles: '... too fat.'

For a moment I'm stymied but finally burst out with: 'I love your fat.'

There's a silence in which her blush grows deeper. But she keeps looking at me—her blue eyes. A bus starts up somewhere nearby.

'You don't,' she says at last and lifts herself off the seat. 'Think I better have a cup of tea.'

I walk out to the front of the depot and step off the concrete into the dark. I keep going, on up the road, the stars out on the horizon growing brighter as I go. I'm still chewing on the Cherry Ripe but too upset to enjoy it. I made her blush, an ex-juvenile bikie moll. How could I?

The smell of the grass blows across from the dark. I feel lonely in a big way.

THREE WAYS

Looking back to the depot I see a couple of people talking near one of the petrol bowsers. They seem miles away. I decide I can't go back to the bus. I'll sleep out here and take the next one in the morning.

I walk a few paces into the grass and start to feel an itchy sensation round my calves. It gets so bad after a few more steps I'm forced back to the road. I take my shoes and socks off and see little spearheads of grass sticking in them.

A bus pulls out of the depot and heads my way. I strain to read the destination as it approaches. It says 'Darwin' and my pack's still on board. I decide to let it go and collect it next day at the depot. I step back into the grass so as not to be caught in the headlights but the bus glides to a standstill nearby, like a thing from outer space. The door opens silently.

'I'm staying here, mate,' I say to the driver from my position several metres into the spinifex.

'Get on, son.' There's no argument possible.

As I walk down the aisle, the oldies are having a go at me.

'Trying to walk it?'

'In a hurry, boy!'

'He's got his shoes off.'

I glance up the bus and see two strangers in our seat. 'Pst,' she says from way up the back. She's pointing to a space beside her.

'I told the driver you were up here,' she says and watches as I place my shoes and socks on the floor. 'Don't like to say I told you so.'

'Well, don't.'

She laughs and then gets serious.

'Enjoy yourself out there?'

'Yeah, not bad.' I look into her eyes. 'You should have come too.'

'Aww yeah, what for?' She's playing with the seat pocket.

It must be two or three a.m. I've been asleep leaning against her shoulder. She's awake now, too. She looks across at me in the half-light. Her jowls are crushed and wrinkled but her eyes are still bright. As I rub the sleep from mine, the voices of the women opposite come to me. It's the middle of the night and they're still talking cheese and butter.

'Why don't you stop off at Katherine in the morning,' she says. 'Meet Kim. You'd like her. Come out to the Gorge with us.'

'I don't know.'

'Kimmy's taken the day off work and we're going swimming.'

'Just like in the old days eh ... in the nude.'

'God, you never stop.'

'OK, I'll stop.'

'Don't stop on my account ... but you'd love it out at Katherine. What are you going to Darwin for anyway?'

'I don't know.'

'See!'

She winks at me and puts her head back against the window. I think about her, her languid form, lying on the rocks at the edge of the water. I think about nights with her in a flat in Katherine, Kimmy in another room. I think about her husband.

I close my eyes and begin to fall asleep, in her direction. I snuggle comfortably into her shoulder but I'm sneaky about it. If she wakes up I'll have the excuse of somnambulism. I let my hand slip down onto her lap and wait for a reaction. None. She takes a deep breath, a sigh perhaps. I wonder if she's still conscious, if deep within that flesh her heart is beating faster. Mine is. My hand's like a snake on her lap, ready to strike. I want it to slide up underneath her clothes and suckle its lips around her breast.

We speed on through the night, through the grasslands and the wilderness, through the rutted creeks and rivers, clinging together like a couple of drought-proof seeds, nestled in the arms of the Northern Territory.

Her friend Kimmy was waiting in the red dust.

'Oh God, she's fat too,' Carol said when she caught sight of her. They could have been twins.

'Are you coming?' she said.

'I don't know.'

'Darwin'll still be there in a few days. Most probably.'

I looked at her bright face, her tough red hair.

'Come on, gorgeous.'

At dusk that evening I sat on the cliffs at Darwin overlooking the sea, imagining what she was doing at that moment. I saw her, the sun coming golden through a flywire window. Kimmy sitting on a couch somewhere behind her, laughing. She was laughing too, cooking them an 'easy tea'.

Black Mud and Braille
James Cockington

It was the coldest night in the history of the universe and I was driving from one side of the world to the other, or so it seemed. My grandmother was sick, as she had been for the last decade, but this time it was serious. Serious serious, as Mum described it. I had this instantly nasty thought that if I used my current state of extreme poverty as an excuse to drive to Sydney instead of flying, chances were that she might be dead by the time I got there. Save me another trip for the funeral. Gran and I had always disliked each other with an openness that made me almost like the old crow.

I'd arranged to stay overnight at Ulladulla, where my sister-in-law had a holiday shack. It was sometime after midnight when I arrived, strung out on truckstop coffee, driven half-crazy by the Merle Haggard cassette which jammed in the player fifteen k's out of Melbourne and was on constant repeat. The Kingswood was a bitch at the best of times, but with the bald left rear in the rain it had a tendency to turn sharp left like a shopping trolley. My shoulders were aching and the 'slow, 60K' sign was the most beautiful sight I'd seen since breakfast.

Ulladulla ain't Las Vegas. If anyone else in town was alive it was impossible to tell. Rosie had given me detailed instructions on the back of a dry-cleaning docket, but it still took twenty minutes to find the white wagon wheel that marked the driveway. At least the key was where she said, under the third potplant from the left, being sat upon by a snail. If anything, it was colder inside the shack than out and I didn't have the energy to find the radiator. The smell of dust and Pine-O-Cleen indicated that the place hadn't been touched since Rosie and Spike, her legal shark of a husband, were here last summer.

By now, the rain sounded like World War One on the tin roof. I was too exhausted to unpack so I cleaned my teeth without paste, piled every blanket I could find on top of the double bed, stripped off and crawled into the womb. After ten minutes I stopped shivering and felt my body going numb. Sleep hit me like a Mack truck in the fog.

What happened then was kind of fuzzy, like a three-bong dream or a foreign movie seen through gauze. It could have been ten minutes later or ten days. I knew that something was moving in the room but I wasn't awake enough to react to it in any human way. This revelation pushed me into some kind of limboland where, neither awake nor asleep, I was aware of me watching myself watching the silhouette of someone else moving in front of the window, the only vague source of light in a room filled with black mud. I wasn't conscious enough for fear.

The silhouette appeared to be a woman, judging by the dress which she was trying, with great difficulty, to take off. Next she was trying to take off her pantihose, stumbling each time she stood on one leg. As comatose as I was, I knew what this meant. She, whoever she was, was pissed. Paralytic.

I had no impulse to speak and I was barely awake enough to work out that something was wrong with the plot of what I thought still could be a dream. There was a brief blurry moment of panic until I worked out that if anyone was in the wrong place it was this undressing woman, not me. This naked large-breasted woman, judging by the silhouette, putting on a T-shirt and (another slight moment of panic here) obviously preparing to get into bed with me.

When she did I half-expected her to realise my presence and scream. But it was now obvious that my presence had already been noticed and was even expected. She rolled over and clicked into me like Lego, her right leg forced between my two, as if we had been doing this for decades. I could smell the sudden warmth of her flesh, a mixture of some unidentifiable brand of perfume and, surprisingly in this weather, sweat. Drunk? Dancing? Then the unmistakeable sweet and sour odour of wine and cigarettes, on her breath. She didn't scream. She didn't even speak. With her cold hands and sharp little fingernails she began to explore her territory, which I soon realised was me. As far as she was concerned she was exactly where she wanted to be.

In slow-motion the mouth moved up my neck. In the blackness it felt as large as a whale's. My mouth was instantly filled with her heat-seeking tongue. Her hand found my cock and grabbed it like she owned it. I was already erect. Did she grunt or did I?

We screwed in the black mud of that room for what seemed like days. We fucked by braille. It was the kind of animal sex you only have when you're blind drunk, or in my case, half-dead. Sense snapshots. I can remember the smell of her, the taste of her, the texture of her skin (body hairs erect in the cold) the fact that she had stubble under her arms. There was a series of vague, grey on grey images, film noir set to a soundtrack of psycho rainbeat. A close-up of her mouth, white teeth, slight gap between the front two, lips as big as blimps. Nipples, pubic hair, handfuls of hair (blonde? red? black?), clenched knuckles, fingernails. Edited highlights of a person, but not enough to make an ID in a police line-up.

I think I came three or four times. Make it three times, for modesty's sake. Once, I think, in her mouth, twice in her pussy, once on top, once underneath with fingernails puncturing my forearms. Each time it was like my brain was exploding, followed by a feeling somewhere between orgasm and nausea. I remember being grabbed by the hair and having my mouth slammed over her pussy. She liked this. I spent an hour or so down there. She, I think, was coming more or less constantly. She wouldn't stop and I was in no position to make her. She was in charge and I was surfing in on her momentum, just waiting to be dumped on the beach. They say that everyone has one night in their lives where they win gold at the Sexual Olympics. I won mine with a complete stranger.

I soon entered the layer of sleep normally reserved for the recently dead. Purple velvet coffin sleep. When I awoke the room was filled with what I assumed was grey morning light. I was later to find out it was midday. It was still raining but softly. I had no idea where I was and it was only after I saw the mudguard of my car out the window that the connections snapped into place. Melbourne. My dying grandmother. Ulladulla. Then, my god, last night. That woman.

When I thought of her I tried to convince myself that I had had the mother of all wet dreams. I pieced together as many of the fragments as I could remember before turning to look at the other side of the bed. I was alone. The house was silent and empty. Just me and the smell of Pine-O-Cleen.

The faint echoes of that alien perfume hit me, then a solid wave. The other side of the bed, sheets screwed, pillow scrunched, proved that she had been real. I could still taste her in my mouth. The dull ache in my balls, the desperate need to piss, proved that the sex was not imaginary. I stumbled to the toilet on jelly legs and slumped against the wall, shivering, pissing liquid sulphur for five minutes straight. It hurt like hell. I noticed her bite marks on my forearm. I felt kitten-weak and, for some reason, wanted to cry.

When I came back to the bed, there it was, the final evidence. Wedged into the crack between the mattress and the sheets was the T-shirt I dimly remembered she had worn to bed and removed soon afterwards. That image, her silhouetted against the window, was now as ancient as Dr Caligari. I removed the T-shirt and smoothed it out on the bed. From K-Mart. Size, medium. On the front was a cartoon of Garfield with the slogan 'I'm not overweight, I'm undertall'. It smelt of perfume and sex.

Later, with a cup of instant coffee in one hand and a cigarette in the other, I searched the house for some further clues to her identity. There was nothing. No note, no toothbrush, no lipsticked cigarette butts in the ashtray, none of her clothes in the wardrobe.

Constant flashbacks filtered through a mild morning migraine. The sight of the T-shirt on the bed, flat, empty, made me feel both sad and horny. I had a sudden desire to go back to bed, masturbate and wait for her to return. Whoever she was. Then logic took over. I figured that, like me, she must have been passing through, there only for the one night. Unlike me, she had the energy to get up early, get dressed and leave in a hurry. She didn't feel the need to wake me so I knew she wouldn't be back.

By two o'clock I was in my car and headed north. The rain had slowed to drizzle but Merle Haggard was still jammed in for the duration. Still half-numb, my tongue feeling two sizes too big, I sat there thinking. I thought about her. There were a number of theories but only two held up for more than a minute. Of course it was a set-up. The woman (or girl, I couldn't work out how old she was) was some kind of hooker hired by someone (Spike?) who had told her to sneak in, shut up, fuck me, then split. That would explain how she got in so easily, unless I forgot to lock the door. Yeah, well, a large number of holes in that theory. One, I hadn't told anyone exactly when I was leaving Melbourne or when I would arrive in Ulladulla. Two, this lady didn't use a condom which hookers, even dead-drunk ones, always do. Plus, Spike, cut-throat lawyer and legendary tightwad, wasn't the practical joking kind. Scratch that theory.

Theory two set in around Nowra, and lasted until Kiama. I decided that when I arrived at the shack I forgot to lock the door, so it was possible, well, theoretically possible, that she had been so pissed that she simply walked into the wrong place. Wasn't there a newspaper story about some guy who did this last year and only noticed when the cops arrived. I had this mental flash of her waking up at dawn, seeing to her horror that I wasn't her husband and being so embarrassed that she grabbed her clothes and ran out unnoticed. That theory sat well enough until I remembered the T-shirt she was putting on. Girls don't walk around with a spare T-shirt. She must have got that from somewhere inside.

At Kiama I first had the urge to phone my sister-in-law in Sydney and say, what the hell was I going to say? Do you know who I fucked last night, Rosie, because I sure don't? I got as far as the phone booth when suddenly my curiosity faded. If it wasn't some kind of practical joke then it must have been some bizarre case of mistaken identity. If that's what it was, better to let it ride. No harm done that I could detect. At least I knew for sure that I didn't have AIDS.

It was close to sunset. I got back in my car. The rain had stopped, my migraine had worn off after three Panadol, and the old Kingswood was cruising in third with minimal left steer. I started thinking about my grandmother dying. For the first time I kind of hoped the old bugger would hang on until I got there.

Lovelawn: A Fantasy
David Owen

Rain hardly ever fell in space and Lovelawn was so surprised that he wanted to say something: but he knew better than to talk to himself. The steady downpour of liquid dots fascinated him. He wondered if they made sound or produced scent and what force supplied them with momentum. Then fear replaced the fascination.

Lovelawn jerked himself upright. He continued to stare through the great dome of the Glans. *Rain?* Something was not right. Yet he couldn't be off a charted course. He swung about to seek clarification from the CmndCntrlCntr of Pennis VIII, Braynz. It would know. It would have warned him before now.

Not off course. What then? Lovelawn stabbed an antenna responder and the mystery was cleared. The carol had pierced and was cruising through a Remnant Zone.

Too ironic. Lovelawn swung back and reclined. Had he not inadvertently dozed he would surely have avoided the RZ and now it was too late—but he no longer had fear.

There was no known threat or danger from coming into contact this way with one of the millions of diasporic little oxygenated bubbles which drifted in these remote parts.

All the same Lovelawn remained curious. Pennis VIII had rammed through the casing of this RZ which had therefore burst, terminating its environment. He frowned as his lips turned up. He must have extinguished a Human then. It was a neutral but also comfortless thought. Here he was, a researcher in a carol studying their planetary extinction, and he managed to run one of the survivors over.

Measuring 844.66 metres from Glans through Shaft to Pubend, Pennis VIII was a longer firmer research carol than its predecessor VII, victim of a glomerated viralswarm of mysterious origin. The Species Museum's official record of that incident apportioned everything to it but mistrust—the mistrust of the Museum's thousands of circuit-collar employees who well knew that the far reaches were not safe. Still, Lovelawn had quickly accepted the offer to pilot Pennis VIII. Such chances of vocational elevation were rare and he craved to be alone for a length of time, no matter how dull the work.

But also how unexpected that soon, alone, he had become lonely. A million minutes without reason to say a simple *Hello* was a long time. Braynz admittedly provided a kind of company but its personalised thoughts were too deeply shallow to be stimulating, heartfelt. Also it had a sarcastic binary streak to it which Lovelawn regretted.

Lovelawn had a job and a hobby. He liked the cruising research carol, its size, its comfort, its technological mastery of the finiteless reaches. His routine was pleasurably simplex: Awake. Nutrition I. Conduct Research. Doze. Conduct Hobby. Nutrition II. Sleep. Awake. Nutrition I. Conduct Research. Doze ... The High Fathers of the Museum had carefully pointed out to Lovelawn that the

LOVELAWN: A FANTASY

sameness of the routine, coupled with the uninspirational nature of the research, required the candidate to be of a mental faculty to appreciate such sameness over a lengthy period of isolated time. They had mooted that he might be aloft for a billion minutes, research results depending. It was a moot meant to daunt, but Lovelawn had so strongly disliked his lowly circuit-collar existence that in his interview for the position he gave a perfect answer.

But unpleasantly, by suppurating degree in a creeping way, illicit loneliness got the better of him. He'd therefore sought permission from the High Fathers to undertake a leisure hobby and—after some confusing hesitation—the permission was granted. So now, happily, Lovelawn had nearly completed the intricate and time-consuming data input which would birth him a lifesize Toy Human, as a companion both cerebral and voiced.

Lovelawn did appreciate the comforts of dullness and the High Fathers on the selection committee had seen this in him. He wasn't *different* in any way, so much so that afterwards one had confided in him that he had been given an Nth-Normalcy rating. This was why this hobby-request (relayed via perfect, touchy Braynz through twelve time-warps) had met with stupefied pontification. But in the end they put their faith in his sensibility and permitted him to use the NAHR, the Nominal Archival Human Repository aboard PVIII to construct his Toy.

Beyond the rain-pocked Dome Lovelawn could see very little except dank impenetrable gloom. He thought he could make out a flat silver-tinged cloud far away, in the act of dying even as he squinted at it. He keyed a query to Braynz on the state of the RZ which, presumably, was now coldly disintegrating all around the carol. He read the reply on the screen: *Carol Wet. Worry-Free Interference with Waste Duct 12. Don't Worry. Conduct Research.* Lovelawn gritted his teeth. Of course the thing was wet. It was being rained upon, wasn't it? And he disliked Braynz reminding him of what to do next. But not to worry about the Waste Duct. He swung away from the screen, exhaled in annoyance, stood and walked across to the Viewing Pit. Yes yes yes it was a dull line of research but he had status now. There weren't that many employees of the Museum coasting about the finitelessness as Qualified Researchers. In the Pit he settled himself comfortably and yawned and activated the view-monitor.

The Species Museum occupied a middle level ranking in the ScHeMeOfThInGs. Although its findings were generally of an academic nature these sometimes were of practical benefit. Lovelawn's present research was a case in point: the self-generated extinction of an otherwise intelligent planetary species—albeit an insignificant one—required analysis. Furthermore the diasporic remnant Humans in their RZs needed watching. What if numbers of them were to gather and colonise an empty oxygenated planet? Would they destroy that one too?

So the Museum, despite its reputation for being stuffy and conservative, received adequate funding from the Convocation for Universal Management—C.U.M.—the governing body of EvErYtHiNg.

Lovelawn picked his empty nose and watched three 'caucasian' Humans engaged in a sexual activity in a blue-walled room. There was no sound but the small console at his left elbow was able to monitor their thoughts, by an elementary encephalic decoding, despite the fact that all three had probably been dead for at least fifty-two million four hundred and sixteen thousand minutes—a 'century', as Humans would clumsily have tried to conceptualise such a random block of time. The browny-pink, engorged, shiny penis of the first male was moving regularly in and out of the mouth of the female, who was lying on her stomach on a table. At her other end, the second male was holding tightly on to the base of his thick penis and alternately rubbing its crown against the labial lips then plunging it into the slippery vagina.

The console at Lovelawn's right elbow monitored changes of body temperature in and around the nineteen identified erogenous zones of the Human body (of which, tellingly, the brain was not one. That they experienced chemical rather than intellectual arousal had been one of their many problems ...). Matching the data from each console was tedious and finicky. Nevertheless Lovelawn had already come up with some hypotheses which he felt sure the HFs would embrace. He'd been able to think of nothing else but what he saw on the viewmonitor and this was exactly why Qualified Researchers were required to work in isolation. To concentrate, to analyse, to get the work done.

Now a black-skinned Human male entered the blue-walled room. Lovelawn smiled perceptively. He was always happy to see one of them. The man at the rear of the woman, whilst continuing to 'fuck' her, turned and looked invitingly at the black man who was holding and stroking his enormous penis, to which he began applying lubricant from a small jar on a stool. The man at the rear of the woman positioned his legs more widely as the black first massaged his buttocks then began to enter him anally.

Lovelawn concentrated—for the first time in this particular session the console at his left elbow registered a genuine response. The man entered by the black penis was quite suddenly no longer in control of his orgasmic function. His brain began 'whirling' towards the intense, brief delirium from which fatally Humans had been incapable of withdrawing. Lovelawn knew that the sensation of the black penis had quickly triggered the slow build-up engineered by the labial-vaginal circumvolution. Now, as ever, the caucasian male's brain died a momentary death. Then the encephalic console blipped off. Lovelawn frowned. What was Braynz up to now? Sulking in its Irate Function no doubt. Stupid *it*.

He dabbed at a few break-keys. Nothing. Yet the other console remained operative. Lovelawn rolled his eyes and flared his nostrils in annoyance. Well, he couldn't work now. Irritably he watched the black man slowly withdraw and, squeezing tight his glistening knob, walk round to the other end of the table, where the female's head was. Pressing down alongside her shaft-bulged cheek, and into the dank hair at the nape of her neck, he—

Lovelawn felt hungry. Nutrition II wasn't far off. How could he do his research effectively if Braynz kept getting moody? Then the console did come back to life. Lovelawn stared at it. There was a message: *See The Morrisons Now * * * Cross-Referencing Important.* Lovelawn shook his head. He was dealing here with the non-procreative aspect of Humansex. 'The Morrisons' was the collective term for the visfile containing all the data relating to partner-based sexual intercoupling for primarily procreative purposes. It was a poor file, for research purposes, since the visual data was scant, grainy, as if taken through glass and lace in dark light. So Lovelawn was not enamoured of the suggestion. And he felt hungrier.

Dully he watched the viewmonitor. He knew what each of the two men at the head of the woman were doing but even so—why was the console flashing *Burst-A-Meat?* He dabbed at a query key and exhaled. On yes, yes yes yes, playing tricks again. He read the message: *Apologies Data Input Error: See Mast-Ur-Bate.* Then the viewmonitor cut to a new image in which the female, alone, loomed pinkly

LOVELAWN: A FANTASY

large and the console—well, Braynz—again played up. *Preserve Angel*. Lovelawn angrily poked a finger for an explanation. *Data Input Error*, the console meekly responded: *See Perverse Angle*. It was enough. Lovelawn stormed away. Time to think about his hobby anyway. He'd correlate this data later. Also Nutrition II called. And he still hadn't decided on a name for the Toy.

Lovelawn slept and woke and ate and thought. The High Fathers would be pleased. He'd adduced theories which already were matching the empirical data. His research brief—To Further Investigate the Evolutionary Catastrophe Visited by Human Beings upon Themselves—had initially been daunting until he determined his first theory, from which others were starting to flow. The first theory derived, not surprisingly, from the Propositional Question: What caused the Humans not to combat the Rampant Overpopulation of themselves which destroyed them and their planetary habitat? Lovelawn's first theory had been simply to adduce thanks to the visual data. It was that the means of procreation should not have enjoyed such a powerful chemical reward. Clearly, 'reward' of this type had its place in all those lower earth-planet species unable to communicate by language to discuss the need for procreation and to individually and collectively rationalise over this need. For such lower life forms, the chemical reward *was* the language of procreation; they were one and the same.

Not so with Humans. The fatal error came about when no adjustment was made to this procreation-reward symbiosis, as the Human developed into the domineering, predator-free planetary species. (As a wise old retiring High Father had hinted to Lovelawn, monkey-sex lay at the root of the problems. Masturbating monkeys should have rung evolutionary alarm bells.) This therefore must be the Evolutionary Catastrophe: that the procreational and pleasurable aspects of Human sex were not separated out. Had they been, then tragic self-destruction would surely not have occurred.

All the same it seemed strange to Lovelawn that the urge continually got the better of such a calculating species. Their attempts at contraception during their civilised period had been pathetic. At least they were *aware* of the problem ... and it was by his concentrating on this—the awareness of an evolutionary flaw in themselves—that Lovelawn developed his second theory. In fact the logic of it was almost exciting and—

Braynz alerted him. A small Panicmonitor had begun to flash. Lovelawn walked across to it and, frowning sourly, wiped the dust off its screen. The message read: *Waste Duct Panic-Free Status*. The screen then went blank. In some alarm he returned to the main Braynz frame and fired in a query: *Repeat WD12 Info. Data Input Error?*

No No, Braynz replied.

Lovelawn didn't believe it. Was it playing some game with him again? He knew he would have to go and check, way down towards the rear of the 644-metre Shaft.

He elevated to the *Péage* of the Urethric Highway, alongside which were the Stables. He climbed onto a Horrse and *Péage*. He drove onto the gleaming tubular Highway and accelerated.

The Horrses had been designed for both practical and security functions. They were the internal means of transport about the carol, employing four wheels for driveability and, with the wheels inverted, a climbing-descending hoofed function for the awkward reaches and gullies of the Pubend. In the unlikely event of decompression or some other disaster aboard the carol, the machinated ungulates were convertibles to escape modules. An escapee could get inside a Horrse and depart the stricken vessel with the four legs retroactively positioned as rocket boosters. The head of a Horrse contained a small mainframe drive and the neck carried nutrition supplies. Survival in space in a Horrse was possible for up to one million five hundred thousand minutes; or so the manufacturing company guaranteed.

Stirrupped and harnessed to the mane, Lovelawn sped through the centre of the labyrinthine multi-levelled Shaft. Much of its length was for non-grav aerodynamic purposes, but it also contained guestquarters, datavaults, the ubiquitous Convocation Hall, storerooms, emergency supplies, and safety bulkheads. The Shaft's lower levels contained spare fuel rods, ballast chambers, bilge tunnels and their waste ducts. (By contrast the Pubend, the propulsion system, was simple but monstrously unwelcoming, being a dark spooky cavern of indescribable power to a mere researcher such as Lovelawn. He strenuously avoided the Pubend, secure in the knowledge that it was controlled by Braynz and he controlled Braynz and the Museum controlled him and C.U.M. controlled the Museum and EvErYtHiNg.)

Humming along towards Exit 12 Lovelawn dwelt again on his second theory. It also lay in a fatal evolutionary flaw and was gender-specific: that the male of the Human species had not only been physically stronger but appeared also to have had a greater or more urgent libido. Again, where this combination existed in speechless, intellect-free, predator-susceptible life forms on the planet, that combination was well served. However, it seriously damaged the Human Equation, particularly in the so-called 'century' when its total population doubled twice. Even the simplest student of statistics—as opposed to mere numbers—must surely have been horrified by that. Lovelawn's lips turned upwards as he recalled the same wise old retiring HF gently suggesting that it would have been a good thing had the females of the Human species learnt to eat their male partners after successful procreation.

Now he slowed and turned off the Highway, retracted the Horrse's wheels and clopped the vehicle down the spiral stairway of Exit 12.

He considered: the fact of the male being physically stronger and therefore being able to indulge in cross-gender non-procreational gratification at will, and having also a consistently greater urge to do so, simply compounded the gross evolutionary error inherent in his first theory. Why had that ever come about? Lovelawn still had no real idea. He did however have two 'solutions' for his theories—not that they would help the extinct clever species—but he felt sure that they would please the HFs. And after all there *were* Remnant Humans here and there ... and after all they *might*, by extaordinary universal luck ... it would only take two to couple succ ... and the doomed exponential multiplication would begin all over again! ... Down and around and down and around he carefully led the Horrse until it stepped out onto the clanking underfloor of the Shaft. The Waste Duct was secure. But the air was moisture-tinged and unnaturally cool and Lovelawn knew at once that something was *definitely wrong*.

Back in his seat in the viewmonitor pit, even after a good Nutrition and a lengthy doze, he could still feel the memory of the cold dry-wet air on his skin and in his nose and so great uncertainty plagued him. He'd interrogated Braynz to no avail. It simply kept repeating that WD12 was secure and that the situation remained *Panic-Free*. Lovelawn wondered if a sensory malfunction had been caused by the RZ rain, long since vanished. It would explain the anagrammatical confusions that were still occurring, as when not sixteen minutes ago a monitor had drawn his attention to a *Thrusting Purple Engorged Snipe*—and upon his jabbing a query key the maddening response came up. *Data Input Error. Snipe. Prefer: Penis.*

On cue, Lovelawn squatted in the faecalarium then, because he was so bored at watching Humansex and because of his continuing feeling of panicfreeunease, he decided to break the steadfast rules and cut the research session short in order to indulge in his hobby. After all no-one was watching, were they? And his effigial Toy was almost ready wasn't it?

All the same he walked with surreptitious speed to the Hobby Lab. It was guilt, and he knew so. First the genuine unease, now guilt: he wasn't supposed to have these feelings. They had implanted a Deadener in his cortex as soon as he became a Researcher—in the same operation when they took off the circuit collar. Still, they had warned him about residual emotions and had advised him to ignore them, there being no realistic chance of such residuals being aggravated. Waiting for the doors of the Hobby Lab to open, he assumed by instilled calculation that they were right.

Inside a Kublaidome lay Lovelawn's creative hobby. He was surprised to see just how well it had baked and gelled and unified. Almost done to perfection! He checked a few readings then gazed down through the large clear orb. The male—Lovelawn had decided he wanted one—lay on his back in perfect sublimation, with his hands upon his chest. His eyes were deep blue and his hair a rich golden colour. Lovelawn was pleased; he had been worrying about the hair because the catalogue hadn't included such a colour so he'd chanced his arm and his artistic eye by cross-matching three datahues namely, White, Oxide, and Serendipity Yellow. It was a glorious caucasian result.

Naked and beautifully pre-alert, the lifesize Toy was in fact a head taller than Lovelawn. This was because he'd specifically opted for the well-proportioned type of specimen as he'd seen in so many of the sex visuals. Then Lovelawn focused his attention upon the genitals. Yes, this Toy would be pleased with them too—not that it would 'know'. Only Lovelawn, on Pennis VIII, would be privy to his own decision regarding those genitals. Blue of eyes, golden of hair, cream-coloured of skin, this perfect Toy had a large pure black penis and testicles which, together with their tightly coiled pubic hair, had been named on the datahue chart as Negroid.

Lovelawn stood away. He couldn't wait to talk to it and get it to perform simple errands. Why, in the fullness of time he might teach it to drive a Horrse and go and sweep up Pubend filings. Even better—!—he might just one minute wire it up to Braynz and—

Then he remembered that the poor creature still had no name. He automatically sought the assistance of Braynz and at the nearest console he keyed: *Hobby. Random Name Please.*

The reply irritated him: *Random Is No Name.* Then it added: *Anag Random Meant? Try Moarnd?*

As soon as Lovelawn saw that name—*Moarnd*—he became elated. Yes! That was Moarnd lying waiting in the dome. Waiting waiting waiting to be birthed.

Happily Lovelawn refocused his attention. That's right. He might just one minute wire Moarnd up to Braynz and—

Deeply shocked, though he wasn't supposed to have such a function in such depth, Lovelawn continued to stare. He was immobilised by the warpish effect of what had happened. Nothing ought to have *happened*, but—thanks to the stupid dysfunctional Braynz—now it had.

Braynz had urgently summonsed him from the Hobby Lab back to the Glans atrium. It had been a laser-summons: a critical alert. And now Lovelawn stood aghast in the bright spacious emptiness of the atrium. Staring. At a Remnant Human. Confusions peaked in him. Braynz had almost every available panic button blipping and flashing and counterwailing and yet the Human seemed quite oblivious of or to any noise or distress in the alerted alien environment in which she now stood.

Implanted instinct required Lovelawn to assess IDP, Imminent Danger Potential: he cortex-lasered Braynz through one eye and with the other threw a beam onto the Human. She didn't move. They were perhaps two thousand centimetres apart. She wore a skimpy, curve-hugging unisuit. Still she didn't move, arms loosely by her sides. She was only looking at Lovelawn. Through the beam of his right eye he 'saw' that the suit had an inner pocket. Although empty of matter its outer face contained a looping Human-lettered term. Discombobulation hurtled through Lovelawn. A destructor code of some sort? But via himself Braynz quickly, thankfully, deciphered it as harmless, a typical suit-name label, this one reading: *Karl Karbonfiber*. Lovelawn relaxed tinily. The woman smiled, but he was not convinced by the facial alteration. She carried no apparent weaponry, but that meant nothing. 'Did you get in through the waste duct?' he asked, hoarsely, needlessly. Of course she had! His throat was dry, unused, itchy. She said something unintelligible in reply and took a calm step forward.

'*No!*' Lovelawn shouted weakly, pointing at her. He'd come all over confused, flushed, gelatine-limbed, wary. She frowned and spoke again, now opening out her arms in a clear gesture of harmlessness. * * * *Voice Intruder Scrambled*, Braynz relayed.

'What is you name?' Lovelawn asked. She shook her head.

Name Is 5-22-5-12-25-14, Braynz said. Lovelawn was beginning to experience a terrible acheheadedness from the two-way laser path. The soundless noise of each numeral penetrated like a needlejab. *Inner Wrist Tattoo*, Braynz added. Then: *Sorry. Data Output Error. For 5-22-5-12-25-14 Prefer E-V-E-L-Y-N.*

'Evelyn? ...' Lovelawn said aloud.

This time Evelyn shrugged apologetically and indicated by means of palmed hands that she was very tired. Lovelawn felt sorrier for himself than for her as he deactivated the laser and beckoned her to follow him.

In the minutes following Lovelawn tried not to vary his sleep-wake-nutrition-research-doze-hobby-nutrition-sleep pattern; but he could not stop thinking of her. He'd assigned her to a small guestquarter and by clear visual gestures had instructed her not to wander. Nor did she. Evelyn had clearly understood at once that she could move only between her room and the Glans atrium, via the *Pèage* elevator. She took Nutrition in a small antechamber, together with Lovelawn, and followed him around or else she sat gazing into space. He dared not bring himself to consider what to do with her. At least she *was* harmless. Still, he strictly forbade her any insight into the technical aspects of his research, all of which remained classified Species Museum property. Imagine if she turned out to be a plant! It was a chilling thought, which Lovelawn dismissed, because Braynz would have easily found out by now.

At one Nutrition Lovelawn decided to tell her what he was doing. Her innocent curiosity—which had been increasing as she relaxed into the environment, so much so that she sometimes appeared bored—had given him a playful feeling of superiority. Also, the more he thought of Evelyn the more he wanted to communicate with her. Properly, not just in Dumbladensignlang. So it was that, earnestly, he blurted out: 'I have been researching your peoples' demise. You must be very discomfited by your parableptic optimism to control yourselves. Your collective stupidity.'

Evelyn smiled and did not shrug. Her eyes were bright and happy and Lovelawn liked them, just as he found most fetching her habit of blowing the fringe of her red hair out of her eyes. Emboldened he said, 'Yes, and I have two theories on it so far.' He explained them. She listened politely and laughed once or twice in response to the changing pitch of his voice.

'I also have two solutions. Too late, how sad,' he added sombrely, 'but this is what ought to have happened. Since you were not only predator-free, and not limited to a specific habitat but also capable of pure thought and language, the dual nature of your sexual activities should have been separated out. This would best have been achieved by the evolution in the male of a procreational teste and a recreational teste.'

Evelyn laughed. Lovelawn wanted to laugh too because of her happy reaction. Making her happy pleased him in the oddest way. He hadn't ever felt the like before: his inside stomach glowed.

'As for my second theory,' he said, his nutrition quite forgotten, 'the greater male physical strength and the greater male libido were always a fundamental error in your species. How much more sensible it would have been had the greater libido evolved in the female. In that way your sexual conduct would have been guile-driven rather than protein-driven. That is, a mind over matter principle, in keeping with your Human sophistication in so many other ways. You do understand, Evelyn?' He frowned because she suddenly appeared crestfallen. She spoke rapidly, animatedly. What had he said that she somehow understood? Or was she simply frustrated at understanding nothing? Not knowing, he became agitated. Then he had a good idea. Of course. He could explain his research to her by means other than through the black window of unshared language. The Museum wouldn't care—because it wouldn't know! She was harmless and, more than that now, her presence had placed this unaccountable *glow* in his stomach. It must be some form of Human telepathic placebo deposit: a clever means of signalling friendliness beyond stranded tongues. That had to be it. 'So I'll show you,' he said.

His nostrils were so empty that even in deep sleep he was stunningly reminded of her by her multitude of fulsome saline-like fucaceous skinglowing bodywafted scents.

At the minute carefully appointed by himself Lovelawn invited Evelyn into the Viewing Pit. He made her sit just to one side of him, behind a monitor. He knew exactly what he was doing and he had thought long and hard about it. Of all the dry quadillions of nanoseconds of Humansex he'd watched, one montage stood out as perfect for her; perfect because it included a female with hair, long flaming red hair, strikingly similar to Evelyn's. Lovelawn anticipated a joyous reaction from her, one of powered happiness and wellbeing at seeing a cloneterpart. Also there were numbers of other individuals involved, the sight of whom were sure to cheer her. (Despite their being long-dead. Lovelawn was grateful in this instance that he and Evelyn were not able to talk; he had no wish now to direct her mind to what the C.U.M. Historians called the Billionsdeath, or, the Planet That Was Eaten Alive. Naturally the purists argued that the planet had in fact by a woeful mischoreography devoured *itself*: it made its own mistake. But how could you articulate that to an inarticulate survivor?)

It took Braynz no time at all to find the montage, which was entitled *Waterfall Orgy*. Lovelawn glanced over his shoulder at Evelyn—she sat demurely—and, smiling inside himself, he settled back to watch. He couldn't wait to cast a surreptitious glance at her, at what would surely be a joyful reunion of spirit for her.

Upon the screen occupying all of the wall came the sound of gentle splashing. Splashing made by a tall, sunstruck waterfall cascading with showery lightness into a spreading pool at the edges of which sprouted green foliage, above shingle and moist pale sand, from which ran cosy runnels becoming shallow streams going on their little ways. Upon a large flattish boulder lay spread a nutrition hamper, replete with a variety of open beverages.

Some of the many naked Humans present were coupling, in orthodox fashion, on the sands and in the runnels. Others were watching the couplers, standing near or straddled over them in acts of personal or mutual masturbation. Food contents and liquid containers were being smeared and rhythmically thrust. Closer up, semen and saliva unified as tittering became grinning became groaning. Now Lovelawn felt good as the right moment approached. On an inflated raft in the middle of the gently moving pool, on her back, lay the female with the flame-red hair. Her glistening legs were wide-parted. A male, waist-deep in the water, sucked concentratedly upon her sex. Her long arms were flung back in abandon. Then as he worked she began to bite on one of her fists. She started bucking and the raft device bobbed unevenly—the male had to pursue her with his mouth and it seemed that her climax was thus being agonisingly withheld from her. Arching, writhing, her expression a tantalising grimace, she gripped the male's hair in a frantic effort to clamp him to her crotch.

Lovelawn glanced at Evelyn—and became fearfully concerned for her. Had she turned badly unwell? Her face appeared to be flushed. She sat stiffly, awkwardly, as if she had become a shy little person. But then she emitted a throaty murmur, at Lovelawn. She was sitting on her hands. Immediately he switched the montage off and, stupidly, began to try to find the words to apologise for not being able to communicate with her to tell her he hoped that the waterfall image hadn't somehow contributed to the fact that she looked unwell. All he could do was smile and proffer his empty hands, palms out in supplication.

Evelyn rose from her chair and stood over him. Her scents were overwhelming, her hair brushed against his frozen knuckles. Her breath came in his ear. She bent right over in front of him and said something. Then she put her mouth on his and with her tongue easily prised his lips apart. Her tongue ran over his teeth. She made it stiff and pushed it towards his throat.

Shocked, puzzled and confused, Lovelawn had never experienced anything remotely like the sensation. It went on and on until finally he exploded away in a kind of laughter, because he could no longer breathe. But now Evelyn had fallen to her knees and her hands were searching his lap. He couldn't believe it—but then, she didn't know. So he showed her. He removed his leggings and let her gaze at the button-sized aperture that was his wastehole. Of course he didn't have a penis! Or testicles! Her eyes widened in surprise—and disappointment. Lovelawn slipped his leggings back on. She looked upset. It wasn't his fault. He hadn't invited her to come aboard.

The query from the Species Museum Directorate of Travel Research, SPEMUDITRARE, was terse and direct: it requested information on the alien aboard PVIII. Lovelawn was furious. Braynz! How dare *it* exceed *its* function by unilaterally reporting Evelyn's presence. Lovelawn had hardly ever been furious in his life; he wasn't supposed to be capable of such an emotion. He put the sensation down to prolonged weightlessness but, more than that, he just *was* furious. So it was not difficult for him to be cunning. He fired a return transmission to SPEMUDITRARE explaining that Braynz had been experiencing a minor ongoing D-I-Error fault (Lovelawn included some examples) and had mistakenly confused the almost-born Moarnd for an alien presence.

There being no reply, Lovelawn felt quite justified in his harmless duplicity. The continuing existence of Evelyn aboard the carol remained a matter for his judgment alone. Furthermore he found himself considering a happy probability: that she might well come to prove to be valuable raw material in his research. A live specimen. The High Fathers would be most impressed, since no Remnant Human had ever been taken alive.

But now another matter preferred his attention. At last, Moarnd, ready for birth. Evelyn—who had been subdued since the waterfall orgy confusion—waited demurely in the antechamber of the Hobby Lab. Lovelawn did not want her to witness the birth. So, alone before the Kublaidome, he gazed fondly down at the Toy, breathed in deeply, switched off the incubat cycle and set the Activator Program.

The dome slid back. Moarnd's deep blue eyes closed and opened, closed and opened. He blinked beautifully. The *life-transfer* modem lit up and that was it. Lovelawn took an involuntary step back as Moarnd sat up briskly and swung his long muscular legs out of the dome. His gaze went automatically to Lovelawn. He stood, stretched his arms out wide, and grinned.

'Well, you're alive,' Lovelawn said. 'How does it feel?'

'*Yumyum!*' Moarnd showed his magnificent white teeth.

'And do you know why you are alive?'

'*No!*' He shook his head of shoulder-length golden hair.

'To be my companion of course. Now walk.'

Moarnd walked. He was a joy to behold, a miracle of verisimilitude. Lovelawn felt his pulses racing as the tempo of his heartbeat responded to the success of the thing, a success never guaranteed since from time to time Lovelawn had been obliged to resort to on-the-spot calculations.

'Ask me a question, Moarnd. Ask me anything you like.'

Moarnd frowned. Lovelawn watched him carefully. A pity. He'd rather hoped that his intellect wouldn't be quite so primitive. Now Moarnd's frown became anxious so Lovelawn cheerfully said, 'Don't worry, don't worry. You are my noble savage and can be proud of yourself. I am the brains, you are the brawn.'

'*Verynice!*' Moarnd said. He possessed a rolling, timbrous voice. His eyes sparkled.

'I programmed you to be perfectly happy, Moarnd, and I know therefore that you shall be. But now there is someone who you must meet. She is fascinated by my research and she will be impressed at how I have made you—you see, she is only Human. You must promise me that you will treat her like a guest.'

Moarnd nodded.

'And also,' Lovelawn cautioned, 'she is sensitive. Her name is Evelyn.'

'*Evelyn!*' Moarnd said, grinning.

Anticipating her reaction of awe at his ability to be so cleverly creative—after all Moarnd 'was' Human, though of course not—Lovelawn boldly allowed Moarnd to step first into the antechamber. Hidden behind the man's great physique, Lovelawn peeked through the gap between

LOVELAWN: A FANTASY

Moarnd's right arm and rib cage. Evelyn's eyes had widened in surprise—then delight. Quite obviously, and with her mouth open, she'd come to rest her gaze upon his exceedingly well-hung black genitals with their fulsome mat of impenetrably dark hair. The glow in Lovelawn's upper stomach burned hotly. She was signalling to him the strength of her awe, and he proudly stepped out from behind Moarnd.

The three took nutrition together but Evelyn seemed unhungry, despite Lovelawn's best efforts to coax her. Instead she devotedly watched Moarnd eat and every time he said '*Yummy!*' she laughed in appreciation and clapped her hands. Then she began to feed him what she did not want herself and Lovelawn admired Moarnd's enormous appetite. He ate and grinned and grunted and laughed so much that he became more than perfect. Afterwards, Evelyn led him to a reclining couch and began tickling and stroking his hairy scrotum. Moarnd gasped and lay back—his erection sprang up like a rubber bone beyond his navel. Evelyn wasted no time in stripping herself naked and with her back to Lovelawn she mounted Moarnd and began to ride him. Watching and listening, Lovelawn became unsure of what to do. When Moarnd experienced his first-ever Toy Climax (with a great muffled roar into her neck, his face streaked with her sodden flaming red hair) Lovelawn knew at least that he was really well built.

The very next minute, after an unaccountably restless sleep, Lovelawn could find neither of them. He went from here to there, calling, but heard only the echo of his own voice. Puzzled, he took himself into the viewmonitor pit to do some more research.

He dreamed of Evelyn. He wasn't supposed to be able to

dream. But there, smiling in front of him, she blew her fringe out of her eyes so that he could see them dancing in her face. She bent very close to him and—still smiling— blew him a little pocket of air from between her lips. Then she gently probed at his mouth with her tongue but there was no contact. She moved back. He looked up into her eyes. They were so very serene and full of indefinable promise; they were so very beautiful. And they said that they were his. Ecstatically, in the dream, his heart-organ simultaneously fibrillated and tumesced with incandescent elation, so much so that his very fingertips were on fire. But he didn't know what to do with them. Or with his desperate, almost uncontrollable organ pumping, pumping, pumping.

It happened too fast too subliminally for him but not for Braynz, which had a binary computational knowledge of EvErYtHiNg. Lovelawn kept on seeing Evelyn and Moarnd and nothing was at all wrong until suddenly the balance that never had been was changed and now nothing was right. He'd not had the slightest chance to befriend Moarnd. He'd been so busy with his work ... they came and went ... always *together*. Surely she couldn't be ... was she? *Stealing* him? Lovelawn hadn't the ability to cope with the question which to his dread surprise found its way into him, like a worm. But Braynz had. The ability to cope with the question. Braynz put it this way: *Excuse Data Input Error But *** But But But *** You Are Louse, ja? Sorry. Prefer: Jealous*.

Lovelawn was beside himself with agitated amusement. *Jealous*? He couldn't be if he tried.

Determined to remain rational, Lovelawn did his best not to fret. Of course, Evelyn and Moarnd were like children. But then he could no longer concentrate on his work. He dreamed again and again. The glow in his stomach began to burn with a terribly sad flame. The flame caressed and licked at his heart. It was exposing something. Giving birth to something. Lovelawn lay in agony. Finally, the deep chasm within him yielded up nothing less than that which above all he was never supposed to have known: Sorrow.

She shouldn't have put it in him. He shouldn't have known what it meant, what it was, what it felt like. He lay drifting and tortured, deep in sorrow and sadness, his purpose forgotten. Nothing else mattered but the ache.

In time—so many drifting minutes—Lovelawn rose groggily from the unplanned fate which had become his lot. The slightest instinct made him wince. But one above all now prevailed through the incredible glare of the pain barrier. Lovelawn could not bear it but it was true: *Louse, ja?* He was so filled with *Louse, ja?* that even when his eyes were shut tight they saw only the ethereal image of Evelyn with her swoon-inspiring scents.

Lovelawn lay panting, shallowly, fevered. He didn't know where he was except that the power of PVIII was trembling within him, it being his power. Where were Moarnd and Evelyn? The question had beat too long on his brain. He staggered up. He had only two thoughts. He must rescue Moarnd from her evil clutches. He must save Evelyn for himself, for his broken heart.

He roamed PVIII, going to parts where he'd seldom been. They seemed to be on the move, and he couldn't understand why. Then he fathomed that they must be avoiding him. It was the most crushing realisation. He entered guestquarters where they'd been; sometimes he missed them by so small an amount of time that their holographic images, happy and united, remained behind. Then quite by chance he stumbled across them.

Hand in hand they were walking across one of the *viadoTTis* linking the Shaft and Pubend. He called out, across the long narrow walkway. They looked back. She waved, and therefore so did Moarnd.

'Moarnd, come here,' Lovelawn said. His large noble savage hesitated. Then took a tentative step. Evelyn simply held his hand. Lovelawn watched. 'I want to show you how Braynz works,' he said. 'How Braynz helped me make you. You will be very interested Moarnd. Braynz named you too. Don't you want to meet your maker?'

'*Maker!*' Moarnd said and grinned. Evelyn slipped her hand from his. She walked the few steps that took her back to the Pubend and Lovelawn at least knew now that that was where they'd established themselves; hiding from him somewhere within that cavernous place which he did not like because of its dread unfamiliarity.

'Walk this way.' Lovelawn held out one arm.

Moarnd swung his head around. Evelyn was smiling at him.

'*No!*' he replied.

Brilliant dumbness of purpose overcame Lovelawn. The force of PVIII—which was *his* force—became the answer. To the question of why he had been wronged. It was so simple. But the complexities in the way of that simplicity were as astounding as they were devious.

He lay not long in the Kublaidome. He'd fastracked it and besides, only one part of him needed to be built. He ignored and overrode the logical protestations of Braynz as to the libidonate measure he programmed into himself. And he chose the dimensions as well.

Lovelawn woke with an erection. His tan-hued penis reared up to just beneath his chin. At this full stiffness it had a length of 52 cm and a girth of 37 cm. He got out of the dome and nearly fell over. The scrotum hung heavy towards his knees.

He clambered aboard a Horrse. He set it to maxmachstalliondrive and roared down the Urethric Highway.

Not one minute into the journey and his fearsome libido asserted itself. He hardly had to stroke the giant cock and great plumes of semen shot over his shoulder and splashed everywhere. The relief was ecstatic; but no sooner did the thing droop than it began to rise again and this time Lovelawn tugged it violently in both hands, again and again and again until a hot grey waterfall erupted upwards and made him moan with incomprehensible feeling. Intense excruciating weakness bedazzled his mind and left him crying with powerless joy. In the dimmest possible recesses of his intellect thus magically repressed, a conclusion came to him, as to the meaning of the feeling: but it whipped itself away before he could remember to remember it. All he knew, as the Horrse careered on, was that he wanted more and Evelyn by the meaning of her body lay in deliberate wait. She loved it, he loved her, and Moarnd was not capable of love.

He found them where he feared, in a dank and lightless cavern. They were like half-glimpsed spirits in the gloom, made worse by a cool moisture which thickened the air and dripped in the furthest recesses. Lovelawn commanded:

'Come out, Moarnd, and meet me being to being! You cannot hide her in there forever.' He waited and listened. There was nothing. 'Evelyn is *mine!*' he shouted. 'She always was—you were *never* worthy of her.' The intoxicating lie coursed through him, charging him with an extraordinary energy as he entered a new dimension of what it meant to be alive: he could lie. He had the brute power enabling him to lie, with the conviction that the lie could not be disproved. He roared for Moarnd, for the traitor, to show its toy self.

Moarnd strode across a steamy walkway, naked and unafraid. A dreadful primeval hatred engulfed them as, through the contact of eyes, their souls locked. Each man was stripped to the state of Emperor-Admiral, with no vision other than absolute victory.

But then in a final moment their respect for one another held sway. Lovelawn on high sat ready yet supine. Moarnd's greatly muscular physique seemed to soften, before correcting itself. Lovelawn, holding out one arm, said, 'My friend—think. Why?'

Moarnd therefore also held out one arm. '*Thinkwhy!*' he said, grinning.

Infinitesimal non-time framed and froze them. Then blindingly each pulled in their respective arms and the awesome clash began.

They parried, grappled; each fought with heroic meaninglessness. Upon his Horrse Lovelawn held great sway but Moarnd—the first bloodied of them—had ignoble savagery on his side, on the mossy slimy underfoot of the chosen place of their violent struggle.

All appeared lost for the magnificent-bodied Moarnd and he lay pinned beneath the Horrse's hoovewheels. 'Now think!' Lovelawn sneered. 'Of course she was always mine. You were a fool.'

Moarnd roared: '*Veryangry!*' He pitched the Horrse up off his body with such strength that Lovelawn almost toppled. And so the battle went on, guile countering brute force. They matched it with shouting: Moarnd's the bellows of survival, Lovelawn cursing his intelligence. Until.

Until one lay mortally wounded. Death could be counted drip by coagulating drip, so bringing on the dull grey hue of life most surely departing. But the other's triumph was brief. It became a triumph of loss, of defeat, of empty horror.

And all the while Evelyn had cowered somewhere nearby. Sometimes unable to watch the brutality and also slyly incapable of responsibility in the matter.

She fled PVIII through the Urethric Highway. She had been shown how to convert a Horrse to interstellar drive. At fullspeed she burst through the *Pèage* membrane and at once the Glanshole opened wide: it spewed her out.

Half-clear, she looked back. The thing was erupting. Their unremitting violence must have severed a vital. Burnt flames choreographed outwards to eternity, some vainly licking up towards the fading umbilicus of the Horrse's quad-thrusters which, entwined and spiralling rapidly away, sprayed down their so-called fairy-tail lights.

There were sparks in her eyes. She took one last despairing look, and reined the Horrse away from the setting glow.

Japan
William Yang

In Tokyo Hiroshi and I stayed in separate rooms at a hotel in Hamamatsu. It seemed an ordinary hotel and it cost $140 a night which I later found out was cheap, in fact lodgings don't come much cheaper. After I had travelled six floors in a lift to my room I had certain assumptions, one, that I would be high above the street, and in this I was correct, and the other, that this height would give me privacy. As I undressed to put on the Japanese robe provided by the hotel, a train on a monorail sped past my window. It was feet away. The sound muted by the heavy shutters and the thick window glass scarcely registered but the light from the carriage windows flashed like a strobe. It was startling not so much for its close proximity but for a dislocation in time, I felt I was in the future.

The room was small but comfortable, the bathroom a plastic cube which had been pressed as a single unit in a factory and installed *in situ*. If it was damaged, I thought, you'd have to replace the whole unit. Already there were tell-tale scorch marks where someone had left a cigarette near the basin. I had read in an architectural journal that one of the aesthetics of Japanese architecture was the concept of pleasing decay—the natural weathering of the building materials. An old lived-in house was more aesthetic than a new one (a bit like we consider jeans). I concluded that scorch was not aesthetic, no, not on plastic.

I switched on the TV. There were only six channels. I had expected more. One of them was devoted entirely to baseball and two of the channels showed risque pulp—one a European style costume drama which cut from a sword fight to a bedroom scene and the other an American soap opera where a heterosexual couple swam around a pool. When they got out they started to have sex. He went down on her. A censoring circle around the genital area transformed the image into squares. You could still make it out, but the full experience was spoilt. A warning flashed on the screen in Japanese and English that it was a pay channel and if you wished to watch more you had to press button A—for a charge of $20 you could watch all night.

In the morning I looked out over the flat endless metropolis. Tokyo, Hiroshi told me, is actually seventeen cities all joined up and you can travel from Tokyo Station to Yokohama, the equivalent distance of Sydney to Wollongong, and it's built up all the way. I was in Japan to pick up a photographic award I had won and was staying in Tokyo on my way to the North Island. Hiroshi, whom I knew in Sydney, was here as my guide. Tokyo with its abundant technology is like a city of the future and if I was more impressed by technology I could have got excited, but I wasn't and I didn't.

The Japanese breakfast had finished so we ate Continental: coffee with two thick toasted slabs of white bread with packets of butter and jam.

JAPAN

'Don't they have gay sex channels?' I asked Hiroshi.

He became serious; sex is never a lighthearted topic in Japan. 'No,' he said. 'The channels are used mainly by businessmen staying overnight. They might like to watch a porno movie, since they wouldn't have the chance at home. It's not something a Japanese family would have lying around the house. The husband would find it too embarrassing to watch with his wife.'

'What about the checkerboard grid they put over the best parts? That's a bit disappointing.'

'In Japan, you are not allowed to show nudity or pubic hair.'

'But I've seen full frontal nudity in those Asahi Camera magazines you showed me.'

'They can do it in special cases, if it's artistic.'

After breakfast I rang up Minaru, whose number had been given to me by the Japanese fancier and Sydneysider Jac V, or rather I got Hiroshi to ring him, because Minaru's English was limited and my Japanese dubious. (I had used the phrase, *sole wo kudo sai*, profusely since my arrival in Japan thinking it meant 'please', only to find out it meant 'Give it to me.' No-one corrected me, they were too polite.) By the way, Hiroshi is straight—but he and Minaru talked on the phone for half an hour, which was quite a long time since they had never met and all they had to arrange was a meeting place. When Hiroshi got off the phone he said, 'Your friend, from the way he talks, sounds like a big queen.'

Hiroshi took me to a photographic magazine on the other side of town. The journalist who interviewed me spoke quite fluently but was very apologetic about her English. She said 'sorry' every second sentence. I ended up feeling very sorry for her. Apologising is part of Japanese day to day behaviour but she overdid it. I wondered if all women with careers were like her.

Japan is very male dominated. Hiroshi told me there is a bar where only women go to be attended by hosts. It's a double reverse situation: firstly, men attend the women, which is rarely done in Japan and, secondly, the hosts are all women dressed as men. These hosts pay their women customers a lot of attention. In the tradition of the geisha or hostess, they flirt and flatter. No sex, of course. The clients love it, it's something they never get from real men.

We went shopping. Prices in Japan are usually two or three times higher than Australia. I had already read in the *Sydney Morning Herald* about the $70 rockmelon and I found out at the first greengrocer we visited, but was a bit disappointed because the story was exaggerated. It was a special decorative item with a bit of stem attached, which you gave as a gift, all attractively presented in a wooden box, so it was not really an ordinary rockmelon that you ate for dessert—you could buy those for a mere $30.

We found some clothing stores in Shibuya which had items marked down to bargain prices. Hiroshi couldn't resist buying a bright red tartan coat. 'They were so relieved you bought that coat, they probably had it on their shelves for years,' I said. Tokyo is full of grey clothed people. Hiroshi with his long hair and bold manner really stood out.

I never knew Hiroshi's sexual persuasion for most of the four years that I had known him in Sydney. He was a photographer and I met him at parties. I had seen him at gay parties, and certainly he took a lot of photos of gay people, but I never assumed he was gay, neither did I assume he was straight. He did show excitement at women's naked breasts but I put that down to a weird Japanese cultural trait. He was indefinable, he just didn't give off a sexual identity. Jac, who used to invite Hiroshi to his parties, would debate with me Hiroshi's persuasion. Jac was convinced he was gay and one day asked him outright. 'Hiroshi, are you gay?' Hiroshi did not answer the direct question, he just evaded it—a very Japanese response. Asians favour oblique approaches, so Jac and I remained unenlightened. The question was suddenly resolved in an unexpected way. We were at an exhibition of Hiroshi's photographs when an Australian girl I vaguely knew came up to me and introduced herself as Simone and explained she was Hiroshi's wife. 'Hiroshi will be angry I've told you, he doesn't like people to know, but I don't care, I tell everyone.' I was stunned at the time, but now observing the Japanese, I can see that Hiroshi was just acting like a typical Japanese man. They leave their wives at home, they earn the money, they go out alone and they never talk about their wives.

Hiroshi has a strong attachment to food, he imbues it with a mythical quality. There is a restaurant in Osaka, his home town, to which he promised to take me, which served a noodle soup, the best in Japan. When you eat this soup, he told me, you will never forget it, it will haunt you, you will dream about it.

We had dinner at his favourite restaurant in Shibuya. Their speciality was pork cutlets which I don't like so I pointed to a dish of dry noodles that someone was eating and ordered them. They arrived, looking beautiful, served on a rectangular wooden dish with a pale blue bowl of thin sauce. I poured the sauce over the noodles with a flourish only to see it seep out across the white table top. The dish didn't have a bottom, it just had slats across it. 'You're supposed to dip the noodles in the sauce,' said Hiroshi as we mopped up the mess.

We walked through Shinjuku. Hiroshi pointed out interesting places. At this place you can hire a room for about $200 a hour if you want to bring a girl there and that place is like a massage parlour, the girls will soap you up and rub you in the right parts. Hiroshi explained that these places were originally called *toruko* (Turkish Baths), the word *toruko* coming to mean massage parlour. The Turkish ambassador complained, the name was banned and now they're called Fashion Massage Baths.

Minaru and his friend Masa were waiting at the door of the Kingsman, one of the oldest and most famous gay bars in Tokyo. It lets in women and foreigners. Tonight, however, the Kingsman was quiet so we went somewhere else. Shinjuku is full of thousands and thousands of bars. Most are small, some extremely small seating as few as six people, and only a small percentage are gay. This next bar, GB's, also admitted foreigners. There was no cover charge but you had to buy a drink just to get in and that cost $10, which is a reasonable price. They told me about places where the drinks are $60 each and that wasn't even top of the range. 'Who can afford to go there?' I asked. 'Businessmen with expense accounts,' I was told. About half the people in the bar were Japanese and the other half Caucasian. The decor featured framed black and white photographic prints of Hollywood movie stars, male and female, of the thirties. Music played but it was not loud, the ambience was Western and familiar.

Minaru was slender, with a stylish haircut which curled up on his head, expressive eyes and a slightly effeminate manner. Masa was stocky with a round face and a businesslike appearance—straight acting would be the description, but then most Japanese were. Later I told Minaru that Hiroshi had thought, from his voice on the phone, that he was a 'big queen'. He shrieked at this, then blushed: it had never occurred to him that he appeared like this although it was quite obvious.

I found out they were radical for Japanese gays. Minaru worked for the health department and was involved in HIV education but their programs were very limited. Most

Japanese gays were closeted. For the first time that year a gay man and a lesbian had come out on a TV show similar to *Hey Hey It's Saturday*. (I later saw the tape and the compere asked the gay man what he did in bed. He replied that it was an unfair question to ask just because he was gay, the compere wouldn't ask the same question to a straight Japanese. He said sex is a private thing and people don't talk about it in public.) The younger generation of Japanese were much more open to gays and lesbians. It was something of a craze for young straights, mainly girls, to go to dance parties where the atmosphere was gay and the floor shows featured stereotypical glamorous gay men. Neither Minaru nor Masa had come out to their parents although their flatmates knew.

We went to a gay book shop situated on a street corner, its wares spilling onto the footpath. Most of the books and magazines were in Japanese which I, of course, couldn't read. There were further frustrations as Japanese videos won't play on Australian machines. Half the videos were Asian, the other half Western, mainly American and German. There weren't a lot of titles, but they seemed to have Jeff Stryker's full catalogue and little else, and the Japanese ones featured some intricate bondage on the covers.

Minaru gave me the address of a sauna, Jin Ya, I could visit. He and Masa had not been lavish with information because they said neither of them went to saunas, and I believed them. We said goodbye and Hiroshi and I set off for the sauna. Hiroshi wasn't going to stay, but he needed to show me the way.

Yes, I'll confess, I'm a steam queen. The first sauna I went to was in Bondi Junction, it burnt down years ago. I went more often when I was younger and got off mainly with Caucasians. A taste that I haven't always had is a liking for Asians, although I have had sex with them at times, but only when there wasn't anyone else. They were never my first choice and usually I was never theirs. Most of the time we'd avoid each other.

I had to go through this thing of coming to terms with being Chinese before I could feel really comfortable sleeping with Asians. Now I'm part of an Asian gay group, Silk Road, a support, social and educational organisation. Most of the group are from overseas and the issues that interest them revolve around negotiating the gay scene, which is something that, for them, is very Western dominated and new. Unfortunately these issues do not interest me because I've already done that, I've grown up here. Luckily there are other ABCs (Australian Born Chinese) in the group and I have a lot in common with them. One of the things we talk about is internalised racism. The overseas Asians don't know about this, it is basically a colonial experience. The racism they experience is something external, directed at them, but they don't know what it's like to internalise a loathing of one's own race. Dominic, one of the members, explained that racism is an idea that someone is inferior or has negative characteristics on the basis of their ethnicity rather than objective fact. Racism is taught. It is a product of how different ethnic groups in society interact, particularly the power relationships between them. The powerful shape attitudes. The dominant culture forms racist ideas which are mass circulated so racism becomes part of the social fabric. Since racism is a social phenomenon, it is natural that it is absorbed even if you belong to the group against whom the prejudices run. So you have running inside you an ingrained loathing of the way you look. That is why in the past I had turned away from Asians at the steam bath in Bondi Junction. They had reminded me I didn't shape up to my ideas of sexual attractiveness.

Now I like Asians, sexually, that is. I still like Caucasians too. At first I thought I did it with Asians as a political act, but no, I genuinely like them. And now I was travelling excitedly on a train to Ikabukuro Station and Jin Ya sauna.

After walking in circles for about half an hour we found the lane and a large sign JIN YA in English. What luck. The lane was filled with vending machines (Japan is a vending machine culture, there are more machines than people), but these had a special novelty which I had not seen before, they were filled with porno videos (heterosexual). Hiroshi couldn't believe how cheap it was to get into Jin Ya ($30), he imagined it would cost $200. We found the discreet entrance with its traditional wooden lattice. Hiroshi asked me if I had enough money ($70) to get a taxi home since the trains would not be running and to ring him first thing in the morning otherwise he would worry about me. He then literally ran off, as if he'd catch something contagious if he stayed a minute longer.

The first mistake I made was to walk in with my shoes on. The man screamed at me in Japanese and pointed to a wall of little lockers the size of shoe boxes with glass fronts. That's what they were, shoe boxes. I put my shoes in there and took out the key, then I gave the man at the counter a hundred thousand yen note ($150), he gave me change and I went to walk in. But he stopped me and pointed to a machine. I couldn't work it out. Then I realised he'd only changed my money and I had to put one of the notes into the vending machine to get a ticket. I did this and I found myself in a medium sized modern building of four storeys with lifts. I undressed on the first floor and put on a light blue cotton dressing gown. It wasn't a kimono, it was more like a surgical gown, tied both inside and out, with two separate sets of strings.

On the bottom floor was the bathroom with showers, an area with stools and tubs for personalised washing and a large Japanese bath with swirling very hot water. I immediately checked out the steam sauna. It was small and obviously not a place to meet people. Already I had seen some naked bodies in the bathroom. The standard was very high, trim bodies everywhere. One of the young men was close to athletic perfection. I lingered in the hot water tub watching him soap himself, then fearful I would faint from the heat, I got out. Everyone was modest. When naked, no-one flaunted themselves.

Next to the bathroom was the TV room with chairs lining the back wall. Eiderdowns and futons had already been pulled out and made into beds by people sleeping on the floor. On a cheap looking TV screen, a Japanese couple had sex in a plot format that was a copy of your average Western porno video; you know, kissing, sucking, arse licking and fucking. What I wanted to see was something uniquely Japanese. Again there was that annoying censoring circle over the interesting bits. One of the segments was bondage which I watched with interest.

I have this theory about bondage which could be naive, but here it is. Two cultures in which bondage is a common practice are the English and the Japanese, and both are extremely repressed. In environments such as these one has to struggle for expression, and in the case of sexual expression, one has to fight to break out of the bonds of cultural containment to achieve an orgasm. Hence the rope is the physical manifestation of the cultural metaphor. Bondage and leather is a method of physical restraint to achieve the elusive orgasm. I was hoping to see some good bondage videos in Japan to test my theory, but the segment that came up in the Jin Ya TV room was rather limp and featured nothing like the intricate display of knots I had seen on the cover of the video at the bookstore. So I was disappointed.

Later I was to witness the screening of a Western video

and half the audience walked out. I thought that the imported product might not be censored but it still had the squared circle. The quality of the original video was so bad you could scarcely tell which parts of it were being censored. No masturbating went on in the TV room and if there were erections they were well concealed. There was a definite vibe but no overt cruising.

On the first floor, men sat in a recreation lounge drinking beer and other beverages from vending machines. A lot of talk and socialisation went on and I wondered if the people knew each other beforehand or whether they had just met. A foreigner, a *gai jin*, watched baseball on the TV. I assumed he was American, however, I did not rush up to him and say, 'I'm a Westerner, do you speak English?' Oh no, I was happy in my disguise, I had not said a word and no one suspected.

On the third floor were special private rooms which you could hire. For how much extra I don't know. There weren't many people here, apparently you fished down below and brought your catch upstairs.

All the action was on the second floor, the main area. There were no cubicles, just three big rooms, bare, apart from a pile of eiderdowns, futons and pillows. Men bedded down, apparently asleep. On closer examination I noted that some people were embracing under the covers, and in one case the covers were pulled up to reveal two pairs of thick hairy Japanese legs, slightly entwined, which I found very sexy. This was the big revelation of the Japanese sauna, people came here to sleep overnight.

When in Rome ... I picked up a quilt and made a bed for myself in a spare space. The room was rapidly filling up with supine bodies. On my left was a person who was apparently sleeping and on my right was a couple who were embracing. As I lay there I worked out how the Japanese cruise. It is by eye contact. As we slept or feigned sleep others would come up and peer into our faces to see if we were awake. I guess having one's eyes open was the big signal. It was quite bizarre to have all these people come up to stare at your face while you pretended to sleep. There was a steady stream. An old man, the only one there, was the most persistent. Most of the people were young, twenty or thirty.

The couple next to me started to fuck. It was slow, intense and very contained. These guys were chunky, on the side of sumo wrestlers, but not that fat. I'm not sure if they used condoms but there was a period of fumbling before one was penetrated so I assumed or at least hoped they did. They were very close to me, our heads only feet apart. It seemed odd that in Japan where everything is very private I should be in a situation where I was practically part of the action. I like a bit of voyeurism, remember, I'm a photographer.

The person next to me tossed around, he never made eye contact, nevertheless I decided to make a move. Actually I felt unsure of myself because I had no idea what to expect. He did not reject me, but neither did he encourage me. At times he moaned with pleasure but he never got fully erect, nor did he ever become fully awake, yet he was not asleep. I was able to take off his gown and roll him around. At first I found this extremely titillating (he was quite good looking), but as it went on for quite a long time, I found the passivity off-putting. I wanted some sort of interaction but there was none, so I stopped. At this point language would have helped but I had nothing to offer.

The place was quite full now, all the futons had been used up. A young guy came and lay down beside me. He didn't have an eiderdown so I threw mine over him as well. I thought of a Japanese novel I had read, *The House of the*

Sleeping Beauties. A woman owned a special house which specialised in young girls, below twenty. Older men came to the place to lie with the girls who remained asleep, drugged. There was one house rule (and the Japanese are very good at keeping to the rules), you could not do anything distasteful to the girls. The men came there to sleep, to remember and to dream. I had always wanted that story to be different, to have more action, for the men to do something distasteful, but it never went the way I wanted. Now in this room among these sleeping men, listening to the shuffle of feet, the rustle of the eiderdowns, the soft moans of ecstasy, the flapping split curtain in the doorway and the distant whirl of the lift door down the corridor, I understood that story.

    I awoke with a start, I opened my eyes and saw a person with his face quite close to mine peering into my eyes which I shut again. I felt the person retreat, the pull of the eiderdown on my legs as he walked off. What had actually woken me was my neighbour's hands on my cock. The skin of his hand was tough. I lay there in a half-dream state savouring the experience. He persisted, I responded. I traced my hand along his arm which revealed a firm but not bulky muscularity and I guessed he was some type of manual labourer. He had knotted both the ties to his gown which took me a while to undo, but I was not in a hurry. I rolled him around taking off the gown and he co-operated although he never opened his eyes. He had a beautiful body, trim, defined, reactive, and it convulsed when I licked his nipple. He pushed my head onto his cock which was already erect.

    He did not handle me quite the way I like, he was a bit rough, but I am not complaining, it made him seem more deliciously rough trade. Although he was prepared to reciprocate, there was a tendency for him to just lie there. We both came in each other's hand but I felt I had never fully awoken him to a conscious acknowledgment of an orgasm. I realise now that was expecting too much. The veil of sleep was something he could not fully lift, because it allowed him an escape, he could drift off into forgetfulness and in the morning deny that it ever happened. Thus is the stuff of dreams.

Early in the morning he got up and I followed him to the bathroom just so I could see him in a better light. He lacked the perfection I had imagined under the eiderdown and he was older than I thought but he was still young and very spunky. He wiped the dried cum off himself. He did not acknowledge our intimacy.

I looked around just once more before leaving. In the downstairs TV room the video had been switched off and the room was full of people sleeping on the floor, while others slept in the chairs. Someone was jerking off into the urinal while wearing the special scuffs that are provided just for the toilet. Upstairs the *gai jin* caused a sensation—he fucked one of the boys in a completely brazen way. Something of an exhibitionist, he had thrown off the cover and everything was completely visible. The boy taking it up the bum still pretended to be asleep. A small circle of Japanese stood around watching.

During the long taxi ride back to the hotel, I thought about Japan—what a hidden place it was. Everything so formalised, the whole culture ritualised into strict surface form, while individual desire was buried deep. It was there but never seen, like the Japanese tattoos where a whole body can be covered with designs but the head above the neck and the hands beyond the wrist were left untouched. A person could have a normal appearance in clothes and yet be deeply marked. Everything seemed behind a veil. I couldn't stop thinking about those sleeping men at the sauna, their desires hidden in a dream state. I wondered, too, what were the thoughts of the circle of Japanese men as they watched the *gai jin* brazenly breaking the codes of behaviour. Did they think the veil had lifted? Did they think: is this real life, is this really what it looks like without those little coloured squares?

My Feminine Side
Mark Mordue

It was one of those strange days. Overcast and drifting, lidded. I was twenty-one years old. I'd gone down the coast to Moruya for the funeral of an ex-girlfriend's father. And I wasn't over the ex-girlfriend at all.

I stayed with a couple of other friends, a pretty kooky pair. The guy used to wear white suits and white hats, very much like Elton John on the cover of *Greatest Hits, Volume 1*. Not a look you normally see much of in a small town like Moruya.

'Elton' had this vision of himself as something of an avant-garde photographer. His favourite subject at the time was men's penises in all kinds of abstract formulations, a florid Robert Mapplethorpe of the south coast. Needless to say this dandy about town cut a rather gay figure among the truckies, bikies, surfies, farmers and hippies.

His girlfriend was no slouch at alien style either. She wore pink miniskirts, furry boots and outfits that must have come out of early '70s musicals like *Hair*. She also wrote epic poetry inspired by Tolkien.

The two of them used to smoke pot and sometimes work on the poems together, speaking their own language, a kind of high, squeaking Olde English that got more garrulous and out of control the more stoned they became.

Most of my friends aren't like this. Even now this couple stand out for being unusual. The important thing about them is a girl they introduced me to—for only they could have done the introduction.

Their new flatmate looked like a younger, sexier Chrissie Hynde, a real dynamo. I couldn't figure out what such a happening, super-intelligent girl was doing in Moruya in the early '80s. She had Sydney, if not London and New York, written all over her.

It's no understatement to say I noticed her. But then just about any guy would. Even so, I was embroiled in my unrequited love for my ex-girlfriend, my inability to understand why she went out with her new boyfriend—he was so boring and conservative the logic of it eluded me like an insult—and the funeral itself.

At the funeral I longed to be a supportive presence, to wrap my ex-girlfriend in a blanket of tenderness. But even then I recognised my supportiveness was really a pressure on her, that it held an urgency coloured most by my own needs, and even, on the day, my selfishness. It was me who needed the connection. Me who was angry at not being able to touch and hold her.

After the church service there wasn't really a wake, except for the close family. I was outside the circle of my old girlfriend again.

My evening was free, so I ended up with 'Elton' and 'Hair' at a wild party full of bikies and hippies. 'Chrissie' was there too.

I had not seen her all day, but with the funeral, the frustrated emotional energy, and the greyness of the weather, a sexual energy seemed to sleep in the liddedness of my feelings. I could sense my attraction to her, the way too, she appealed to me, directing energy at me—bristling and raw beneath the affable and polite gestures.

And yet something about what was happening between us felt out-of-kilter, though I couldn't put my finger on it. At the party, she hung invitingly close, standing quietly beside me for a while before I lost track of her amid the revelries. Elton and Hair disappeared. And I ended up staggering home through the lonely streets of Moruya at about 2 a.m. It didn't seem to matter in the end. I was happy to let myself be carried away. There was that final sense of being released to myself in the empty cool streets, of being free from everyone, and free from my own needs.

I was fixing up my makeshift bed on Elton and Hair's couch downstairs when there was a knock at the door. It was Chrissie.

She had locked herself out, and gone over to a friend's house to kill time before trying to get in again when someone was home. Things seemed to move with an automatic agreement or understanding. We had a glass of wine and a smoke, chatting away pleasantly before we finally started kissing and rolling around the floor.

After quite a bit of this rolling about I managed a rather breathy 'Let's go upstairs'. We laughed as if the whole day had been wasted pretending to deny this, going through the motions that finally led us where we both really wanted to be.

Her room was simple and spare, with wooden bookshelves crowded with cool literary books as well as a few that indicated a fascination for the dark side of life: postmodern theses on S & M; obscure art magazines devoted to all kinds of peccadillos, like Stellare, the performance artist who hung himself from a ceiling by fishhooks, or Chris

Burden, who had himself nailed to the back of a Volkswagen and got someone to drive him around a small suburb for a few minutes before releasing him.

As interests go, they were fashionably twisted and arty. It was the early '80s, the beginning of an age when physical distortion was regarded as powerful and dangerous.

In some inarticulate way at the time, this irritated me. I felt predictably offended and bothered. But my primary interest was Chrissie, and a pretty straight up-and-down heterosexual experience. So I didn't worry too much about philosophies and arguments about fetishism.

She was olive-skinned, dark-eyed, and spectacularly fit. By now we had our clothes off and had slid between the sheets, but she did this odd thing of leaving an overhead reading lamp on just above our heads.

Perhaps I've neglected to make it clear that by now (in my foolish youth) I had smoked some particularly strong marihuana. It was like toking on an acid trip. So the fact I kept getting this funny, unreadable message at the back of my mind, an uncertain blinking charge of the synapses, wasn't all that surprising.

The reading light shone over her face as my hands moved feverishly down her breasts to between her legs. I was out of it, young and relatively inexperienced, and I began to have trouble finding her vagina—which was rather embarrassing, to say the least. I lacked panache. It was much worse than just fumbling over a bra strap.

In the meantime her face seemed to be changing. I studied it like water, stupefied. It was as if one second I was looking at a girl, the next it would waver into the face of a boy. Back and forth. I started to blink as this kept happening, my hands fumbling between her legs with less and less intensity.

'What is it?' she said challengingly.

'Oh ... er ... oh ... er, I'm sorry, I've had this really strong pot and this probably sounds weird ... oh God, I'm really out of it ... you see, um, well ... Are you a boy?'

Chrissie looked back at me, not angry, just emphatic. 'I am a woman and I have always been a woman.'

Eh? I thought to myself. What kind of fucking answer is that? 'I am a woman and have always been a woman.' The phrase went round and round in my head, and when I asked her again she said it again. It didn't have a very convincing ring to it. But she did have the body of a woman. She was a woman. And yet things weren't quite right.

'Well, er ... it's just ... like I can't sort of quite find your ... er, well, your ... er, vagina. I can't find it.'

Just saying the word 'vagina' made me feel embarrassed. Then Chrissie took my hand and jammed two fingers up between her legs. It was not an erotic experience for me. It *was* there after all, but it felt kinda funny. And I just half-sat, half-lay there beside her, my fingers inside her like someone had shoved them into an electric socket, looking at her face changing—boy/girl, boy/girl, boy/girl ...

Finally I extracted my fingers and sat on the side of the bed, my head in my hands, confusion reigning. 'Look you'll have to excuse me ... I'm not sure if this is happening ... I'm very heterosexual in my mind ... I can't ... it's just that I smoked some very strong pot ... Oh wow, this is ...'

Chrissie listened, making low noises for a while, till I realised she was masturbating. 'What a pity,' she said, looking at me. I was shocked. 'Stop it!' I said. 'Hey! Stop that.' I was embarrassed. A girl had never done that in front of me before.

I explained that I needed to go back downstairs and have a good lie-down on the couch. And she seemed quite blasé about it. I kissed her on the cheek and left, totally blown out, and fell into a heavy, doped sleep. When I woke up the next day I had an early breakfast with her before she went off to work—it was all very husband-and-wifeish. I gave her another peck on the cheek as she left, a gesture of 'no hard feelings' combined with not knowing if the night had really happened at all.

Later I tried to introduce the subject discreetly with Elton, but he just sniggered wisely without giving me a straight response. And so I left Moruya, stunned, but still wondering if what I'd perceived and experienced was true.

A month later I got a brief letter from her saying she was dropping by on a visit to Sydney, and would return a book I'd lent her earlier in my visit. She'd written the note to me on the back of a photostat image that was clearly her at about fifteen, a schoolboy with long hair looking monstrously feminine and in excruciating pain over his own appearance.

At some point or other she must have begun taking hormones and then had operations to begin releasing herself from her male body into a female one. I found myself wondering about the strange, blurred territory between genders, and sexualities, and how I had reacted—my gut response not to follow through with sex, my sensing she was a boy, yet also knowing 'I am a woman and have always been a woman' was a phrase that had truth in it. Nothing fitted into the picture easily, least of all me.

I've often considered the subtle energies in that 'seduction' that first vaguely warned me something wasn't right. That funny feeling in the back of my mind. And I think it was because she, in a way, hunted me down—despite everything about her, the way she approached me was the way a man would seduce a woman, in some unreadable yet *felt* code that put me in a female position. She still approached me like a man who wanted a woman.

The schoolboy picture she had sent was so full of pain, so disturbing, I almost immediately screwed it up and threw it in the garbage bin. It was as confronting as anything I have ever seen. So terribly private. That she wanted to trust me with it, or tell me something, was all the more frightening for me.

Later when she came round to my home, having told me the *exact* time she planned to drop by, I made sure I wasn't there. My flatmate told me 'this "really sexy girl" dropped off a book of yours'. I just said 'Yeah' bluntly. I wanted to escape anything to do with it. And yet something in me felt sad for being afraid, for failing to make the connection.

Every now and then, perhaps once or twice a year, I run into her in Sydney. I pretend that nothing ever happened. And I am so terribly friendly, so regular. I know she appreciates this. And yet the friendliness holds absolute distance in it too—as smooth and undisturbed and blankly reflective as the surface of a pond.

Green Eyes
Angus Strachan

Geoffrey was telling me about rimming. 'It feels great,' he assured me. 'Really special. Honest.'

He wants to rim me. Good and proper. 'You've got a scrumptious bum,' he said.

Geoffrey's beautiful and angelic, with a touch of the satyr about him. We'd been friends for two years and four months. We met singing in a gospel choir. He has soft spiky red hair and there's always a good portion of jockey underpants showing above his frayed and daggy trousers. 'My trademark,' he says; 'Very important.'

When I'm kidding with Geoffrey we both call my bottom 'The pudding!' He finds my term 'The Chocolate Hole' very distasteful. In fact, it makes him angry. He much prefers 'pudding'.

'Will sir be having pudding?' he likes to say. 'You cannae 'ave your pudd'n until you eats your meat,' he says and leers comically at me.

He wants to fuck me. He wants to stick his tongue up my

arse and then he wants to fuck me. Good and proper. My bum's a prize, he says.

I don't want him to. I'm sure it would hurt. He says I don't know what I'm missing.

We went for a walk down at Bondi and sat on the grassy hill above the beach to eat our fish and chips. Then we took the ocean path around the cliffs to Tamarama and Bronte. It was windy and warm and the swell was up. We jumped over rocks and off high sandstone boulders. We edged around rugged cliff faces, our fingers and toes holding us from the disaster below. We yelled and screamed. We played like children. It was intoxicating.

At Bronte we rested on the grass with lousy coffee and chocolate bars. 'This coffee stinks but I like it anyway,' Geoffrey said. We sat on the swings. He told me about being gay and about his suburban childhood in Canberra where his older sister mothered him. She'd recently died of cancer. He cried on the seesaw. He wanted her back.

I told him why I thought I used to drink too much and how I got involved in the men's movement and came to realise I often felt scared of sex. I explained how I could meet a woman and fantasise an entire life with her and have it out of my system within seconds. Geoffrey nodded. 'I do that,' he said.

We walked slowly back, often bumping into each other. We looked at the boogie board riders and at the waves crashing on the rocks below us. We rounded the point at Tamarama. A girl I knew stopped us and said hello. I did the introductions. She was with a boy and she had to go. 'Call me,' she said. I said I would. Everyone says those things. She scared me because I thought she was so damn strong. She wasn't though and it turned out she thought I was.

Geoffrey looked at me. 'You've done it with her, haven't you?' I smiled. I told him I'd slept with her two weekends ago. 'Good on you,' he said. I told him that she'd well and truly rimmed me too. 'You're kidding,' he said. He said the thought of this made him crazy. He wanted to know what else happened.

'Everything,' I said.

'Oh man,' he said. 'I want to rim her. And then I want to fuck her. Then I want to watch you two together. And then I want to fuck you. And then ...'

Geoffrey begged and demanded I tell him the whole story. Every minute detail. Every particular. What was she wearing? What was I wearing? The sheets? Whose place? Night or day? Who touched who? Where? Who said what?

I explained that we'd had great sex that night but then I'd wanted to go home because I slept better in my own bed. She wanted me to stay. That made me want to go more. But I stayed. I said I liked the idea of casual sex but somehow it never felt quite right. 'It's a great distraction,' Geoffrey said. 'Anyway, then what happened?'

In the morning she felt hornier than a harlot, as she put it. She began to lick my entire body. From my big toe to the crown of my head. Which she sucked.

'Sucked what?' Geoffrey asked.

'The top of my head!' I said.

'Incredible,' he said. 'What was that like?'

'Out of this world,' I told him.

She wanted me to masturbate on her tits. And then she wanted me to turn around and sit on her face. I couldn't believe it. Geoffrey said it made perfect sense to him. He said all women liked things anal, it was just that most of them were too scared to try, or else hadn't been shown how to do it right.

She guided me to keep pulling myself off. My cock was

huge and hard. Bigger than it'd ever been before. She was writhing around underneath me. She held one of my peachy cheeks in each hand and shoved her whole face and nose into my pudding. She speared her tongue into my hole. She was groaning very loudly and biting my arse a lot. Huge big bites. I was amazed to hear myself roaring like a lion. What was that, I wondered? It was me! I felt like a gladiator. Proud. Amazingly turned on.

'Jesus, sweet Mary. Couldn't I fuck you, just once. Where is that woman,' Geoffrey said and looked around feverishly. I laughed. 'More,' he demanded.

I came like a rocket. Supercharged. Spurting and gushing all over the place. A torrent of spunk! Everywhere! All over her. All over everything. Even onto her legs. A three or four foot lunge. I just kept coming and coming. She kept going and going. Her tongue seemed to be right up inside me. I was feeling things I'd never felt before in my life. She was fingering madly at her clit with one hand, and with the other she soaped herself all over with my sea of sperm.

'God, that's so beautiful,' Geoffrey said, almost glassy eyed.

I laughed. 'But you're supposed to be gay.'

'So?' Geoffrey shrugged.

I loved him then. Somehow telling him this had eased my discomfort about the experience. I felt validated. And loved.

'So how did it end?' he asked.

We fell asleep, arm in arm in her small Paddington terrace overlooking Trumper Park. The hot morning sun shone through her window. Her body looked glazed and strong and brown. I lay half in, half out of the shadows cast by her curtains. Her sweaty blonde hair covered my face. We fell asleep, breathing easily together.

Geoffrey shook his head. Sadly. Happily. In awe. We

reached the round stone amphitheatre on the Bondi headland and looked out to sea and down the coast to Waverley Cemetery and beyond. We said nothing for a long time. I felt great.

'Thank you,' Geoffrey said and we looked at each other. Really looked. I couldn't stop staring at his amazing green eyes.

I Asked the Angels For Inspiration
Venero Armanno

Last night I dreamed of Rebecca again.

She came in a storm of falling angels. There was a little thunder and a lot of fat rain and the scent of wild roses. The rain pounded down. It beat on my iron roof and made cold waterfalls from the age-rusted holes of the guttering. It made my hands shake when they touched Rebecca's face. She lay beside me in my bed and she comforted me and she said, *I heard you this time.* She cradled my head. *This time I had to come.*

And there was that scent of wild roses again.

I looked at the river, at the sea of roses, at the angels falling from the black sky and into the white river. The wind blew me cold and Rebecca reached out for me. I brushed her hair from her forehead and she closed her eyes.

I said, 'I better answer the telephone.'

Don't, Rebecca whispered, and her voice was as gentle as the song of a choir of Christmas angels. *Don't, it's supposed to be a secret, you'll spoil everything again*, and she was gone into the two-thirty morning.

Through the din of the rainfall, the telephone. Again.

Stumbling through the cold house, wondering why it was a sin to feel such longing, I navigated the darkness—badly. Forehead against a door jamb, knee against a coffee table, and none of it really necessary for the kitchen light was on and Paul and Magda were in there squeezing oranges. Why hadn't they saved me from this; why hadn't they left me to sleep with my Rebecca? Fuck the casual cruelty of those who help us pay the rent. Paul and Magda were in T-shirts, their bare arms and bare legs brown as cowhide. Among not many other things they shared a passion for beaches.

Sour in the mouth and crabby in the heart I stood by the telephone and stared at Magda's legs—which I do a lot of.

Tall, foreign, dirty as an unwashed potato, I'd had a werewolf's desire for Magda since the day Paul had taken her from a Noosa beach to his New Farm bed.

'Why don't you answer the phone?' I said.

Four hands ran with orange juice.

'Leave the thing,' Paul said. 'They'll give up in a minute.'

But I can never leave it.

On its spindly supports the old house was rocked by rising winds. The wooden walls trembled. I trembled. The place was about to be blown off its ridiculously high stumps and out into the Brisbane River, where we would be washed away until we met the sea. I put my hand on the thrumming receiver and Paul said, 'Go back to bed, you fucking idiot, you know who it is at this time of the night. Why do you encourage them?'

The house quivered.

Why do I encourage them?

I ASKED THE ANGELS FOR INSPIRATION

Because of the dreams I have, Paul, because I know I carry a stone in my heart, Paul, that's why.

As if I could ever explain that to him—but Magda smiled at me and then she returned to the hand-juicer and a mountain of valencias. Oh, Magda could look into a man's heart as easily as look into a stinking garbage bin. Her gift was to look without curling her lips in disgust. How had Paul managed to keep her so long?

The ringing ran out.

I said, 'Well, I forgot to take the receiver off the hook before I went to bed.' Lingering, watching Magda's legs. She came into better focus. Legs the colour and texture of expensive magazine photo essays. I was no longer sour. But hardly sweet. 'Sorry it woke you,' I said.

They came by with their glasses of juice.

'The telephone didn't wake us,' Magda said. 'We have been sleepless.'

The rain fell hard but the noise was not enough to drown the new ringing of the telephone.

'Tell 'em to be fucked,' Paul said.

They smelled of stale sex and oranges, the sleepless Paul and Magda. Why couldn't I squeeze oranges with Magda while Paul was left to dreams of a ghost named Rebecca? There were goose bumps along Magda's thighs. She knew I was looking. I moved to the windows and pulled them fully shut.

'Go on.' Magda smiled at me again. 'Don't be ashamed. Answer the telephone.'

So I picked up the receiver.

It was as it always was. Silence. Space, the final frontier. Nothingness or eternity in my telephone line. No sense of a Being, but there was a Being. Two-thirty in the morning was this Being's time of day.

'Goodnight,' I said, and put the receiver down.

Magda walked by and put the two empty glasses in the sink. She poured a generous glass of juice and handed it to me.

'This was your stalker?'

'This was my stalker.'

I wanted to lean close for the scent of her hair, for the scent of oranges, for the scent of spoiled sex.

She went to the couch and she and Paul cuddled there. They might very well have been about to copulate there. I took the glass into my bedroom, bolted the door and bolted the juice. I turned out the light and lay down. Outside, the elements howled. I waited under the bedclothes for Rebecca to return, but the bitch wouldn't return. I tried to lure her with randy thoughts but only the rain kept me company. Its insistent fall against the iron roof lulled me. *It is a lie to say I am lonely. I am only alone.* And as longing as my stalker. With every passing night and day, the same sin.

Those two-thirty telephone calls had started a few months earlier. Whose life had I crossed back then? I had no idea. Who was it who wanted me? I couldn't imagine. Was it Rebecca? If only. The rain cried out.

Rebecca. Rebecca.

Holiday mornings. The telephone won't ring. Coffee and newspapers and the sunshine of a Brisbane day. Sit, waste time, watch the minutes drag. Fester alone. This I like.

I have a bad habit.

I like to video-record *Rage* most nights. With the Long Play option you get six hours of old and new music videos. I like to put the tape on when I vegetate around the house. It's my soundtrack for reading the papers, cleaning the toilet inside, sweeping the path outside.

The morning was humid. From the rear windows of my house I could see the river. Ferries quietly steamed against the current; off a jetty a man angled for catfish; at the closest bank a group of kids stood with their bicycles and smoked cigarettes. In a neighbour's weedy yard a fat black cat rolled onto its back and exposed its belly to leaden clouds. I sipped my coffee and read claims about Bill Clinton's sexual appetite.

I blame the endless funk feature on *Rage*.

The house started to sway, this way, that way, this way, that way, just like in the old Smiths' song. Ten-metre supports at the back of an old wooden house will let you feel most vigorous movements. Sylvester was singing in his curiously appealing falsetto and I was at the dining table swaying as if on a rocking ship. The house was moving, moving, moving to an insistent funk beat. Why the fuck was I surprised?

For Paul had the libido of a randy mutt. He was always ready to mount a willing schoolgirl, a tree trunk, any available shin bone. I'd known love once but my housemate had known enough copulation to keep a cricket eleven happy into their dotage. Or was it in fact Magda with the unquenchable fire? The house rocked, the table rocked, my eyeballs rocked. Generations of funk passed. We dabbled in the sixties and the seventies and the eighties, even into the Reverend Al Green's current piece of gospel-drenched funk, but the rocking hardly abated. I turned the television up louder and went and stood in the furthest removes of the house.

Nothing worked.

But I guess I had to admire Paul and Magda's dedication. Paul's even more so. Why is it that only the most worthy and undeserving of men suffer from PE? Paul must have been as numb as a gum shot full of novocaine. Even as that thought crossed my mind the screaming started. I know not to be fooled by this. Experience has taught me this only signals the end of Paul and Magda's foreplay.

I packed together a few things and fled before I lost my mind. From a corner telephone booth I rang Henry.

And he arrived at the street corner, at the top of the cul-de-sac that went down to the New Farm ferry jetty. Where I cowered from life and libido.

Henry said, 'G'day!' and I scrambled in.

His ugly Cressida was rotted through with rust, like the guttering of my house, which the landlord couldn't afford to fix. Neither could I. I lost my last job for stuffing up one too many times a Pearl Jam lead break and ending it with an unhappy *ker-plunking* of strings. Now no other band wanted me. Somewhere, sometime, some prick had called me *Leadfingers*, and of course it stuck.

End of a career.

Henry's car picked up speed along Brunswick Street—no prostitutes were out yet—but had to slow down in the Valley. The mall and the streets and the shops had long-since been festooned with lights and coloured streamers and Christmas bells. Families were out in force; where the families prospered the prostitutes failed. As we rattled by the market-day mall we saw crowds and heard music and saw children with their faces to the glass of art school Christmas displays.

'Boy,' said Henry. His contacts were giving him trouble and he worried at his eyeballs as he drove along.

I was glad to be out of Fortitude Valley but then there was the City. Ann Street to the bit of freeway that leads to Coronation Drive. The City was busier with Christmas lights than I could have imagined. The world was out shopping. What do you do when you're broke and the three-to-five-year-olds in your extended family have no idea what the word 'dole' means?

'Drive faster,' I said.

'Fuck off,' Henry said, and worrying at his eyeballs like a dog at a flea he nearly swiped a grinning pedestrian. 'Should have hit her,' he said.

And what can you do when the marketing men have your name and number, what hope have you got when a database remembers better than you what it is you love?

We went to the RE beer garden and festered the day through.

People came and went from our table, mostly to talk to Henry. Self-deprecating, almost nauseatingly sincere, and the only person I knew under sixty-five who could do the rhumba and the tango, he had the knack of making young women at parties fall in love with him in five minutes and contemplate marriage in ten. He was taller than me, funnier, better looking, and when we played tennis could actually hit a backhand. He didn't have a regular girlfriend. That levelled us a bit.

'Do you know what date it is today?' I hinted, always between drinks.

Henry popped his lenses and put on his glasses. His eyes were big and startled. 'Close to Christmas?'

We sat in the beer garden and listened to a fucked acoustic trio and at intervals rubbed suncream over our arms and necks.

Magda had met Henry once at drinks. During the evening when Paul was out of earshot and Henry was within earshot she had said to me, 'Your friend Henry Carter is a man I will very much like to fuck with.' Maybe I'd envied him since that night. A little later and with a little more vodka in her Magda had said, 'But you are not very old and yet you are very soft in your stomach.' Maybe I'd wanted to smack Henry in the head since then, who knows?

As the sun went down and my head went similarly, inexorably, down toward the table, I remember asking again: 'Do you know what the date is today?'

Henry gave me a strange look. 'What's gotten into you?'

'Too much beer,' I answered.

And both our heads went down and we had a nap and because it was Henry, nobody even thought to throw us out.

By nightfall we were propping each other up in the busy bar next to the Rum Boogie cafe. I can't remember how we got to Fortitude Valley all the way from Toowong.

'What you don't see,' I was telling him, 'is that tennis is a metaphor for Life.'

Henry was watching a young woman in a black dress. Her dress was one or two sizes too small. Her lips were incredibly red. A gaggle of stockbrokers circled her. Because Henry is a polite man he nodded at my meanderings.

'John McEnroe, the Australian Open, 1992, against the German goliath, Becker. Becker was number four in the world at the time and he'd beaten McEnroe in all their previous encounters. You with me? McEnroe was thirty-three and feeling it and Becker was twenty-four and just about on top of the world. McEnroe, all touch and not much power. That fluidity, that anticipation, that magic, but against the German? Not a chance. But he beat Becker in three sets. That night Becker left the court a humbled man.'

Henry looked pained to have to listen. He said hopefully, 'Want another drink?'

'Wait. Wait. You see, the magic was with McEnroe again. He kept fighting. He refused to die. He couldn't win but he did win. Then he went on to have that fucking amazing five-setter against Emilio Sanchez. And he won, but it took just about four and a half hours. How did he do it? Wasn't he supposed to be worn out? Wasn't he supposed to be at the end of his career? This is what I'm saying. When you're down and out, why do you have to stay down and out? When you're dead why do you have to stay dead?'

I ASKED THE ANGELS FOR INSPIRATION

Henry's big eyes shifted from the shark-encircled young woman to me. 'What is the matter with you today?'

I looked into my glass. 'I used to play in a rock and roll band. I used to take drugs and write songs and dream about making love to Jean Seberg.'

'Why don't you just find yourself some babe?'

'You find yourself some babe.'

'Okay.'

It seemed a decent idea. So we moved on to find Henry a babe, but first all we did find was some old friend of his.

The bloke was in his twenties and drunk enough on beer and vodka to see past a man's blood and bone, just as Magda could without booze. We were in The Beat and the electro-dance thump was as it had been since 1985. What had changed was that many of the men in their leather shorts and singlets and muscles now had girlfriends. It wasn't a predominantly gay club any more. Anyway, Henry's friend leaned against me, slurped vodka, took one look into my face and said, 'You're the unhappiest soul I ever saw.'

'Who the fuck is this?' I asked Henry.

Henry said to his friend, 'Today has a special significance for him but he wants to be mysterious about it.'

His friend said to me, 'Tell us about it.'

I said to him, whoever he was, 'Why don't you get fucked?' And to Henry, 'You too.' And to the girl standing by me, 'Want to dance?'

So we danced.

She was wearing a sweet white dress that matched her sweet white hair and she looked a little like Madonna from the days when you wanted to fuck her rather than smack her one. But later when I was in the toilet the blonde was in there as well with her dress hitched up around her hips and a quarter-pounder pointed into the urinal. You take your chances. When I emerged Henry and his friend both said, 'Look, just tell us about it.'

I said, 'I'm not telling you a thing.'

Henry said, 'Okay, I've had enough of this,' and he and his friend exited The Beat. His friend fell over once but caught up. I caught up as well. We stopped in at another busy bar. Henry had a job so he said, 'Okay, I know it's up to me. What are you having?'

I said, 'Crown lager.'

His friend said, 'Stolly. Get 'em to give you a double.'

Henry disappeared.

Henry's mate said, 'The problem is you like to carry your problems around with you, but they're only baggage that you can choose to lug or leave behind. You don't want to leave 'em behind. You love 'em. They're what make you you. Still, you coulda left your baggage at home just tonight.'

I stared at him, not inviting him to continue.

'You have a choice, a clear choice. You can be weighed down—or not.'

'Thank you.'

'The problem is too many people associate depression or sadness or misery with depth of character. Can you believe it? But you're no deeper than your average check-out chick or grave-digger. This misery of yours is an open invitation for someone to come out of the crowd and save your fucking life. That's why you love it so much. But nobody's gonna save you. Especially not a girl. Unless she's fucked in the head—and that'll really be where your depression starts. Try shaking one of them girls. Can hardly be done.'

'Who the fuck are you?' I asked as Henry returned with our drinks.

Henry said, 'This is Gordon. Gordon's kind of a poet.'

'Kind of a poet,' I said. 'Kind of a fucken drunk. And he

I ASKED THE ANGELS FOR INSPIRATION

smells.' I drank my beer and Gordon drank his vodka. He tried to roll himself a cigarette but it went on forever. I rolled it for him and jammed it in his mouth and lit it for him. I said, 'I had a girl and she left me three years ago today. I met her three years before that, on this day. Six years ago this day I met her and three years ago this day I lost her. She was the first and the only girl for me.'

'So?' Gordon said.

'Tomorrow I'll have been without her longer than I was with her.'

Gordon said, 'Count your fucken blessings. How old are you?'

'Nearly twenty-four.'

Gordon started to laugh. And Henry, expecting me to pour out my heart, or thump Gordon, moved on. We trailed him down the Brunswick Street mall and he couldn't lose us.

It took Henry ten minutes in The Site to find a babe. Or maybe a babette. She was about seventeen and a friend of Gordon's. So it wasn't Henry's pulling power, anyway. Through the cigarette smoke and the smoke machine smoke, and through the neon-lit dark as well, Gordon and I watched the blossoming of nightclub romance. Dancing with the million other dancers, drinks at the bar, covert conversations with each leaning towards the other's ear-hole— Gordon and I drank with heavy bitterness.

Gordon said, 'You know, you should get yourself a new girlfriend. You might lighten up.'

I said, 'I wish I was Henry.'

Gordon said, 'I've never heard so much shit.'

I said, 'Well, what about you?'

Gordon said, 'I don't know about sex. It never made me happy. Sometimes I get obsessed and sometimes I die for a root but most of the time I know it won't make me happy.

Women complain with me. Women get pissed off with me. I just come too soon.'

'My housemate could probably give you lessons,' I replied. 'He never comes.'

The name of the young woman with Henry was Helen. She had long brown hair and very trusting eyes. She wore a black halter top and a brown skirt and out-of-date black Doc Martens. She seemed most comfortable with her arm around Henry's waist. I liked her. I said to her,

'What do you do, Helen?' and in the electro-beat she mis-heard me for she hollered back, 'Oh, Curve and Suede, really. I think the Pet Shop Boys have always been fun but this latest one, it's just the pinnacle. I still love *Died Pretty* though Peno shouldn't enjoy showing his dick so much. Chris Bailey's made a welcome return and who would have thought that after so many years *REM* could make such a beautiful album? I hate Guns 'n' Roses and Nirvana more than anything. I didn't go and see U2 but "Lemon" is the best David Bowie song David Bowie never did. And I definitely didn't buy tickets to *The Girlie Show*. How can that woman have any allure left? And that diamond in her mouth. It just looks like she's got a really rotten tooth.'

We all agreed that was true.

I said, 'I saw U2's concert. It was a stormy night. Brisbane summer, after all. All around all that technology and all those screens and all those people there were all these lightning strikes in the distance. It was like armageddon. I remember thinking, "Gee, they really *are* big." And the duet with Lou Reed, that was really something.'

Henry said, 'U2 supping at the cock of corporate rock.'

Helen looked at him with the beginnings of that thing that happens between men and women on nights like these. We got onto books. Helen said, 'I've been reading a lot of

Nietzsche lately. And Henry Miller. Do you think it's funny they go together so well?'

Henry was smiling. Well he might. I wanted Helen so badly I could have thrown up there and then, but he had her all right. A recurring nightmare I have is that one day I'll really fall head over heels again, only to find the object of my desire's favourite albums are *Bat Out Of Hell I*—and *II*.

Henry said, 'No, Helen, I don't think that's funny at all.'

I guessed it was love, then.

Everyone wanted to go back to my place.

Gordon said, 'Any beer or vodka at your place?'

'No,' I said.

'Fuck,' he said.

Somehow we knew we'd be crazy to try to drive home. We counted out our money. I had seven dollars, Gordon thirty-five cents, and Henry a twenty and some change. Just enough for a cab fare and one bottle of cheaper fire water. Helen looked at us as if we were the world's greatest losers, but Henry was already somewhere near her heart. She came with us.

Out in the street, hailing a taxi for us, Helen's eyes glittered when she looked back at me and said, 'You should cheer up. Think happy thoughts.'

She smelled of roses.

Gordon carried around the odour of beer taps and dolour, Henry the sweet scent of success, me the whiff of death, but Helen, sweet Helen, she just smelled of the world's most beautiful flower. How had we latched onto her?

In the street, with sloping drunks and sad-eyed blacks, with daydreaming cops and sloe-eyed whores, we all latched arms and waited for a taxi.

Magda and Paul were screaming in their room. This time it

was the type of screaming normal people do. The house wasn't swaying at all.

I said, 'Let's put *Rage* on.'

Everyone wanted to do that. We turned it on and turned it up loud and over the *The The* retrospective we heard Magda and Paul redefining the terms of their relationship. It went like this:

This Is The Day and Paul was a worm who bolstered his piteous ego with a fat bank account;

The Twilight Hour and Magda was a slut;

Giant and Paul's BMW was an all too obvious extension of his (tiny, she shouted) penis;

Infected and Magda was a fucken slut;

Sweet Bird of Truth and Paul had never come to terms with his emotions or his sexuality. To him love was sex. Sex was life. Life was an epic search for a root. A root gave his life meaning and substance. A good root made him his own personal deity.

'It's the truth,' Henry said.

'You're about to know,' Gordon said.

I said, 'I quite like *The The*,' yet I was only speaking to Gordon because Henry and Helen inexplicably vanished. A wink of an eye and they were gone. The bottle of fire water was down to less than half. Vodka. Very fine. My ears were ringing and there was a discomforting sense of otherworldliness about my own house. How much time had passed? I said, 'Where are—?' and Gordon tilted his head toward the bedrooms.

'Maybe she's giving him a blowie.' Very politely he said, 'Got any beer?' His rollie had gone out and he was having difficulty getting it going again. I lit it for him.

'No beer. Drink the vodka.'

'. . .'s making me sick in the tummy. I smell coffee.'

'You're imagining it.' But I smelled coffee too. I stood

up, swayed, staggered. Gordon, lotus position on the carpet, put out his hands and propped me by the thighs until I had my balance. It took a while.

Meanwhile—

Slow Train to Dawn and Magda told Paul the worst thing she had ever done was to give her body to him (this was a line from 'Cruel' by PIL—I never knew Magda was a music fan; yet again, an interesting woman with someone else. I couldn't be more depressed).

—and I was falling toward the kitchen.

Someone had indeed made a fresh pot of my Lavazza. I poured a mug of it for Gordon but Gordon had gone to sleep on the carpet. His rollie had dropped out of his mouth and was burning a small secret hole in that carpet. The bottle of vodka had overturned and the carpet had sopped most of it up. I hated that baby-shit coloured carpet anyway. On the television—*The Mercy Beat* and

> *I was just another Western Guy*
> *With desires that couldn't be satisfied*
> *So one day I asked the angels for inspiration*
> *And the devil bought me a drink*
> *And he's been buying them ever since*

—and I watched a while and straightened the bottle and picked up the burning butt. In his sleep Gordon muttered *Cynthia, my darling, my darling* or maybe it was all just in my romantic imagination and he was nothing but another boozy *disparu* of this world.

I thought of Henry and Helen and the many bedrooms.

The wind was up and the house rocked ever-so-slightly. This meant he was probably giving her a gentle one in my bed. It was two-thirty in the morning. I knew this to be so because the telephone started to ring. I went down the dark corridor and threw open the door to my own bedroom. There, there, there they were, in my own bed. Except that they were over the covers, they were drinking coffee, and they were playing cards. Had I ever come across a more nauseatingly innocent scene?

Helen said, 'Join us for some rummy.'

Henry grinned up at me, 'Come on.'

I pulled the door shut and leaned in the corridor.

Why should I be so threatened by one man who proves himself better than me? Once upon a time Rebecca and I had lain on that bed late into the night, had listened to music, had drunk coffee or coke or champagne, had played mah jong and scrabble and chess. Now—the corridor belonged to me.

And the telephone.

The ringing was insistent. This Being who seemed to understand longing and loss needed me.

I went to the telephone. I knew what would be waiting there. Through the windows I could see the river. I said, 'Hello?' For that's the game we liked to play. I liked too the familiarity of the emptiness and of the silence and of the breach in time and space. It seemed right. Henry and Helen playing cards in my bed, Gordon asleep in front of *The Violence of Truth*, Paul and Magda fighting or fucking their way into oblivion, and my Rebecca, lost forever in lovelessness for me.

I said into the receiver, 'Come on, Rebecca. It's you. It has to be you.'

Silence, and for the first and last time a breath, and the line was dead in my ear.

We went down to the river, Magda and I, for we were the only two left in the house who might communicate. Paul had thrown on some clothes and had slammed out of his room and had driven to parts unknown in that powerful German extension of his penis. Henry and Helen were two sleeping angels in my bed. Gordon, rudely awoken by Paul's departure, was drinking again, bleary in front of the television. I doubted if he took in very much. My last sight of Gordon, at least for that night, was as he tilted in front of *The The*'s elegiac video to *The Kingdom of Rain*. Only the lotus position stopped him from once again falling sideways onto the carpet.

And then there had been Magda, in the dark, in the corridor, crying.

So we walked together in the windy night.

New Farm Park smelled of roses. No wonder, for the southern hemisphere's largest rose garden grows there. Under the fat old moon all the roses were in bloom. Only that moon lit the rolling hills and the sweep of the vast parklands. Magda and I walked amongst the rose beds. Magda ran her hands along the fat blooms and petals. Over the reds and the pale pinks and the whites, Magda's hands danced. Then she picked a rose and stepped on it and led me down the green banks to sit by the winding river.

The surface of the river glittered. The day made it muddy but the night gave it magic. The air was sweet and the river was enchanted and the moon was the colour of snow. There were no stars. Here and there came the sounds of the slapping of water, as if some sad muddy mermaid was climbing from the river to sit on a polished rock and lick herself clean.

Side by side, Magda and me, under a huge tree. I've never learned the names of trees. We leaned together. To me Magda would always smell of stale sex and oranges. She took my hand and she put it on her breast and I took my hand away.

Magda said, 'You know of that song that speaks to Montgomery Clift. That song that tells him to "just let go". This is what you must do.'

I said, 'If I let go, I'm alone.'

Magda took my hand and she kissed it and I took it away again. She said, 'Just let go.'

I leaned my head on Magda's shoulder.

Oh, why does it take as little as a look to make me fall in love and as long as a lifetime to make me forget it?

Magda wouldn't take no for an answer so I let her hold my hand. No sad-eyed mermaid sat on any rock, yet in the space and the silence we watched the dark glitter of the river for a long time, as if we believed she was there. Or about to appear, our mermaid, full of grace, out of the black waters.

A fruitbat flapped overhead and screamed.

Surrender
Roger McDonald

Whenever the young teacher Dorriel Marquette walked past the post office he saw Camilla Jason-Smith watching him. She wore a white angora sweater and tailored tartan slacks, and had long ash-blonde hair and a pale narrow face like an Irish wolfhound. She was sixteen, the youngest daughter of a Riverina grazing family, the Martin Jason-Smiths of Bulgamarra.

She had been away to school in Moss Vale but was home that year, with little to do, apparently, except come to town with her mother and sit on the post office steps where she met girls her own age from families who could not afford to send their daughters away. Her open stare made the young teacher feel there was something he was expected to do in relation to this girl and her family, a social role waiting to be filled. He hated the feeling and rejected it before it was ever voiced.

The local high school with its population of young teachers was a centre of social life. Scandal, gossip, and infatuation were to be found there. After Australia Day each year a batch of new teachers arrived on the train from Sydney. They were scorned or desired for their differences in a place where the horizons were open as the sea, and the night sky pulled thoughts upwards into oblivion. Late at night the smashing of glass and shouts of raw anger in the streets echoed the emptiness of the heart. No wonder there were suicides and shootings, poisonings and drunken bashings. Young farmers parked their utes under pepper trees outside the school and made truculent contact with possible future wives, spirited women who spoke French, flatting together in Railway Avenue, who after courtship and marriage would have to be corrected from their mistakes, who'd had serious lovers and were rumoured to have had abortions and were ready for compromise in exchange for a kind of peace before they turned thirty, but still had got to be idealised somehow, before they could be courted—all this driving the young farmers mad.

Sometimes, in this town, a bolder girl would say to a young male teacher about a friend, 'She likes you.' This could mean nothing, or it might set something going, a confused meeting, a love affair with a country schoolgirl maybe. There was life here despite the heavy heat haze, the languor of the Olympic pool, the lonely sound of train whistles, the stunned drunkenness of the still nights. Dorriel Marquette wanted someone, but it wasn't Camilla Jason-Smith. He didn't know who.

After school each day Marquette went back to the bar of the Golden Sheaf Hotel to drink beer with teachers his own age. The woodwork teacher, who taught only boys, talked continually about the senior girls and named them, wetting his lips—Margaret Whiteley, Jill McCutcheon, and Alison Routley, bursting from their bras, giving a man the eye. The woodwork teacher told Dorriel Marquette, who had these three for English, If only it was him, he'd show them, they were all sluts. Dorriel Marquette stared into his beer. This bad-mouthing was all bullshit, it got in the way of what could happen between people, what was to be found. These girls had crushes on him and were avid students, they would get As and first-class honours in English and Latin. In the privacy of his hotel bedroom Marquette wrote poetry containing fragmented images of ruin and despair. He longed to be broken in to life. He wanted no young girl's idealism at all, but was rapacious in himself, a libertine in waiting. At the bar of the Golden Sheaf, when he heard the name Camilla Jason-Smith spoken by the woodwork teacher, he turned to him sarcastically and said, 'What's the word on her, then?' The woodwork teacher replied that Camilla Jason-Smith had leukaemia. That she was going to die.

One afternoon Dorriel Marquette was at the post office. He met Camilla Jason-Smith for the first time. She twisted her hands as she spoke. Her voice was flat and conventional. Her smile had been learned in deportment classes. That she had leukaemia was dreadful. But it would not touch Marquette's heart. They did not talk about her illness. Camilla Jason-Smith talked about rugby, polo, and associated social events. She talked about boys she knew who had been to Marquette's school in Sydney. She mentioned Warwick Ogilvy who was taking out her twenty-two-year-old sister, Miranda. She said that Miranda lived for the moment and she envied her. Also that she loved her, but could never understand her.

Warwick Ogilvy and Dorriel Marquette had been students together in Sydney. Ogilvy was born to gallantry. He was the boy mothers swooned over on behalf of their daughters, and he got lucky all the time, in Dorriel Marquette's estimation, in the back seats of cars, on beaches after dances—anywhere.

Dorriel Marquette envied Ogilvy his charm, but despised him for stupidity. Ogilvy scorned his old schoolmate because working in a government school slighted class values: Marquette had to be a socialist. Recently Ogilvy had told Dorriel Marquette about a good thing he had going, a woman who would fuck him in the morning, make his lunch, go caddying for him at golf, and fuck him again when they got back to his place. So that was Miranda who lived for the moment. Dorriel Marquette started thinking about her and couldn't stop. Her sister Camilla told him in a piping voice that the local girls thought he was handsome and she had to agree with them. She spoke as if trained for everything, with no instinct underneath. Dorriel Marquette felt terribly sorry for her. What could he do? He excused himself and said he had to get back to the hotel for tea.

Lying on his bed smoking, watching car headlights sweep across the plaster ceiling of his narrow room, he wondered about Miranda. He wondered what she looked like. They had never met but his feelings followed her down through a gloom of dusk where touch and longing were everything.

He received a printed invitation to a party at the Jason-Smiths' place, Bulgamarra. Mrs Jason-Smith scribbled on the bottom that Camilla would be delighted if Dorriel would be her escort for the evening. *Would* he be so kind? He went with a cold feeling in the pit of his stomach. This was how it felt to be kind. Camilla met him at the door. They went to her father on the verandah and the men drank beer. It had no effect. Ageing farmers with red faces were everywhere. They had been Spitfire pilots and bomb-aimers in the war. The younger section of the party spilled over into an old barn, where there was dancing. Warwick Ogilvy was there. He worked selling airtime for a Wagga radio station and had stacks of new releases to play. He had the Beatles in German. He had the Rolling Stones. Marquette danced with girls from his English class, jiving, moving with his pupils through every nuance of reaction. He was only four years older than they were. He was pleased at being able to be with these girls so naturally, instead of having the pupil-teacher role forced on him. He was released to desire them or not. He could choose. He had already decided to resign his job. He had broken with his girlfriend in Sydney. While he danced he was watched by a young blonde woman with the saddest mouth and most melancholy grey eyes he had ever seen. She was talking to Warwick Ogilvy and nodding in Dorriel Marquette's direction. So that was Miranda. She was asking about him. Marquette felt sick with desire. Her silky blue dress clung to her lazy curves like a shimmering skin. With a hand on her hip, she seemed to wilt despondently, and Marquette's heart went out to her like a runaway train. She held his eye and then she turned away. Stunned as he felt, later he found himself talking to her. They talked easily and naturally, and laughed a lot. After a while they went outside and sat on a stone wall. When they came back inside Warwick Ogilvy winked at Marquette and said, 'Go for it, mate.'

From then on he was unable to think of anyone or anything other than Miranda Jason-Smith. She drove him back to the hotel that night in her car. They talked outside for an hour. He wanted to cup her face in his hands and kiss her wide downturned mouth with its flat lips, and touch her. He wanted to ask her to his room. None of that happened. At three in the morning Dorriel Marquette said goodnight to her and she drove off. They met several times over three weeks. He was in constant excitement and dread when he was with her. They did nothing together except talk. He told her his dreams, his plans. Many of them were wild and unlikely, only thought-up on the spur of the moment. People saw them together in the milkbar, at the pictures, in the park. It reached him that Miranda had a name for going around with different men. The plain-minded people of the town thought she had not given much time to Warwick Ogilvy before switching blokes. It slighted them that a good-looking young teacher from their local school was going around with a squattocracy slut. Their daughters were always talking about him, how nice he was. In the staffroom one day the woodwork teacher asked Dorriel Marquette if he liked old coats.

One evening that was just the same as all the other times he put his arm around Miranda Jason-Smith and they started kissing. Clumsily he banged his head against her in his hunger, and bit her lips, and held her head between his hands, trying to see if her eyes were any happier, and when he saw they were not, he experienced a longing for her that made him feel like vomiting up his life. On the next Saturday afternoon, when the upstairs corridors of the hotel were deserted, she came to his room. They barely talked. She took off her clothes and lay back on the bed. The sad welcome of her smile was all Marquette wanted from this life. She said she loved love. He ran his hand up her legs and thrust himself inside her. As he started moving he tried to speak. He said he loved her, but the expression sounded artificial. She said that she was safe. They were remote from each other, each had a task of driven pleasure, and when he erupted into her she bit her own fingers and shook her head, looking sideways. Dorriel Marquette wanted her again. He did not speak any more, lying at an angle to the side and watching himself slither from her, shining with wetness. The room reeked of sap and tidepool. Dorriel Marquette did not wonder what the pleasure was for her. She had him ride her. He felt more remote from her than he had felt sitting in her car, talking about films and plays. Yet all the time he was lost in the gravity of her expression. Her looks made his blood heavy. She told him to stop, she was burning, the bed was awash, he must let her up, please. She stood naked beside the bed looking down at him. Her expression was just as sad as the first time he had seen her. He wanted her just as he had then. Stickiness ran down her legs from tufts of saturated hair and dribbled on her shiny knees. It trailed from her as she walked across the room. 'Just look at me,' she said. She asked for a towel, and escaped down the empty hotel corridor to the bathroom, where she showered and washed her hair, and emerged combing it. She told him she was sorry, she had to go. There was a Little Theatre performance in Wagga. She had a role in it. She had to drive there, a long way. Dorriel Marquette did not see her again before he went away for the school holidays.

In the city about a week later Dorriel Marquette discovered pus oozing from his cock. He went to a doctor who told him he had gonorrhoea. The doctor sent him to a venereal specialist in Macquarie Street, a fat old man who asked him to bend over while he poked a surgically-sheathed finger into his arse. The doctor had not fully explained what he was doing, or Marquette had not understood. Deep inside him the doctor touched a part of him and semen dribbled from his slack penis. The action caused a slithery stolen pleasure. He had not asked for it. It shamed him. The doctor took a sample over to a microscope. Marquette felt violated by the doctor's actions and his man-to-man gloating attitude. He tried to extract every detail from him about his relationship with Miranda Jason-Smith. He called her the woman. The doctor assumed that Marquette did not love the woman. He called her a slut. Her name and address would be forwarded to a government registry of gonococci carriers. A chart could then be drawn, like a family tree, of everyone who'd had her. The doctor implied such charts existed. Dorriel Marquette hid his contempt. Through the holidays he was required to come back to the surgery for a repetition of the humiliating test. The doctor told Marquette that he was lucky to have learned a lesson, but Marquette did not know what lesson he should have learned. It was love. That was all. He wrote letters to Miranda Jason-Smith but screwed them up. He did not know what to say. There was nothing to say. He just wanted to be with her. But when he was with her, he knew, it would be bad. Having her was to end up wanting her more than he started out wanting her. He was not finding the pleasure with Miranda Jason-Smith that he had with his other girlfriends, getting interested in them, finding out details of their lives, comparing likes and dislikes, sharing pleasures and anxieties. He had been through all that. It was love sickness now. This was what infected him more than any physical disease. Surrender.

The doctor told Dorriel Marquette not to go near women again until his course of treatment was finished. But he went round to the city house the Jason-Smiths owned in Woollahra and Mrs Jason-Smith answered the door. She was overjoyed to see him, thinking he had come to see Camilla. He was shown upstairs to Camilla's bedroom. Camilla had become ill again since the night of the party. Marquette thought bitterly of jumping over the bannisters onto the marble flooring below. Either that or of walking straight past the sickroom door, through an open window at the end of the hallway, and down a drainpipe to his freedom. He had only meant to be kind. He went into the bedroom. It was not terrible in the way he expected. Camilla was wasted but her eyes shone. What had seemed stupidity in her nature Marquette saw as bravery. Her manner was so bloody brave. He wondered what she knew about him and Miranda. Whatever she knew and whatever it meant to her, it was something she accepted. They would put her teddy bear in her coffin when she died but she would not go to the grave a child, even though then dustmotes danced in a sunbeam through the window curtains, she said, 'Look at the dust fairies.' She was heavily drugged. Marquette had seen the party through as her escort. The sham had been cruel. Here she was, glad to see him, acting out the part of a young girl welcoming a favourite boyfriend to an innocent bedside chat. She fell asleep. He left the room.

Downstairs, Miranda was in the kitchen wearing a short tennis skirt that showed her white cotton undies against the smooth flesh of her inside leg. He wanted her. She leant against the refrigerator drinking iced water. She was with a man named Charles, a lawyer, also in tennis clothes. From Charles' behaviour, Marquette knew that Miranda and Charles had not slept together. Charles said wasn't Miranda gorgeous. He said they were to be married in the New Year. Miranda corrected him languidly, 'We're going to have to delay it a few months, sweetie.' Miranda would be on a long course of antibiotics, as he was, thought Dorriel Marquette.

Outside, Miranda drew him aside. 'Christ, I'm so sorry. I gave you something I only just found out about myself. It doesn't show up as obviously with us. You don't see it. It takes longer to knock out. I haven't a clue where it came from. Really I haven't. I feel awful giving it to someone I loved.' Miranda stared at him with her luminous gravity. 'One day I'll see you with someone really beautiful. I'll go mad from jealousy. I really will.'

Dorriel Marquette did not go back teaching or to the town in the Riverina. He rented a room and lived on his savings, trying to decide what to do next. He lay on his bed in the mornings, when it was cool, listening to the whine of cranes on the docks and the shouts of wharfies. He was lazy. He wrote poetry and smoked cigarettes. His poems were about lost children, inconclusive battles, old houses and deaths. People lived their whole lives in states of shock. Dorriel Marquette watched the long muslin curtains on his window twist and writhe. He tried to imagine what it was like growing up a Jason-Smith. He tried to imagine what it was like being Camilla, striving to understand Miranda all the time. He thought he would give up on it eventually. That's what he would do. Just surrender.

When a Man Realises He's Bad
John Birmingham

The thing is, most men labour under the delusion that they are basically good when in fact we are basically bad, programmed for mischief and evil from our very first days. When a man understands this he comes to freedom. I came to freedom on Christmas Eve at the foot of a rumpled bed in a huge, decaying old Queenslander. It was explosively hot in that dark little bedroom and a young woman lay just in front of me, close enough to reach out and touch had I felt like it—which I didn't. She had drawn herself up into a tight foetal ball and I stood back with my hands in my pockets, regarding her long, shuddering sobs and cries with a sort of wry, empowered detachment. I loved her desperately, you understand, and it felt good to see her this way.

She'd done me wrong, this girl, put a real hurting on me. I'd never known anything like it and don't suppose I ever will again. At that moment I was enjoying the fiction of breaking up with her. Really, quietly, getting off on it even though she'd actually put a bullet into our relationship a long time beforehand. A weak little thing, it had twitched and thrashed about on the floor and neither of us had had the sense to finish it off until now. I'd pushed my way into her room—perversely hoping to catch her with someone—tossed a poorly wrapped Christmas present at her and started in on an hour or so of carefully crafted emotional torture.

I had originally intended to say my piece and escape with some dignity after a few minutes. But as she curled into a bundle of woe at the foot of the bed something weird happened. I started to feel good. Started to walk with the King, as they say. I was behaving badly and really enjoying it. Truth be known, it was giving me a bit of a woody. I felt stronger than I had in weeks, not just inside, but outwardly, as though my profile had somehow pressed hard into the scenery of the room. Such a change from the timid spectre I had presented to the world the past few weeks. Such a pity nobody was there to see it and applaud.

Guess I should explain. You'll be wanting all the details, of course.

When I met her I thought she was Irish. She had these green eyes. And piles of dark, wine-coloured hair. She wore cheesecloth and hung rubber bats from her bedroom ceiling. Kept a skull with a candle melted on top by her bed. We first kissed under a dinner table while Guns 'n' Roses screamed out of a really old, cheap Sanyo and two of our friends tried to sleep off three helpings of her awesome lasagna. She was beautiful. After we went to bed for the first time we had cheese and pepper on crackers for breakfast. She taught me how to drink Tequila slammers, how to listen to the Pixies' *Surfer Rosa*, how to move safely through a room where everyone has recently risen from the Dead. I cooked chicken curries, used her toothbrush and made a bucket bong from which we pulled a thousand cones. It didn't last very long and when it was over I fled interstate.

But back to this performance on our last morning. I've forgotten exactly what I said to affect her so badly. It was probably just a lot of bitter bullshit anyway. Hardly worth repeating. I do remember being taken with the sound of the word 'dog' though. I've got a really vivid, digital standard memory of lashing her with the phrase 'You treated me like a dog' maybe six or seven times over the course of an hour. Really whipped into her with it, you know. And she cringed and curled up, just like a dog on the end of a chain. It's kind of shameful to think about it now.

Fact was, however, I'd always been a bit of a prick. The acid bath of this relationship just stripped me back to basics. Even so, it was kind of surprising. I'd always known a few blokes who would have been known as cads or bounders in more genteel times; just never considered myself among them. I never considered myself a brother of Scotty, the champion deflowerer of naive schoolgirls. Never thought I could match it with Marty, an obsessive collector of women, cross-matched by alphabetical and geographical reference; started with Anya from Amsterdam and was joining the dots on his way to Zoe from Zimbabwe, even had a database set up on his computer to keep track of his progress. And I never *really* put myself on the same team as Robbo, a full disclosure man whose enormous sexual appetite seemed to be driven mostly by a need to entertain his mates over drinks. Robbo it was who knocked up his high school maths teacher. Robbo it was who bedded a novice nun. And Robbo it was who liked to demonstrate his remarkable ... uhm ... *control* by getting naked, cradling a bowl of milk in his lap and drinking up every last drop ... but not with his mouth. Now *there* was a guy who knew he was bad. A man who had come to freedom. He once told me about how he had been rogering some poor blonde thing, motoring away, making her head bang into the wall with every thrust. He was drunk. Spastic drunk. Sweating and spinning out and giggling to himself as this girl's head banged into the wall again and again.

It seemed to go on for hours. He was starting to tire. Starting to get muscle cramp. And still nothing had happened. An incredibly hot ball of tension had built up in his groin but it just wouldn't burst. He gritted his teeth and clenched his buttocks and pumped even harder.

And then a geyser let loose. Bursting. Gushing. Surging. Rushing. On and on and on and on. And on. He was beer-bleary and brain-fogged with sex but he knew there was something wrong. He withdrew and clambered unsteadily to his knees. His condom was growing. It was the size of a football and still growing. He had time for a confused and drunken grunt of 'Huh?' before the engorged rubber launched itself across the room on a high powered stream of urine. Good old Robbo. Nearly sprained his ankle running to tell the lads about that one.

Funny thing was, though, nobody thought the worse of him for it. Not even the unfortunate blonde on the receiving end. He had a way of telling the story, you see. Had this raffish charm working for him. Even women seemed to think it was pretty funny and I think it was basically down to his complete lack of shame. A really weird sort of innocence informed his whole routine. It wasn't so much a psychopathic disconnection from the consequences of his actions as much as a full-blooded celebration of them. He understood, down in his meat, that guys are just bastards being natural about things, which is why babes dig them so much.

A lot of guys get themselves all torn up over this. Especially sensitive undergrads on their first swing through Simone de Beauvoir. I saw one of these guys recently at this

WHEN A MAN REALISES HE'S BAD

Egyptian restaurant. It was a pretty cool place, had really great food, but it had this belly dancer. I hate that belly dancer shit. Just hate it, you know. There isn't a white man alive feels comfortable in the presence of a belly dancer. But there's about half a dozen of us there, all late twenties, all established couples. So there is zero sexual tension, it's a dead issue. All we want is a feed and to be left alone by the belly dancer.

Sitting at the table next to us is this young white male. And he's got a date with this incredibly horny-looking Arab girl. A real seven veils character, but only sixteen years old. One of those girls who can actually give you chest pains because your heart constricts when you first see her and you realise that you will never even say hello. And this poor bastard had a date with her. He wasn't good-looking. Had no charisma. Had nothing going for him really. Except a pair of balls. He'd done the one thing that no other man had done on this particular night, he'd asked her for a date. Got past her awful, intimidating beauty and put the question. At first I thought, 'Good on you pal,' because I'm not even jealous. It's not an issue.

But after a while I realise it's just not going to happen. She wasn't very impressed with this middle-eastern restaurant. That was his first mistake, operating on her territory. He should have taken her out to a dance or a pub, hooked into a bit of surf and turf. But he's tried to make her comfortable, tried to do the multiculturally correct thing, and now all these fried donkey dicks and roasted grasshoppers are turning up and he's just losing it. After ten minutes they ran out of small talk. And then the belly dancer sees him. And these belly dancers are cruel women, you know. They can smell your fear. And she flies over and starts giving it to him, the belly dance thing, and he's hopelessly embarrassed. He's sitting there burning up. His girl goes off to the toilet. He can feel every eye on the place watching him. The whole fucking joint knows. I'm sitting there feeling for this kid. It was like a bond, you know. A brother was hurting. And I'm thinking if only there was some way I could do the Vulcan mind meld. Like reach over and grab his carotid or something, effect a direct transfer of knowledge and power, pour out all my hard-won knowledge, years of bitter frustration and fucking it up until I got it right. I wanted to give it all to him. But I couldn't, of course. We finished eating and we left. I kept looking back as we walked up the street. I was praying that she would lead him from the place, take him in hand, take him home and do incredible middle-eastern sex things to him. But I know that just didn't happen. I know he probably dives into shops to avoid meeting her gaze on the street now.

I used to be the same way before I was bad. Before I came to freedom that is. I went through a phase of tying myself into a tangle of neuroses over these completely marginal issues. Like, should I pay for dinner? Do you kiss on the cheek or just brush the lips chastely to establish your credentials as a non-date-rapist? Is it acceptable behaviour to start a fist fight with a guy who gives your date some lip on the way to the restaurant? What form of words are appropriate before grabbing a handful of breast? And on rising from the dinner table with an erection does policy really require an enlightened man to shuffle around like a half-folded flick knife? Whatever. I don't lose a lot of sleep over these things now. I woke up on an interstate train a few weeks back with a massive erection—sometimes known as a Travelling Horn, stood up, stretched and turned around to find a whole carriage load of schoolgirls and their attendant nuns agog at this indiscretion. What to do? Well, a long time ago I guess I would have turned grey and dived back into my seat. But now I simply scratched my arse, nodded

WHEN A MAN REALISES HE'S BAD

to the head penguin and strolled off towards the bar car. Because I'm bad.

There was some hard road travelled before I got to that point, and I'll tell you about it, I promise. But I've got to say I didn't come to this point completely innocent. None of us do. It's true that I came to freedom on that Christmas Eve a few years back. But I'd been nudging my way there over the years anyway. For instance, had I not ripped off a church poor box once, desperate for beer money with which I planned to get a good mate's girlfriend drunk and horizontal? Had I not invented a completely fictional young sister only to kill her off in an equally fictional but nonetheless gigantic service station explosion on the Nullarbor Plain so that I could sob to a sensitive young lady and because I didn't want to *spend the night alone?* Yes, it all comes back to me now. We've all got it in us. It's just that we usually need some catalyst to bring out the best.

And mine was this girl, curled up in front of me.

A few days after the scene at the end of the bed I drove down to Byron Bay for a recuperative week-long cone-fest with a good mate. He'd always been a little skeptical about the girl, but he knew the way of things. We talked it out on the way down. Three or four hours of solid roadwork. It's a crock that guys don't know how to express themselves. It's just that they only ever do it around other guys. I remember spending a morning on the roof of a friend's flat in St Kilda, helping him move and paint some heavy furniture. There were three of us up there. All men. All friends from years before in Queensland. It was grey and cold and a mean-spirited southerly was booming up from Bass Strait, making it a bit of an endurance feat to stay outside for too long. But we were all good talkers and stay out we did, getting into the physical labour and the harsh weather and the telling of our favourite stories about women. Not conquest stories. Real ones. About women who'd had the measure of us. Harry, a pallid, night-stalking rock legend in thin, black, stove-pipe jeans, told us about Hillary, a corporate lawyer who'd run a skewer through his soul by marrying a chubby accountant and moving out into the burbs. Evan, an improbably strong, heavy-set graphic designer, confessed to self-loathing at his seduction of an overweight, part-time nurse whom he couldn't bring himself to leave because of a crushing case of guilt. And me? I recounted my hopeless pursuit of the lovely Joanne, which came to an end the day *she* suggested we go away on a holiday and I couldn't unlock my jaw to reply because of a black fear which swelled up inside my chest, a fear of eventually, inevitably losing her. It's kind of a pity that women never get to see that shit—it might give them pause to think—but then again, maybe it wouldn't. Men understand these failings in each other implicitly. Women usually just think it's pathetic.

Anyway, Tim and I were headed down to Byron a few days after Christmas. We had a big bag of smoke in the back of the car and a house rented just outside town with a bunch of girls we knew. We weren't fixing to hit on any of these girls. They were old friends. Tim just figured I should hang out with some babes who weren't going to gut me at the first opportunity. He'd come out of a bad scene a year or so back himself, a real medusa scenario—you know, head full of snakes—so he'd been there. I was one tender puppy on that road trip. The sense of power which had filled my bones at the foot of the bed back in Brisbane had turned cold and sour about fifteen minutes after I'd pimp-rolled out of the front door. Timbo was a hardy, barrel-chested sort of character, but he understood. We talked about guy stuff for the first hour or so; sport, politics, drugs. He broached the topic of women shortly after we'd stopped for a chocolate-covered banana in northern NSW. Asked how the girl was going.

'The big splitteroo,' I shrugged and then fell quiet, because you don't want to spill your guts, do you?

Tim nodded and eased into a recounting of his twelve months with the snake woman. He'd had to fight off the attentions of three or four other guys to get to her and he was kind of bemused now that he'd even bothered. Kept smiling to himself as he told stories about her. She was European, a Pole or something like that, second generation, and poor old Tim had turned himself inside out trying to cater to her multicultural whims. He dragged himself around an endless series of folk festivals and family outings and tried to ignore the increasingly complex and arbitrary little psycho-dramas by which she spiced up their emotional life. It took a secret attack on his flat—after he'd dipped out of a visit to a Polish film night—before Tim, standing amid the rubble of upturned tables and slashed cushions, realised he might have made a mistake chasing this particular piroshki. He ditched the flat, moved way across town, and didn't go out for six months.

It made me feel a little better. The girl on the bed hadn't cut up my clothes or anything, only my feelings. And of course I gave her back almost as good as I got. And in that weird kind of way, I enjoyed it. I remember careening around my house a few days after the torture scene on Christmas Eve. I remember this moment of absolute clarity. Like Marlon Brando at the end of *Apocalypse Now*. Martin Sheen has arrived, all fucked up and confused and ready to do him in and Brando is just sitting there mumbling good naturedly questions, 'Are you an assassin?' and trying to explain the pure crystalline nature of horror, and how it shot him through the head like a diamond. Or something like that. In my confused state it made perfect sense. I remember stalking around the house slapping my own forehead at the purity of the experience I'd just gone through with this girl. She had fucked me up. And I had fucked her back. Completely, totally, irrevocably. There were no half-measures or weasel words. There were no fists. There were only feelings. For a very short time we had loved and then we had hated. It was really pure shit.

I rang her that afternoon. I felt like I was in the eye of a storm, or maybe experiencing one of those moments of clarity that only madmen and drunks know of. Looking back now I'm still amazed at my absolute calm. It was almost blissful. I had to get to her before it passed, as I knew it would. She was surprised to hear my voice, as you can imagine. I didn't stay on long. I told her I had to say this now while I still could. She waited nervously.

'Thanks,' I said. 'Thanks for everything.'

I hung up. Feeling strong.

That was a few years ago. We're friends again now. In fact I saw her just recently. But I had to make sure that I didn't find myself staring at the soft bow of her mouth while she spoke, or dwelling on a mote of light reflected in her dangerous green eyes. Even so, things are cool. There was a rough patch when I couldn't bear to look at her. In fact I moved interstate so I wouldn't have to. But being burned is being cleansed and I owe her a lot. Through her I learned, as de Beauvoir once wrote, of virtue, lust, renunciation, devotion, betrayal and tyranny. I found all those things in the world and then, I found them inside me. And I came to freedom.

Running Hot and Cold
Chad Taylor

The old carpet slouched in the door.

'You brought white.'

She said it flat, without tone or inflection. She read the label slowly, rotating it against the hallway bulb, and the light shining through the bottle turned her skin green. 'Don't you like it?' he asked. 'I could get something else.'

She considered. His weight shifted from one foot to the other, then back again. Finally she let the bottle fall. 'White's good.' She smiled. 'I like white.' And motioned him into the room.

His footsteps sounded loud on the floorboards. Ripping up the carpet had left lines of broken staples maybe fifty years old. The wood was dark as chocolate.

'So, are you happy?' he asked.

'I don't understand.'

'With the house.'

'Oh.' She slipped past him, digging in the kitchen for the corkscrew. 'Yes.' She gestured towards the cat that glared at him from the windowsill. 'Pussfeller likes it. Don't you? Eh?' She made kissing noises. He remained unsoothed, as did the cat.

He spoke for a while about foundations and studs. The wine tasted bitter, he thought, but then again he knew very little about wine. He caught himself before he leant on a stack of brown cardboard boxes: the lids had been marked FRAGILE in red ballpoint pen. 'You should unpack these,' he warned, 'instead of leaving them lying around.'

She shrugged. 'Probably.'

'Before you know it you'll be here six months with everything still taped shut.' His eyes followed the rim of her glass.

'Do you like my hair?' She had slicked it flat across her forehead, like an old-fashioned photograph. She was wearing a man's white shirt with the sleeves rolled up, and the tails covered her body to mid-thigh, front and back. Her legs were bare. Her sandals buckled at the ankle.

'I like it.'

'I got so dirty, cleaning,' she regarded the ceiling. 'I put my bathing cap on.'

He laughed. 'And your togs?'

She shook her head. 'Nothing.'

'Nothing at all?'

'Nope. Just the cap, then you get in the shower and wash everything off.' Nonchalant. 'It's the only way to clean ceilings. Weren't you taught that?'

'Who'd teach me?'

'I dunno.' She smirked. 'Anybody, really.'

He switched on the oven light. 'Mutton.'

'Yup.' She filled his glass again. 'You want to get out and let me finish cooking it?'

He raised a toast. 'To the new house.'

He found the bathroom at the end of the hall, opposite the bedroom. He did not switch on the fluorescent. He watched his shadow washing his hands in the mirror, in the half-light. Then he picked up his glass and went into the bedroom and sat down on the unmade mattress.

He smelled perfume. There were more boxes in the corners and beneath the window. He listened to the squeak and clump as she opened the oven door, and the fat spitting as she turned the meat. 'You want me to carve?' he called, and waited. She hadn't heard. He held the glass between his knees and looked down at his shoes. Good wood on the floor. It was a good place. He tipped his weight back, then forward on his toes and stood up, stretching. He could still see himself in the bathroom mirror. The wine was going to his head. He drained the glass. 'You want me to carve?' he called again, and she heard him this time.

The dining table was almost as big as the room.

'Asparagus.' She stood the plate on the table, green stalks swimming in cream. 'Adds salt.' She smiled quickly at the thought and drew her chair close, ushering in the next sentence with a short bob of her head. 'Makes your piss salty.'

'Makes it stink.'

'It's not that so much as the salt strengthens it. The flavour.' She began to say something else but stopped herself. 'Excuse me,' she laughed. She pushed her empty glass across the table. He saw that her fingernails were broken, the skin pads grazed white. 'Would you mind?'

He poured.

'I'm glad you like my hair,' she said later. 'I thought it might have been a bad idea.'

'Let me see it again,' he said. She turned her head.

'No,' he corrected, 'closer than that.' She leaned forward over the empty plates. He reached across the table and took the back of her scalp in his fist and tipped his knuckles, carefully judging the tension. 'It's good,' he confirmed.

She gasped: 'It's shorter at the back.'

He shifted his grip. 'Here?'

'Mmm.' She drew in her top lip.

His laugh wasn't a sound so much as an exaggerated breath. She opened her eyes to him, her shoulders hunched. He let go. She blinked and sat back, pressing her palm against her cheek. 'There's dessert,' she said, as if she'd just remembered. 'Apricots.' She got up to fetch them.

He stood up and walked to the bathroom again. This time he turned on the light and saw a pale man in a cheap shirt, slightly bored by the routine. Dinner had been slow, really, too slow for him. He looked at the mattress across the hallway and wished she'd taken time to make the bed instead of charging in and ripping up the carpet for two days. He shut the door and unbuckled his belt, and when that was done he took off his shirt and his shoes and socks.

After a time he heard her footsteps coming down the corridor. 'Did you see the shower?' she called, her voice muffled by the wood.

'What?'

'The shower.' She came in apricots first, pushing open the door with the rim of the bowl and placing it in front of the mirror. He watched her reflection, soft in the dark stripe of the hallway. She was naked now, except for her shoes. She chose an apricot and leaned on the door to eat it. 'The shower,' she said. 'Look.'

He looked at the walls and then down at the metal basin: the floor had been marked with dozens of tiny dents. She pointed the bitten fruit at her delicately laced ankles. 'Someone wearing heels in the shower,' she said.

'Who?'

'The people before me. She. Him, I dunno. Mmph.' She spat the fruit stone into her palm and set it carefully next to the basin. He watched it rock on the formica.

'Was that good?'

'Oh yes.'

He reached up and put his hands around her sides and pulled her towards him. He was fascinated by her skin. He touched it, licked it, bit it. He enjoyed foreplay as if that was where he expected it to stop—at the skin.

She was easy to lift, balanced on her left hand, reaching out and turning the shower taps with her right. He raised her up against the shower head and the water fell in gulps, drumming on the basin. She shut her eyes and said something about the water stinging.

For a second, her knees were sandwiched exactly between their shoulders. As his cock touched the beginnings of her cunt she let go and pissed in a fine, straw-coloured stream. He held her tight and still. The water and her piss ran down in two streams on either side of his balls. And then her legs fell and he was inside her, and the noise was incredible—the water in his ears and the shouting and the impact of their bodies against the cubicle wall.

They dried each other with the same towel and sat watching the steam collect on the walls. She sat on his stomach and ran her hands over his chest and fed him apricots, and when they finally grew cold he lifted her into the bedroom and they fucked again on the mattress, their hands lost for a grip on the slippery factory quilting.

She lay face up in the darkness, with his arm across her. 'My orgasms are all so different with you,' she said. 'I feel like I should give them names.'

'What would you call that one?'

'Beatrice.'

He felt warm in the sheets, but the sheets themselves were cool.

'Sometimes orgasms are hot,' she explained, 'with a centre, like a bomb's been dropped. You get warmer and warmer. And other times they spread out from my stomach in a wave and go through my fingertips and my toes ... And sometimes they are sudden. Quick. You want another because you feel you've missed the first.'

He had been told this before, and was still intrigued by it. Her orgasms were as varying as his were consistent. Every time fucking was the same: a hunger, an initial wetness, then repetition, then a hunched, frantic twisting, a splitting noise in his head ... and then extreme relief, a tonnage removed. Afterwards he wanted to roll away but she held him close, insistent. In those minutes she wanted him so much while all he wanted was a glass of something cold. And yet this was the base stuff she turned into so much jewellery. His sex was an unbearing vein in which she blossomed. Flowers in the dirt.

'What would you name your orgasms?' she asked.

Smith, Smith and Smith. 'I wouldn't,' he said, sitting up.

There was a bottle of flat ginger ale in the refrigerator. He drank some, standing the empty tumbler on the bench. Then he went back to bed and took her in his arms and kissed her on the cheekbones and the sides of her eyes and her eyelids and the base of her neck—never on her mouth, not until his cock was hard again and inside her. She had a third orgasm. She said she would call it Petronella.

Two weeks later he smashed her pelvis. He did it inadvertently, with the back of his car. She was walking up his driveway as he was reversing down. She waved but he didn't see her. The car was travelling at eight kilometres an hour when it hit her. She wanted to scream but could not: she instantly went into shock. All he heard was the thump and even that was nothing—it could have been the wheel going over a stone for all he knew. But something he saw from the corner of his eye—the white of her shirt, maybe, or her face—made him stop and get out.

The impact had thrown her onto the grass, and knocked

the earrings from her ears. Her pocketbook lay three metres away. Her mouth was open and her eyes were wider than he ever recalled seeing them, dilated, bulging. She grasped at the air and then lurched up on her elbows to look at her left leg which was sticking out from her side at a perfect ninety-degree angle. And then she voided herself, her urine jetting on the cement. He reached out to her, collecting the shambles of limbs and blood and fresh warm piss, and began moving her towards the house.

He set her down on the basement floor, near the place where his car dropped oil. She seemed even paler compared to the black greasy mark on the cement. She was still panting but her gaze was steadier now. Her hands explored his jacket, probing beneath for the flesh, the warmth.

'Sorry,' he said.

She laughed, but the laugh got away from her and turned into more panting. 'Ouch,' she said.

Sometimes in the past he would find himself avoiding her gaze. But now he wanted to look. He remembered a playground game: you had to hold hands with someone and not break your gaze for two minutes. At first there were giggles, then nervousness, then a feeling of extreme discomfort— aggression. And then the feelings fell away, and the two players became friends. He cradled her head.

'I have never had feeling for you,' he began. 'Not truly.'

'Doctor.'

'I just put up with things.'

'Doctor.' She was describing a picture in her head. 'Hospital.' Something white and safe. Warm, but with cool sheets.

'Don't try and sit up,' he told her, laying her head back on the ground.

'Doctor,' she said again.

'I'm not going anywhere.'

He paused for a second, wondering.

He fumbled with her buttons for a brief second and then discarded the idea. He did not want to look at her body. This was no time for caressing, for regarding her nude. He had finished looking. As he leaned above her he realised what he wanted to do. While she lay pale.

Something in his stare communicated it. She was dizzy from the impact, beginning to dream. And in shock, her body chemicals had kicked in. The pain was leaving and taking with it its outward signs. Trembling. Reflex. Speech. Soon it would be too late.

He stood back. He reached down and began unbuckling his belt. She smiled.

He was slow with her, infinitely gentle. This time they made no sound. Her eyes rolled back in her head like a broken toy.

It had been—what? Seconds? A minute? And then the panic came.

He sprinted upstairs to phone and the ambulance came and they lifted her into the back. He sat with her on the way to the hospital. She swayed in the cot, her eyes opening a crack with each corner and bump in the road. As they drew up over the diagonal yellow lines of Emergency he crouched down at the head of the stretcher. She was straining to make out his form. He put a hand on hers, his fingers on the tubes taped to her wrist. Her hair was wet and her eyes were very dark. The cement floor had left an imprint on her cheek. He leaned close to her ear. 'Violet,' he told her.

'Violet.'

'What?' The ambulance boy looked up. 'What'd you tell her?'

'I said, "Violet".'

'That her name, is it?'

He shrugged. Then the ambulance drew to a stop and someone threw open the doors.

That night when visiting hours were over and he was finally asked to leave, he returned to her house. He examined the bills on her dresser before writing her a cheque. He dusted the four empty shelves of the bookcase. He cleaned the dishes. There were still boxes in the back room so he unpacked them. He found photographs, which he looked at, and letters, which he read. He pulled out the drawers of her dresser and stared inside, thinking. He looked at the shoes in the wardrobe.

His hands smelled of dust. He took a shower and dried himself and climbed into her bed. He fell asleep.

He woke up gasping and tried to understand why. Although the room was dark something had flashed through his head. His face was wet. He heard the cat drop to the floor and run out of the room. He put his hand to his face and yelped. Something hurt terribly, like a hot edge. He scrambled across the bed and flicked the reading lamp: there was blood smeared on the light switch, and his hands, and his jaw. His body made a noise, an involuntary squeezing of air from his lungs that was neither shout nor moan. By now the pain was intense. He made it to the bathroom and took a breath before looking in the mirror. When he did he saw three red lines running from his cheekbone to his chin, spattered and ragged behind the fatty white of the exposed skin. The blood was pooling in his collarbone. The cat had stepped across his face, and damn near tore his eye out. He looked around for the animal, and then for something to throw at it, and then slumped to the floor, too afraid to hold his head in his hands.

The cat sat and watched him from the dark room, its eyes unblinking and green.

Baby Oil
Robert Drewe

Anthea had been living with Brian in Paddington for almost three years when she began an affair with Max in June. Anthea and Max met on a fashion shoot in Noumea. He was not the usual photographer her magazine used for fashion assignments, but Gunter was in Mauritius for *Vogue* and Max stood in. By the time they boarded their U.T.A. jet for Sydney a week later they were talking, rather surprisedly for such people as they recognised themselves, of being in love.

This affair was different from the other encounters Anthea had experienced while living with Brian. One afternoon at lunch soon after their return from New Caledonia, tanned and dreamy and still out of tune with the weather, she invited Max home, into her and Brian's house and, by extension, into her, their, bed.

In the past she had joined her lovers—a very catholic assortment with a rapid turnover—on afternoons at the Hilton or, on the rare occasion when one was single, at his place. In the spirit of frankness which marked the beginning of their affair she had told Max all this. The squalor of the bachelor flat had even added a *frisson* then, Max guessed, but only before the act—and there would never have been a return visit.

Anthea admitted to Max that her willingness to make love to him in her own bed was an indication of her strength of feeling for him, their spiritual and physical closeness. Their star signs were also terrifically compatible.

'We're kindred souls,' she said, kneading his buttocks in the lift going down from the New Hellas after lunch. She had also mentioned (rather defensively, he thought), 'I believe my body is mine to do with as I like.' Brian, a daily political cartoonist whom Max had never met, worked long hours on several publishing projects, and she travelled constantly, so the opportunities to uphold her belief were numerous.

Max could understand why someone wanted their lovers away from the domestic hearth. But having decided to break her usual rule she showed amazing *sang froid*, he thought, in drawing him urgently by the hand into the bedroom and onto the bed beneath a framed skiing holiday photograph of her with Brian, both beaming in red sweaters, cosy and radiant in the snow.

She was even more ardent than in Noumea. Her practice showed, her lean, whippy skills by no means subdued by the presence of Brian's accoutrements around them: pens, opened mail, coins and keys on the bedside table, Brian's *New Statesman*s, *Guardian Weekly*s and *New York Review of Book*s stacked beside it, even a pair of Brian's red underpants hanging on his wardrobe doorknob. If she suffered any pangs of conscience at these souvenirs, at the juxtaposition of Brian's happy picture and Max's naked body, it didn't show.

BABY OIL

It occurred to Max that as Anthea had obviously planned for them to return here after lunch this particular afternoon, but had not removed the more intimate traces of Brian's occupation, even the rather blatant note of the discarded underpants, that maybe she got a kick out of it. Or perhaps she was just a sloppy housekeeper. Anyway, the combination of this selective insensitivity and her carnality held enough intrigue for him. And Brian's bits and pieces didn't unduly concern him; perhaps, if he were honest, they even added a spark.

He was right, there was a perceptible change in her lovemaking now; not in her techniques exactly, but she was slightly less romantically swept away, even more lustful than under the Pacific palms. The face was not expressive with tropical wonder. She had changed up a gear. Her in-bed personality now was one of impassive sexual hunger. She burbled sweet obscenities, her body was warm and responsive, but there was something almost neutral in the eyes.

'Just wonderful, my darling,' she said afterward, fetching them tumblers of Chablis. Max sipped, and flipped through a *New Statesman*. Very dull layout, no photographs to speak of, a couple of anti-Thatcher cartoons. Brian was presently in Alice Springs or somewhere doing a book of drawings of Aborigines. Presumably she washed the sheets before his return. Maybe while she was at it she could throw in the bloody underpants.

A little later, for the encore, she reached up to the bedstead for a bottle of baby oil. Slowly anointing them, she whistled softly at his pleasure. She had obviously made a speciality of this. Under a film of oil her tan glistened. On her brown breasts the nipples were big silver coins, then their slippery cones darted everywhere—even the backs of his knees, the soles of his feet didn't escape their touch—until he couldn't differentiate between tongue and nipple.

Anthea glided knowingly over him, they slid together, undulating like an ocean swell, rolling and curving towards shore. Owing to the wild buffeting of the bed Brian's coins and keys rattled and danced.

As their affair intensified over the next weeks Max spent a lot of time in Anthea's bedroom. Emboldened by the intensity and intimacy of lunch they would kiss on restaurant stairs, hail taxis with incautious exuberance, and she would draw him home to Paddington. He succumbed gladly to the force. What could match the thrill of the cab ride along Oxford Street, thighs pressed conspiratorially together; the anticipation as she fished in her handbag for the key? Max's senses sang, his hormones fizzed. The teasing abandonment of the kiss inside the door! Her fellatio attacks on him in the hallway! (The sensual relaxation of her lower lip almost floored him.) His heightened perception amazed him. Her textures, smell and taste were uniformly exquisite.

It went even further than Anthea. Max's general attention to detail was never more acute than in the opening minutes of their afternoons together. Even as he entered the bedroom and began undressing every corner of the room instantly registered on him. He noted the current disarray of male and female clothing or any minor adjustments to the furnishings since his last visit—the addition of a TV set in front of the bed, for example—which hinted at domestic conviviality. Conviviality was the alleged keynote of the Anthea-Brian relationship. Implied was plain old friendship rather than romantic sexuality. That was all right; Max could live with conviviality.

'He makes me laugh,' she'd volunteered to Max. 'That's all.' He knew better than to pursue the matter. He was never quite sure what women meant when they said that. It sounded platonic but he suspected it covered the whole range to one hundred per cent sexual. Women were so wonderfully dishonest and dismissive when it suited them. In the face of this treachery Max quite often felt more in league with the husband or boyfriend he was cuckolding than with the woman in question—equally, eternally ignorant of the extent of female fraudulence.

Objects still registered on his consciousness as he climbed into bed—even the bed coverings themselves—and created their own spun-off meanderings. The erotic suggestion he'd got one afternoon from black satin sheets, for instance, was partly allayed by the realisation that they were *their* satin sheets and that at one time at least they had thought black satin sheets would be a sexy thing to experience.

'Kinky,' he joked, the day of the sheets.

'A bit of a cliché, aren't they?' said squirming, sliding Anthea, slippery enough as she was.

The oil plus the sheets made purchase difficult. The sheets did not return.

'I love you,' she told Max often, whenever he looked serious.

'I love *you*,' he repeated.

The State Department gave Brian a trip to the United States for being a pace-setter in his branch of the media— and to keep him on-side. Max rejoiced. His afternoons with Anthea quickly formed a pattern. They managed to meet about three days a week throughout August. They would rush to bed and make love. Then Anthea, pulling on one of Brian's T-shirts, would totter downstairs and bring them up glasses of wine. Once, returning to bed, she stretched to remove the shirt and Max saw for an instant the light catch the shine of his moisture on the inside of her thigh. The image of this peaceful interval remained fixed photographically in Max's mind when they were apart: their quiet bodies settled obliquely across the bed as they murmured and sipped wine and laughed softly. He ran a finger along her vulnerable hip. A cool breeze played with the net curtains. The cat rearranged itself in the laundry basket.

Before long she would take his glass from him, reach for the baby oil and slyly, languorously, begin Stage Two.

Cool rain. Drops as distinct as purity fell on his thirsty skin. Sighing, Max reclined as she dripped oil on his penis, spread oil on her nipples with a studious familiarity and then caressed herself with him. Her New Caledonian tan had faded; she was the shade of peaches. The silken delicacy of her touch approached no touch at all. Though her lubricity made it redundant, Anthea passed him the oil to caress her thighs. He dropped some oil into his hand—one droplet—and his heart jumped. The bottle was empty. Two days before it had been a quarter full. Squeezing hard, Max forced out the last drop of oil. He let it fall in her navel.

Perceptibly, even against Max's inclination, Brian's possessions and knick-knacks began to get on his nerves. It became an effort to use the bathroom, to shower after their love-making, with Brian's *New Yorker*s stacked by the lavatory, his *Eau Sauvage* on the shelf, the ubiquitous red underpants hooked over the doorknob. In bed he would look up from her face or breasts or thighs into the tanned faces of the amiable skiing duo. Her hair was longer then, darker, her face rounder. He hated the Anthea in the photograph. He made love with great passion and they both cried out with equal vehemence. Afterward she gave him a quizzical look but said only, 'I love you.'

One late August afternoon when Anthea left the bed for the bathroom, Max, compelled, took Brian's pen from the bedside table and marked the oil level in the current bottle. Its label said:

**Johnson's
Baby
Oil
PURE—MILD—GENTLE
Johnson & Johnson
200 ml**

Max made a small spot of ink alongside the J for Johnson's at the top of the label. Replacing the bottle, his pulse racing, he saw the oil as suddenly volatile, with a sheen like gin.

It came as no surprise to him, though set his heart beating in his throat with a delicious, frightening anguish as if to choke him, to note two days later that the oil level was well below his mark. It was actually between the B of Baby and O of Oil. Following their afternoon in bed, a feverish, almost savage exercise that left them both drenched and shaky, Max again marked the oil level, now just above the P for PURE.

Three tense days passed before they could next go to bed together. Max had hardly slept. Each dawn, jogging red-eyed and heavy-limbed along Bondi beach, he decided resolutely to end the affair. Each morning she rang his studio cheerily to say, 'I love you.' He resisted saying it.

'Tell me you love me,' she wailed.

He had trouble visualising her at her shiny green desk, a cigarette going between her bright nails, talking like this. 'I love you,' he said.

'Good.'

On the third day when Max entered the bedroom the bottle may as well have been the only object in the room. They could have been fucking on bear skins or broken glass. The label was turned to the wall but the oil level already seemed lower. The oil was as ominous as a sultry sea at dusk, tropically translucent before a storm. Its diffused whorls hid sharks, stingrays, venomous transparent mysteries. Max's senses almost exploded. As soon as Anthea went downstairs for the wine he snatched up the bottle. Of course the level was down, way below the P, almost to the next J.

When she returned he was subdued, flaccid as a jellyfish. 'When did Brian get back?' he asked, almost strangled by nonchalance.

'He didn't.' Then she said, correcting herself, 'He comes and goes,' blushed and sniggered softly, a noise midway between embarrassment and coarseness, the most unattractive sound he had heard in his life.

She picked up quickly. 'Why do you ask?'

The essence was right out of him and he let it go. 'No reason.'

'I love you,' she said, staring into his eyes.

As the oil dropped on him he watched her face, impassive except for a small moué of sensuality. Fury revived his spirit and they collided in lust and high emotion. Coins and keys spun and jangled beside them. Later, while she went to the lavatory, he marked the bottle. The tiny dot, between the J and the 200 ml, took his final strength.

Max and Anthea had a passionate lunch at Doyle's, overlooking the slick spring Harbour. Behind clouds a pale sun hung over Watson's Bay. They held hands on the table, drank two bottles of Chardonnay, kissed in public, overtipped and caught a taxi home to Paddington.

Max hadn't even undressed when he grabbed up the oil bottle right in front of her to examine it, stare at it. On the other side of the label, was a clearly inked cross which accurately recorded the present level in the bottle.

Still
Christopher Cyrill

'Three plates,' she says. She is standing behind the kitchen counter. 'Did you get up and eat again last night?'
'No,' I say. And then I try to be sure. 'No.'
'I didn't either.'
Melissa and I stare at the third plate and the bones left after the meal. A small tangle of capsicum lies beside the bones. The bones have been snaped in half and the marrow has been sucked out. Even the cartilage has been eaten. A glass crusted with milk at its brim stands beside the plate. Neither of us touches it.
Last night I cooked chicken cacciatore. I used a bottled sauce, which I had bought from the supermarket. I then dumped the empty bottle in the glass recycling bin out the front of our apartment. I cut thick figure eights of capsicum and rings of onions and added them to the sauce. 'Homemade,' I said to myself. I turned down the gas stove and lit a cigarette. I held the cigarette over the food and watched the ash lengthen. Then I dusted the ash into the palm of my hand.

At about five o' clock I poured my seventh bourbon, lit another cigarette and waited for Melissa to get home. She had left for work at the shoe store earlier than usual yesterday morning because a shipment of new running shoes was coming in and she and the other girls had to clear away the old model. I had awoken and showered as she was leaving. Then I sat at the kitchen counter and pretended to work. I reread the page of notes I had written the day before and reread other pages which I had written weeks or months earlier. Some of the pages were filled with long sentences written over and over again yet somehow left unfinished, sentences that described the trains that passed on the horizon of our street, trains that seemed to run along the roofs of houses. Other pages were filled with drawings of teeth and tombstones and dogs or odd phrases such as 'Ying/Yang tattoo' and 'abortionist near gas station'. Yesterday I had started to drink early and just to fill a page I transcribed from an encyclopaedia the birthdates of painters and Nobel Laureates, anything about anyone just to fill a page, just to have something to read the next day, hoping that something in those facts would reveal to me a fiction. About six months ago I won a prize for a poem I had published in *Stork*, a local journal. Melissa had hated the poem.

'Don't write about me,' she said. 'Write about anything, just not me.'

When Melissa got home she looked at the glass in my hand, glanced at the bottle near the stove and then she walked into the bedroom. She closed the door behind her. I hated her for closing the door. I felt like throwing the glass against it.

'Listen, if you're sure it wasn't you, then someone has been here,' she says. And she says it in her way, the way that makes me feel guilty.

'It can't be,' I say.

The front door is padlocked and chain-latched from the inside but the bathroom window, which is the size of a car window, is ajar. Our apartment is on the second floor and to get to the kitchen someone would have to walk through our bedroom. I check my wallet and Melissa checks her purse and her glory box. Nothing is missing and the most valuable thing either of us owns is Melissa's opal ring, which is on the bathroom sink. I check my folder of notes and the kitchen cupboards while Melissa finds a rattle among the boxes in the wardrobe.

'This is ridiculous, Black,' she says. She always calls me by my surname. 'We're looking for something that has gone. If someone, this "dinner guest", has taken something then it's not anything we'll miss. Why couldn't he have just taken the fucking TV so we could be sure?'

'Sure of what?'

'That someone was here.'

'And how? Did a dwarf, no wait, an acrobatic dwarf, a dwarf on a fucking trampoline or some kid come in through the window?'

'Then explain this to me.' She points at the plate with the rattle.

I can't, and I feel like I have to say something but I say nothing. I light a cigarette. Melissa clicks her teeth together and holds herself.

I met Melissa about two years ago at an Italian restaurant on my sister's twenty-fifth birthday. Gwen and I are twins and look a lot alike except now that I have straight hair and she has curly hair. When we were babies I had curly hair and, to hear Dad tell it, I was often mistaken for a girl. My sister now lives in London with my mother and teaches art part-time at a college in Brixton. My mother divorced my dad when we were thirteen. Gwen and I stayed with Dad.

At the time I thought that Dad needed us more because he was still in love with Mother. I often repeated the phrase to myself, 'still in love.' Dad kept their wedding photo on his bedside table for a year after she left, next to his dentures and harmonica. Once I asked him why he didn't move the photo.

'I am here because of then,' he said and I felt as if he had meant to say something else. And not long after that the photo was gone.

On the night of her birthday Gwen introduced Melissa to me by calling her 'Melissa from uni'. Gwen had another friend named Melissa, whom I never met and whom Gwen referred to as 'Melissa the singer'. I sat across from Melissa during dinner. I didn't talk to her. I looked her in the eye whenever she said something. While everyone at our table was having dessert I walked to the bar of the restaurant and stood where she could see me from the table. Leave it up to her, I thought. Before she came and stood beside me at the bar and before I bought her an apple cider, saying that it was my dole day, I drank shots of bourbon and imagined my hands on her face and her waist and my face in her hair and the excuses and apologies I would make to Gwen who didn't like me dating her friends.

At the bar Melissa and I played 'Rock, Paper, Scissors' to decide who bought the next round. The bar staff stared at us and smiled and let us keep drinking while they cleaned up. Gwen had left them the rest of her cake. Melissa was wearing a long sleeveless dress and she hadn't shaved under her arms. I kept touching her arms. Later we pressed against each other in bed but nothing more, we were too drunk. A month after that she moved in with Dad and me and Gwen and a week later Gwen moved out.

Melissa clicks her teeth again, as if it helps her think. She presses her right hand against her spine. She rarely smokes but she asks me for a cigarette. She looks scared and she looks tearful and she exhales smoke in short breaths. I look her in the eye for the first time in a long time and for what seems like the first time this morning, I wake up.

I start to think of the things that Melissa has probably already thought about. Someone has come into our flat while we slept. Someone has walked through our bedroom, heated some food, eaten at the counter, poured one or two or three glasses of milk. I picture this person, this man, standing above our bed. He holds a knife or an axe or a gun. He has turned on the gas and set fire to the curtains and as the gas creeps towards the fire he is touching Melissa, her hair, her breasts. I try to remember if we made love in that half-awake way that she likes, that she starts with her hands, and I can't remember and I can't ask her but I see him watching, joining in.

'Don't think,' I say. And I mean something else.

Last night Melissa and I ate silently. I picked a chip of bone out of my teeth. I had a headache after eating so I poured myself a shot of bourbon and swallowed an aspirin with it. She drank four or five glasses of water and then went to the bedroom and dressed in pyjamas. I hate her when she dresses for bed. I undressed and lay beside her and she looked at me as if I were a stranger. I ignored her. I remembered that Dad's Birthday was coming up and I wanted to buy him a camera and I wanted Gwen to pay half. Then I tried to remember how many times I was photographed last year. I was photographed at a wedding and by *Stork* and by Dad the day Melissa and I moved into the flat. I started to think that perhaps people are photographed less as they grow older. First there are baby photos, then photos on seesaws or at parties with relatives, annual school and high school photos, graduating university, marriage, photos of their own children. Then I thought that perhaps the older you get the more photographs people take, as if every moment must be recorded and remembered, unless you are famous or infamous or marry many times and then I decided I would never marry Melissa.

I started to wonder how I had come to be in bed with a woman whom I knew I wouldn't marry. I knew that I could find in family photo albums at least one photo of myself in every year of my life, like random stills taken from a cartoon. I knew I could arrange these twenty-seven snapshots in a line beginning with my sister and me in my mother's arms and ending, after various ill-at-ease poses on playgrounds, in classrooms, on cricket ovals and stages, with a photo of Melissa and me standing in the kitchen of our flat. Yet there would be incidents that would remain unrecorded, the meeting in a restaurant and Dad wheezing as he carried her boxes into my room and his hand trembling as he signs the cheque for Gwen's deposit. And also Melissa's mother spilling wine on my hand and grabbing the waiter by the belt and other restaurants and bars and birthdays and a wedding, Melissa crying for a whole day, an anniversary we both pretended to forget and throughout a feeling I could never name, like having left something in a taxi or tram or train and not wanting it returned. I imagined that if in my sixth or seventh or eighth year I was not photographed, I could only prove my existence to myself, and then only through memory, through repeating 'I am here because of then'. I wondered how, if in a time I forget love or forget that I had once loved Melissa, I would prove to some stranger or simply to myself, that I once had a lover whom I argued with over rent, who was once a friend of my sister and whom I had once fucked on a park bench, except by a photograph, which shows only her cutting vegetables while I fill an ice-tray, a pose that could mean we were cousins or friends or brother and sister.

'I think it was a woman,' Melissa says. 'Because of the way the capsicum is put to one side. It's absurd, I know it's absurd.'

'It was a man,' I say. But I start to think it was a woman.

'I want to call the police. And tell them that someone came here and stole food and nothing else and we don't know how she got in unless she was a dwarf or a kid and we don't know if it was a she ... and Black, don't drink tonight, I mean, you couldn't even remember if you had got up.'

'It wasn't me,' I say. And I am sure.

'I know, I'm sorry.'

'Ring work and say you're sick. Don't say anything else. I don't know, I don't know what has happened or how or what.'

I hold her while she calls. I touch her shoulders and smell her hair and feel under her pyjama top and leave my palm on her belly button. She hangs up and kisses me. She touches my palate with her tongue. I touch her hair, her breasts.

It is afternoon when I wake. I turn and look at her. I close my eyes. 'Melissa,' I say. She wakes. She touches my face. She gets up and walks into the bathroom and washes her thighs with a sponge. She closes the bathroom window and walks into the kitchen.

'Three plates,' she says.

And I don't want to hear what she is going to say next.

Natural Healing
Alan Close

Down at Bronte Carl saw a guy with no leg hopping down to the water. It was midweek and the bloke stood out. He was very graceful. He sprang forward on his leg with his arms pumping at his sides like a cumbersome piece of nineteenth-century machinery run by steam. Apart from that he looked normal, except he had no leg.

Carl leant down to try to see up his Speedos but he couldn't see anything. No stump, nothing.

Halfway to the water the guy stopped for a rest. He got down on his haunches and balanced himself with both hands out on the sand beside him. In this position he looked like a big gawky bird, all limbs, not human at all, of another species.

A few moments later he was over the hump where the beach fell away to the surf and was gone.

Carl looked back to where the guy had come from. A girl was sitting on her towel watching his progress. She must be his girlfriend. She looked nice. She looked like a nurse, or maybe something natural—yoga, or herbs, or something.

As he watched she yawned and lay down on her stomach and reached behind her to undo her bikini strap. She lay her head on her towel and closed her eyes. Her breast, flattened beneath her, was secret and white. Carl wondered about the character of a girl who would be with a guy with no leg. There'd have to be some commitment there. Carl tried to imagine them having sex. He tried to picture the logistics, to work out what concessions would have to be made when you had sex with a guy with no leg. He wished for a moment that he didn't have a leg, or Janelle didn't. Then they could be sure of something. What it was about each other they liked. Why it was they were together at all.

When he closed his eyes he saw himself getting up and going over to talk to the girl.

'Hi. My name's Carl,' he'd say. 'I just wanted to tell you, I think you and your boyfriend look good together. I think you look like a nice couple and I think it's great that you love him although he's got no leg. That's all. I just wanted to tell you.'

She'd look up at him, shading her eyes from the sun.

'Thank you,' she'd say, blushing.

'Won't you sit down?' she'd say, gesturing to the sand.

He'd look around, and say, 'Yes, thanks. I will.'

They would talk, and while they were talking the guy with no leg would come back from the surf. His girlfriend would introduce Carl and they would shake hands and Carl would repeat what he'd told the girl. Then the bloke, like his girlfriend, would thank Carl and they would talk about what it was like having no leg, and Carl would ask point-blank how he had lost it and the bloke would tell him. There would be no embarrassment. In due course Carl would take his leave, and with a cheery wave come back to his towel, his heart thumping with excitement at the naked communication that can be achieved when the usual layers of small talk and social circling are dispensed with.

He opened his eyes suddenly from his imaginings and looked about him. He felt good, fulfilled and worthy. The sun sparkled off the blue sea. A plane banked in over the headland with its belly glistening and its undercarriage down for the approach to the airport. It looked so fat and slow Carl imagined it dropping right out of the sky, causing a massive disaster in the streets of Coogee. He would be first on the scene, hauling survivors out of the fiery wreckage. He would refuse to be interviewed on TV and would turn up to receive his bravery award from the Governor with his hands still bandaged. After that his life would change. Someone would see him on the news and ring up and offer him a job. He didn't know what sort of job, but it would be perfect. It would utilise all the skills he knew he had but couldn't readily identify.

He would be happy, and through the job find true love with a woman who was beautiful and interesting and with whom sex would be eternally spontaneous and varied. He pictured the house they would live in in the country, the kids they would have, the vegetables growing in neat lines in the garden. He could even see the dust motes circling in beams of sunlight in the hallway.

His mind ticked over contentedly. He could feel the trust and security in his belly.

Then he noticed the guy with no leg again. He was standing on the sand down near the water, wavering on his one leg, looking around with his eyes shaded. Water glistened on him. He was out of breath from the surf. Carl sat up and glanced over to the girlfriend. She hadn't moved. Carl looked back to the guy and whispered, 'That way, mate. Over there.'

The guy worked out where he was and started springing back up the sand.

He reached his towel and crashed down, sprinkling his girlfriend with water. She sat up laughing, remembering to hold her bikini top around her. Her teeth were white and strong. As he towelled his face and torso the guy talked, and she listened, doing up the straps of the bikini behind her. The guy made swimming movements with his arms and pointed out to the surf. He threw his hands up in the air and laughed and his girlfriend laughed back. While he was towelling his back she leant forward on his knee and kissed him. Carl lay flat on the sand watching. He could imagine their tongues moving wetly over each other's lips, exploring gums and teeth.

Carl had been with Janelle for three years. They had never really fallen in love like you're supposed to, but started off sharing their flat and after a year became lovers. They had known each other from before when they were both in the same food co-op in Glebe and used to sit on each other's loungeroom floor packing boxes of vegetables together. They had kept track of each other's lives and over the years had seen each other through several major relationships.

Janelle had even been married. She turned up at Carl's thirtieth birthday and told him she was breaking up with her husband. Carl had to move from his place and they decided to look for a flat together. They discussed the danger of getting involved and made a vow to not let it happen, Carl all the while staring at the gap between Janelle's teeth and imagining her naked. Janelle kept seeing her husband but then she found out she was pregnant and they broke up finally. During this time Carl was there for her. He drove her home from the clinic and put her to bed. He liked the role of brotherly protector. He gave her two Disprin and switched off the light and came in later to watch her sleeping. Her mouth was open and there was a dark patch on the pillow where she had dribbled.

But that was before.

They were the easy days, the delicious days of anticipation and restraint. Now they lived in the same bedroom things had changed. On paper Janelle was the perfect partner. She was pretty and supportive and enjoyed her job, teaching English to migrants. Carl worked part-time mowing lawns with his friend Barry. Barry talked about setting up a little cafe down at the beach, although so far nothing had come of it. Barry wanted Carl to come in as a partner but Janelle told Carl that Barry was a dreamer and he had as much chance of starting a cafe as he did of entering the Melbourne Cup and winning it on his own. Carl didn't know what to do so he didn't do anything, just waited to see what would happen.

No-one believed Carl and Janelle could be having troubles. But Carl knew he was quite capable of maintaining his sunny exterior while inside he had a heart of darkness. He knew something was wrong. He knew that what was happening to him came not from Janelle or anything concrete to do with their relationship. It had been in him for years and only now was bubbling to the surface, noxious and putrid, like gas escaping from an ancient animal decomposing in a bog.

When the guy with no leg and his girlfriend left the beach Carl followed. He leant against the low wall outside the change rooms while they were inside. He had his sunnies on, and although he felt inconspicuous the lifesavers and surfers hanging out in front of the kiosk kept stopping their conversation and glancing over at him.

The guy with no leg came out first. He looked around, then started swinging towards Carl on his crutches. They were the aluminium sort, with hoops for the forearms and hand supports out the front. They creaked every time he put his weight on them. Carl moved aside and the guy wheeled himself around and leant back on the wall.

'Thanks,' he said.

'No worries,' said Carl. He glanced quickly at the empty leg of the guy's shorts.

The girlfriend emerged from the change rooms and came over smiling.

'Okay?'

'Okay,' the guy said.

They headed across the grass to the bus stop. After a while Carl followed.

A bus was waiting. The guy hopped towards it, his girlfriend behind him with the bag of beach things. He transferred both crutches to one hand and heaved himself into the bus. The girl didn't move to give him any assistance. She looked away and only turned back when he was up. Carl figured it was something they had talked about and agreed that there were certain things the guy preferred to do by himself.

Carl bought a ticket to Circular Quay and made his way down the aisle to sit at the back. The bus pulled out and the engine strained for the climb up the hill. The couple were together in the middle of the bus already looking down into books.

They got off on Bondi Road. A little girl standing on her seat watched the guy hop up the aisle and said loudly, 'Look mummy, that man's carrying his legs.'

The driver looked in the side mirror and swung the big

NATURAL HEALING

steering wheel to pull out. Carl turned around. The couple were heading into a milkbar. He got off at the next stop and walked back.

As he approached the milkbar the guy crutched out of the shop straight into his path. He had a big smile on his face. The girl followed with a smile just as wide. They must have just shared a joke. Carl stopped and they stood facing each other, the guy looking Carl right in the eyes.

'Whoops,' the guy said.

'Sorry,' said Carl. He hugged his daypack to his body, his heart racing. The girl had a white milkshake container in each hand. She stared right at him.

A woman passed by pushing a stroller.

'No, Jason, you can't have any lollies until you've got all your teeth,' she said to the kid inside.

They watched her pass. The guy on crutches turned to Carl. 'Now that doesn't really seem fair, does it?' he said.

The girl smiled at Carl and laughed.

Carl went into the newsagent two doors down. He picked up a copy of a cheap tits magazine. A headline said A CHICK WITH A DICK OR A MAN WITH A CLAM? Underneath was a grainy photo of a naked girl at a beach with what looked like a penis emerging from her pubic hair.

'Bullshit!' Carl said out loud, and the newsagent looked up from behind the counter. The photo was obviously faked. He held it away from him then brought it up close. Surely no-one believed this shit? He shook his head, and turned the pages of the magazine, but couldn't stop himself coming back and examining the photo to make sure.

He could see the couple over the top of the magazine. The guy was lowering himself onto a bus seat, his crutches beside him. The girl stood over him with the milkshakes. He took the milkshakes from her and she unslung herself from the bulky beach bag and sat down beside him. He gave her her milkshake and reached his arm around her. She nestled into his shoulder. They knocked containers and sucked in silence, their heads bent together. It was so private and intimate Carl had to look away.

He replaced the magazine and browsed along the row. A few minutes later he looked up and walked quickly out of the shop. The couple were a hundred metres ahead. They turned down a side street and into another street off that and then stopped at a front gate and disappeared out of view.

Carl waited a minute and then continued down the street. The house was a single-storey semi with a plastic Santa still pinned to the door.

That morning this thing had happened. Carl and Janelle had been having sex and Carl's mind had gone off.

'What's happened?' said Janelle.

He said, 'I don't know. I started thinking of something. Sorry.'

Janelle looked him in the eyes. After a moment she said, 'It doesn't matter. Just help me then.'

Afterwards he started reading his book. Janelle lay behind him.

She moved in close and hooked an arm and a leg around him.

'Tell me you love me,' she said.

His eyes stopped moving along the lines. He looked past the book to her rack of clothes, her shoes jumbled together underneath.

'Just tell me,' she said. 'Say anything. How do you really feel about me?'

'Carl?' she said, after a minute.

'I heard you,' he said.

The rich aroma of their lovemaking wafted from the bed.

Usually he couldn't get enough of this smell. This morning it nauseated him.

She said, 'Is it that hard to answer? All I need is some reassurance.'

He said, 'I'm thinking about it.'

She said, 'Well, Jesus, if you've got to think about it ...'

He said, 'I think you're a much better person than me. Definitely a better person than me.'

She said, 'Is that all?'

He rolled over to look her in the face.

'He said, 'Jen ...' and then stopped as she grabbed at the opportunity for contact and searched desperately from eye to eye. Then suddenly she threw back the bedclothes, jumped from the bed and stormed from the room.

'Why do I bother? Why do I even fucking bother?'

Carl didn't move. He lay staring at the blue sky framed in the window. He listened to the shower running, then heard it being turned off, and then the rasp of the towel rack as a towel was dragged off it.

Janelle came back in. She hadn't dried properly. Her back was still wet. She stepped into a pair of underpants then pulled clothes from coathangers. She dug her arms through their sleeves, turned to examine them in the mirror, and unbuttoned them impatiently, wrestling them off into a pile on the windowbox. Carl watched her, the bedclothes pulled up under his chin. After she left he stayed there staring out the window.

When he went into the kitchen she was sitting at the table with her muesli. She looked smart, like a young thing in the ads having an on-the-run breakfast. Except she was crying. Big tears rolled down her cheeks and dropped onto the varnished surface of the table and stayed there. Her hair was still wet. She looked sexy.

He leant in the doorway naked.

'I'm sorry,' he said.

She looked at him as she chewed, her spoon hand resting on the table, shaking. The other hand was around her glass of water. She even ate her muesli soaked in water. It was a hard, spartan little meal.

'What I can't get over,' she said, 'is your coldness. The whole thing is so cold and loveless and empty. Why am I kidding myself with you?'

She shovelled another spoonful of muesli into her mouth, watching him as she chewed. She clutched the spoon in her hand like a weapon.

'I don't need this, you know. I can live without this. I don't need your suffering. There's a whole world out there waiting to be lived and even if you don't want it, I do. I think what I've been through with you. All your shit. And I give you so much. I'm always there when you need me. But when I need some support? Where is it? All I get is a kick in the face. A cold shoulder. Worse than that. A cold nothing.'

She pushed her chair back noisily and went to the sink and ran water in the bowl.

She said, 'I mean it this time. This time you're not going to slime your way back in.'

Her eyes were hard. He looked into them. He could feel the fear on his face.

He said, 'Jen, I'm sorry. I really am. I don't know what it is. If I knew I'd tell you. Maybe everyone goes through this. Maybe it's like this for all couples. Maybe it's something we all have to go through. I don't know. If I knew any one thing I'd tell you. I don't know which way to go. I don't know what to do. I feel as if I'm nailed to the ground flailing and struggling but I can't escape. As if I've been cut off at the knees and I can't move. But the one thing I know, the one thing I'm not doing is deceiving you. I don't know what's going on but whatever it is I'm not telling you any lies.'

He stood in front of her naked. Her hand rested on the tap. She held her glass up to her lips. She turned and threw the water down the sink and walked out of the room.

It was Janelle's yoga night. Carl left her a note. DARLING, OUT WITH BARRY. WON'T BE LATE. He clicked the door closed behind him and padded down the stairs. His gymboots felt light and springy.

When he got there the house was in darkness except for a light at the back. Carl glanced up and down the street and stepped over the low gate. A passageway with a paling fence down the middle separated the house from the one next door. He edged down the fence in the dark, almost slipping in an outside drain. He could hear the traffic on Bondi Road. When he reached the lighted window he found the bottom of it was head high. Very slowly he raised his eyes above the windowsill. Across the room the couple were in bed.

They were reading. They had a lamp each, on tables beside the bed. This was the only lighting. The rest of the room fell away into darkness and looked empty. The floor was bare boards, with a rug at the end of the bed. Piano music came from somewhere out of sight. It was a Beethoven piano sonata. Carl felt ice in his stomach. He and Janelle had a tape of this very music. How many times had they laid like this couple with this exact sonata tinkling them to sleep?

He felt light-headed. Woozy. He leant his head against the warm bricks and pressed his hand against his chest. His heart was pumping like an express train in the night.

The couple had a sheet over them. The girl was turned

away from the guy, the sheet pulled up under her armpit. The guy was sitting up. He held his book in his lap and with the other hand stroked the girl's arm. She had a hand under the sheet behind her. The guy looked down and said something and moved some hair away from her ear.

The girl turned and leant up to kiss him. She pressed herself against him. Her muscles strained to hold her and the length of her backbone stood out in the hollow of her back. The sheet lifted and her book slid off the bed and hit the bare boards with a clunk. Carl strained to read the title. He'd been right! The book was called NATURAL HEALING FOR YOUNG LOVERS.

The guy edged his book out from under her and let it slide off the bed and slap to the floor as well.

'Hang on,' the girl said.

She twisted around, the sheet around her lap, and pulled open the drawer in the bedside table. Her breasts shuddered. The guy reached over and started playing with one nipple until it was erect. Carl watched the girl's eyes. She smiled and kept scrabbling in the drawer. She didn't have young girl's breasts. Her breasts had started to get heavy and soft and her nipples were large, ready for a child or a craving lover.

The girl brought out a diaphragm box and a tube of spermicide. She took the lid from the box and blew powder from the diaphragm. She closed the box and put it on the bedside table and held the diaphragm up to the light.

The guy's hand kept moving under the sheet.

The girl rolled back towards him and covered his body with hers.

'Hang on,' she said, more insistently this time.

She sat up and leant forward, and found the tube of spermicide in the folds of the sheet. She undid the cap and ran the tube around the rim of the diaphragm and put a dab in the middle. She screwed the cap on and holding the prepared diaphragm carefully with the tips of her fingers put the tube back on the table.

The music on the tape had ended. Silence crackled in the room.

'Whose turn?' the girl said.

The guy smiled. 'My turn.'

Outside Carl moved his feet and swallowed. His mouth was dry.

The guy took the diaphragm carefully and his girlfriend threw back the sheet. For the first time Carl saw where the guy's leg had been. There was nothing. No stump, anything. Just a big scar. His cock stood to attention beside it. He was like a model in a museum, cut away to reveal the workings inside.

The girl lay with her legs apart. Carl felt his eyes flitter.

The guy eased himself down and squeezed the diaphragm together and Carl watched it disappear. The guy had his tongue out between his lips in concentration making sure the diaphragm was in the right position. His girlfriend had her hand on his shoulder. She giggled.

'Quite sure now?'

'Just about,' the guy said.

Carl had never seen another couple do this. They did nothing different from the way he and Janelle used her diaphragm. Everything was so similar between them! A massive reassurance spread into Carl's stomach. He wanted to call out, to stand up and say, 'Hey! Hey, you guys, guess what ...!'

And suddenly then he imagined Janelle at home, sitting at the table with a bowl of miso soup and the morning paper. He saw her taking sips from the Chinese spoon and imagined her leaning forward to read an item at the top of the page. His heart flooded with remorse for the way he'd treated her that morning. He almost laughed. What was his fuss about? Suddenly it all seemed nothing.

He wanted to run home and apologise and take her in his arms and make it up to her.

'I do love you,' he would say, covering her with kisses. 'I do love you.'

'Is that right?' the guy with no leg said.

'Feels right,' the girl said.

At that moment there were scratchings from the front of the house next door, and voices, and floorboards creaking. Carl glanced around. His bladder wanted to open. He clamped it closed.

The guy swung himself off the bed and started hopping towards the window, his dick wobbling about like a blind animal sniffing the air in front of him.

'No need to give the pervs a free floorshow,' he said over his shoulder.

He was only a few feet away. Carl stared into his eyes. The guy still hadn't seen him but when he reached up for the cord to the blind his face changed totally. In the house behind the lights came on, bathing Carl in brightness. A picture entered his mind, of Janelle turning up at the police station to bail him out. She'd be worried and exasperated and angry, grasping in her mind for explanations of how things had come to this. He saw himself standing with his hands on the bars of his cell and the look on her face as she walked towards him, his eyes burning, his heart full.

Matchbooks
Matthew Condon

1

The Bowl

I didn't think anything of the matchbook bowl at first. What is there to say about a matchbook bowl? It just sat there on the sideboard, a big, round, crystal bowl that had come with Jordan when she moved into Parthenon Place.

'What's this?' I had asked her.

'My matchbook bowl,' she said. 'A little hobby of mine.'

I would have preferred to put my hand-carved Indian salt and pepper horse on wheels in the middle of the sideboard. I loved that little horse, the way its torso was cut in half, and slid out sideways revealing its hidden intestines of salt and pepper. But when Jordan moved in she really moved in, matchbook bowl and all.

I had never lived with a woman before. It wasn't an easy transition for me. I enjoyed my own space, my litany of rituals and habits and idiosyncrasies. I think everyone should be able to hold onto their rituals, no matter what. It is the rituals that define you, that furnish your character. In that respect I was well furnished.

Jordan, too, had her own way of doing things. The difficulty was her rituals totally absorbed mine. They crashed over every one of them, diluted them, and washed them away. Fine, I said. This is what it's about. Compromise. You have to have a bit of compromise about you. So I compromised.

I, in fact, compromised myself into non-existence. Within days of Jordan arriving there was virtually not a sign of my own life, the trinkets that adorned it, the mess that followed in its wake. ('You're like Pig Pen,' Jordan often said early on. 'You know, in the cartoon. There's a big trail of dust and dirt that follows you. You know?') I thought this unfair. I flossed. I used moisturiser on my skin. I had a wide range of aftershaves, soaps, nail clippers, brushes, lufers and foot odour pads. As far as guys went, I was pretty meticulous about my hygiene.

Jordan, though, set new standards in cleanliness. She was obsessed by it. Not only that. Everything had to be in its place. The tea towels, the crockery, the paintings on the wall, the dish rack, the little wooden chicken on top of the stove, the iron, the ceramic seahorses on the bathroom wall, the wine glasses in order of size, the saucepans, the magazine rack, the number of magazines on the coffee table, the coffee pots, the bread basket, the sideboard decorations.

'Nice bowl,' I had said to her.

'It's from Sweden,' she said.

'You could put a fish in it.'

'No, Ick,' she said, looking pitifully at me. 'Have you never seen a matchbook bowl?'

'I don't believe I have.'

MATCHBOOKS

She laughed lightly here. 'It's something I picked up from the American magazines. It's the in thing.'

'Oh,' I said. 'The in thing.'

'Yes, silly,' she said.

I felt very unsophisticated, having never heard of a matchbook bowl. But there you have it. I doubt she had ever heard of an Indian salt and pepper horse on wheels.

I cradled it in my hands as she replaced it with the bowl. I loved that horse. Jordan just looked at it with sympathy, as if it were the ratty toy of a child. She shook her head at it. I grabbed it even tighter. I went and put it on my bedside table to let her know how much it meant to me. The next day I found it on the window shelf in the lavatory. This was where Jordan had designated it to be. Next to the plastic mushroom smelling of pine needles, and her floral tissue box.

It might seem trite, but it took me a long time to come to terms with my salt and pepper horse with its garland of gold nails and squeaky wheels parked beside the air freshener, stuck forever in the water closet with its murky variety of smells and noises. Things have their place, as if they are naturally drawn into a particular space. Over time objects then claim that space and when they are removed from it, the space is no longer whole, but empty, almost sad, without them. That's how I felt about the horse. Cut off from the space it rightfully owned. The horse lost its special lustre in the lavatory. The glow had gone from it, or so I thought, its unique spirit still there on the sideboard, underneath Jordan's massive Swedish matchbook bowl.

It was half-full, the bowl, with matchbooks from all over the world. Jordan had not been to all the places on the little cardboard flip-tops. There were places there that a beautician at the Salon De Beauty could not have possibly afforded to go—The Ritz in London, the New York Oyster

Bar and Grill, a cocktail lounge in the Caribbean, a paella house in Malaga, Spain. The life tentacles of a beautician at the Salon De Beauty on the Gold Coast only extended so far. She had let it be known in her circle that she was a matchbook collector, and so these tiny souvenirs found their way across the world and into Jordan's glass bowl.

It was when she started collecting her own local ones that I began to get suspicious. It changed everything, that bowl with hundreds of small coloured sulphur heads. It blew everything up, and ultimately led the wooden horse back to its proper place.

2

The Bar Venus

Jordan and I spent a lot of time together. I liked it that way. I liked to know where she was, what she was up to, how her day was going at work, what she thought of an idea that had only just, seconds before, come into my mind. It was what had driven some women away from me in my past. It was not out of jealousy. I didn't develop that strong contact in order to keep tabs on her. It was something within me, a need inside me, that I had never been able to shake.

I bought her a mobile phone so we could always keep in touch. Her girlfriends thought it quaint, that little yellow phone she kept in her handbag. She did too. For a while. Then she started turning the phone off. I didn't mind that either. She was a busy woman. She had priorities, obligations, business. When I couldn't get through sometimes I had to laugh at myself. Why are you ringing? Why do you have to tell her what you had for lunch, whom you saw in the street, how you were going to make a small fortune renting out unsold penthouses to Japanese honeymooners on the side, or how you had this brilliant idea, see, this masterstroke, selling cassettes of bird noises and pub sounds and the creaking of the Australian bush at airports as a novelty for potentially homesick overseas travellers? It can wait. I'll tell her later, at home.

But it didn't work like that. If I got the message that her phone was switched off I'd try the number over and over, ten, twenty, thirty times before I got through. I became obsessed with it. I'll just call ten more times and then I'll give it a rest. I'd mark the calls off on my blotter, like a prisoner scratching the days on the wall of his cell. That was me. Hopeless. It's a miracle she didn't leave me for that alone. Others had departed for less. I didn't mean any harm, though. That's the point to remember. I was in love. I did it out of love. It was love that was the basis of all my actions.

One Friday I got home early and decided to cook the dinner. I'd have it nice and ready for Jordan when she got home. I went further. I set the dining room table. I brought out Jordan's precious damask tablecloth. I took her best cutlery from its box, slid the appropriate knives and forks and spoons from their individual plastic wrappers and arranged them with the aplomb of a waiter. I chilled the champagne, let the red breathe, prepared my ingredients in neat piles in order of cooking. While the pots simmered on the stove I went and changed into my old tuxedo. I went over the top, even for me. I didn't understand, then, why I had gone to such elaborate lengths to make this dinner special. Why something told me, on that Friday evening, to go all the way. It is impossible to see the pattern of things when you're in them. It is impossible to discover the reasoning, because you're not looking for a reason. You're not trying to work out a pattern. You only see it later. Only then do you learn that things happen for a reason.

Jordan was usually a little late at the end of the week.

She had all those ladies wanting to be beautiful for their Friday nights, or a Saturday wedding, or whatever. That's the way it happened in the Salon De Beauty.

I put on my Beethoven piano concertos. I was no classical buff but I knew Beethoven's piano concertos went down well with fine wine and candlelight and a meal. I knew it would soothe Jordan. 'It's so soothing, that stuff,' she often said, before the soothing wore off, and it became repetitive to her.

Still, everything went to plan. Perfectly. The entrée was ready the minute she walked in the door. The sonatas were warming up. And picture me. In my tux. The hair oiled down, like in the 1920s. I stood by the dining room table, as suave as I could stand. Then I remembered the candles. I fumbled in my pants pockets. No lighter. In my jacket. Nothing. Jordan was fiddling around in the foyer. I ran to the matchbook bowl. I dipped my hand in it and pulled out one of the matchbooks. I ran back to the table, lit the two candles, and shoved the matchbook in my pocket. Phew. I'd made it.

Finally she walked into the dining room.

'Sweetheart,' she said, looking all loving and motherly.

'Madame,' I said. 'Your table is ready.'

'Ohhhh,' said Jordan softly. 'It's so sweet.'

'Would madame care for an aperitif?' I flicked a serviette over my right wrist.

It was a triumph. For once everything combined—the meal came out like a dream, the wine was superb, the piano notes weaved their way around our goblets and our candles and our intimate chatter. Jordan was suitably soothed.

We had a bath together (though I'm not entirely fond of baths) and went to bed and made love and everything was fine.

I found, then, I could not sleep. I was still excited by the evening, how well I had pulled it off, how happy Jordan seemed, and the residue of all that stayed with me.

I slipped on my tux trousers and tiptoed out to the lounge. It was milky with the lights from the adjacent apartment block. It was, I discovered, still only about nine o'clock. I found my cigarettes on the coffee table and went out onto the balcony. Life, I sighed to myself. How fulfilling the small moments can be. Between two people. It was love that had always amazed me. How love can exist in a look, in a hand, in the curve of an eyebrow, the curl of a lash, the dip of a hip beside you. How I loved love.

I took out a cigarette and wondered what I had done to my lighter. I never usually mislaid my lighters. Only around my friend Wilson, who, for some odd reason, collected them like a bower bird. He could go out with his journalist buddies of an evening and come home with a dozen lighters in his pocket. He just picked them up and pocketed them. He didn't do it deliberately, I don't think. I had never gotten to the bottom of Wilson's lighter fixation. But I hadn't seen him in weeks.

I felt my pockets and there was the matchbook I had taken from the bowl earlier in the evening. I had already used one match lighting the candles and worried about using a second for my cigarette. Jordan liked her matchbooks pristine. It was, she said, an intrinsic part of their value in the collection. It would not be a true collection if matches had been used from them willy-nilly, scorching the back of the flip-top, creasing the pretty pictures and words on their covers.

But what the hell, I thought. I had already used one. And I could hide it deep down into the bowl later. She'd never know, I thought.

I lit the cigarette and closed the matchbook. I took a long draw, turning the matchbook over and over in my hand. Love, I sighed.

There was a party going on across the way. I could see women in evening dresses milling around on the balcony, sipping cocktails, moving their hips to the music that I could only hear snatches of. I was glad to be out of that scene. I was, in that sense, grateful to Jordan. Chumps, I said to them quietly. Chumps.

I looked down at the matchbook and in the glowing light could make out a heart on its little cover. A sign, I thought. There is no coincidence.

I brought it up to my face to read the lettering. Bar Venus, Gold Coast Hwy, Surfers Paradise. Ah, the new bar everyone was talking about, I thought. Any new bar, I found, was something of serious discussion amongst my colleagues in the real estate trade.

I looked at the heart for a long time. It had only been open a week, the Bar Venus, from what I was told.

And I knew I had never been there.

3

The Velvet Booth

I sat in the velvet booth in the corner of the Bar Venus for three hours and fifteen minutes. I had, as company, my new pack of Wee Willem cigars and a succession of bourbon and drys. It was a nice booth as far as booths go. Comfortable, dimly lit, with a good view of the rest of the bar. I must admit I'm not big on bars. Only when I travel on my own do I seek the warmth of bars. There is something about foreign travel, about being completely alone, that unlocks in me the capacity to sit in a bar on my own. It is feeling a part of something, of the life of a strange place, through proxy. I have never gone for a drink on my own on the Gold Coast. Never. When you see people drinking on their own in your home town you see them as lonely. That's the way it is. There are two ways of looking at it. Always. There are two ways of looking at everything.

I asked the waiter for a book of matches, which he promptly supplied on a white saucer, and I sat in that corner of the booth and tried to absorb the vibes, tried to pick up any trace of Jordan's movements in the Bar Venus.

I studied the matchbook with the red heart on the cover. Had she been here with her girlfriends and forgotten to tell me? Had she come at the invitation of a man? She could have. Then I began to see it in another way. Maybe she had dropped in merely to souvenir one of their matchbooks. It was, after all, a new one to add to her extensive collection. Or perhaps a friend had been to the bar and pocketed one especially for her. Collectors often had a wide network of spotters on the ground, did they not? I remember my great aunt who had the largest collection of spoons in Brisbane, possibly the world. Everybody knew of her collection. Friends of friends of friends brought them back for her from all corners of the globe. Even I had picked up a couple for her on my travels. So why shouldn't Jordan have a wide-ranging, all-encompassing team of matchbook suppliers?

'Another drink, sir?'

'Sure,' I said.

What did it matter anyway? What if she had had a drink with a colleague? So what? It was how I had scored some of my biggest deals. Chilled sake had led to my greatest triumph to date. They still talk about it in my circles. How those little ceramic thimbles carried Icarus into the big league. So why not Jordan?

I began to feel comfortable in my velvet booth in the Bar Venus. I started smiling at everyone who passed, nodding, lifting a finger of welcome from my bourbon tumbler.

'Hey,' I said, quietly. 'How you doin'?'

I noticed a woman who looked a lot like Jordan. I smiled.

'Another drink, sir?'

'Abbbbbbsolutely,' I told the waiter.

I began to feel all warm and cosy in the booth. I couldn't get that stupid grin off my face. I waved to the Jordan lookalike.

She whispered to the man sitting on the bar stool next to her, and he came over to the velvet booth.

'You got a problem, buddy?'

I didn't understand the question. My grin widened.

'What's so funny? You find me funny?'

That's when I started laughing. It started as a giggle, then it just picked up its own momentum. I couldn't stop it. A tank barrier couldn't stop it. I worked my way steadily towards a howl. The darker his face became, the more I laughed.

He didn't ask me any more questions. And he did find something to stop my laughter with. His fist.

I became the first patron to be thrown out of the Bar Venus.

4

On Hobbies

Jordan didn't seem too enthusiastic about the 1,000-piece jigsaw I bought her. She had dropped to her knees in the lounge room when I presented her with the gift-wrapped jigsaw, delicately slid off the green ribbon and carefully removed the green silver paper. She loved gifts, did Jordan. And I loved giving them to her. She went back in an instant to being the child at the base of the Christmas tree. Her face lost all its adult experience and problems and accumulated wisdom. Her eyes widened. Her mouth opened just a little. A little tear came to my eye whenever Jordan opened a present.

But when the paper gave way to a picture of Buckingham Palace in a thousand pieces the child in the face seemed to flee. It did more than flee. It sprinted off. Whatever it was she had been expecting, a 1,000-piece jigsaw puzzle of Buckingham Palace was not it. She pulled away from it, as if it was hot to touch.

'Oh,' she said flatly. 'How lovely.'

'It is, isn't it?' I said, crouching down beside her. 'Look. Here are the guards with their busbies. And here. See that window there? That's the Queen's bedroom. That's what the lady in the shop told me anyway. It'll be fun, won't it?'

She folded the wrapping paper. She was always one to keep wrapping paper and use it again. Then she stood up, and looked down at the box wrapped in cellophane.

'Yes,' was all she said.

'I'll help you with it,' I said after her. 'We'll do it together. We'll have a special jigsaw night, and do a bit here and there. Then we'll get it framed.'

But she had disappeared into the bedroom, and I was left alone with the palace.

I blamed Wilson. He was the one who told me to get the jigsaw. I had phoned to ask his advice. I wanted Jordan to get a new hobby, I said. This matchbook thing was a silly hobby for a grown woman, I said. She doesn't even smoke.

'Well, let me see,' said Wilson. He was probably stroking his chin at the other end of the line. He always stroked his chin during heavy thought. 'There's always those needlepoint things. You know them? You make a picture out of them. Landscapes. Little girls milking cows. That sort of thing.'

'I don't know about that,' I said. I just couldn't imagine Jordan sitting still in a chair for hours, creating a tin bucket out of thread.

'How about spoons?'

'She's too young for spoons,' I said quickly.

'Too young for spoons. Okkaaaay. Let's see. Does she like the horses?'

'Get serious, Wilson.'

'Right, sorry,' he said. 'Not antiques. Too expensive. Mmmmm. The kids love jigsaws. My kids sit for hours with them. Drives me nuts, but there you go.'

'Jigsaws ...'

'Yeah. They're quite addictive from what I hear.'

'That's not bad,' I said.

'Can't go wrong with a jigsaw,' said Wilson, suddenly the world's authority on jigsaws. 'Hey, let's get together soon for a drink.'

'Sure.'

'Let's check out that new Bar Venus,' he said. 'Heard some dork got thrown out of there last week. Sounds like our sort of place.'

'Dork?'

'Foreigner, apparently. Give me a call.'

'Sure,' I said.

I loved the coast, but God it was a small town.

Jordan didn't take to the jigsaw. We hadn't even finished the patch of blue sky over the palace's east wing on our first official Jigsaw Night, and she was back in the bathroom filing her nails. When Jordan files her nails you know she's bored.

'Come on, Jord,' I pleaded. 'We'll start at the bottom then. Let's do the busbies.'

'No thank you,' she said, filing.

'Okay, okay, the Queen's bedroom then. The Queen's bedroom.'

She raised her eyes. 'Ick. I don't mean to hurt your feelings, but I've never liked jigsaws.'

'Never?'

She shook her head.

'Not even when you were a kid?'

Her head didn't stop shaking from side to side. I knew what she meant. I hated them too. I knelt at her feet.

'Then what would you like? You tell me?'

'What's wrong with you? Why are you doing this?'

'I thought, you know, you'd like something to do, a new hobby, something ... '

'I don't need a hobby.'

'An interest, you know.'

'I have interests,' she said.

'Rather than just those silly matchbooks.'

She stopped filing. 'What?'

'You can't just have matchbooks in your life,' I said. I must have looked pathetic, my hands on her knees.

She put the nail file down on the bathroom cabinet. 'Is that what this is all about? The matchbooks? They're not my hobby, Ick. Matchbooks aren't a hobby. I like the way they look, that's all. What are you talking about?'

'I don't know,' I said. 'I don't know.'

She gave me a strange look and left the bathroom. What was I talking about? What the hell was going on here? I stayed on the shaggy rug of the bathroom for a long time, and picked up some of Jordan's nail dust on the tip of my index finger.

5

The Grand Hotel

Wilson and I sat in the bar of the Grand Hotel and winced at our whisky sours.

'You're paranoid,' he said, his eyes closed with bitterness. 'You've got to learn to loosen up a bit.'

'I know, I know,' I said.

'Be cool,' he said.

'Cool.'

We had decided against the Bar Venus. Or, rather, I had. I told Wilson I didn't want to go to any cheap bar frequented by drunken foreigners.

'She's a good girl,' Wilson said. 'How long you been together?'

'Eighteen months.'

'There you go,' he said, wincing again. 'Bound to happen sometime. These things happen. They keep happening, too, let me tell you.'

'I know,' I said.

'You don't know much for someone who knows so much.'

'I know,' I said. We ordered a couple more sours.

'You've got to learn to trust people,' said Wilson.

'I do trust her,' I replied. 'It's everyone else I don't trust.'

'Got a point,' said Wilson. I didn't remind him that he was the least trustful journalist in a hundred miles. But that was professional distrust, he often told me. That's what gave him the edge.

We sat and talked for another hour. I smoked a couple of cigars and relished the thick smoke, and how it curled into weird shapes in the fading sunlight that came through the window. I went for another one and found my lighter missing. If I'd thought about it I would have known where it was—firmly lodged in Wilson's trouser pocket, along with God knows how many others. But I didn't. I went to the cigarette machine and took a matchbook out of the tray.

'Love a good sour,' said Wilson, looking fondly into his empty glass. 'There's something of the masochist in people like us. People who take to a good sour.'

'True,' I said.

I struck the yellow sulphur-headed match and lit my cigar.

'The mother-in-law must be on them constantly,' he said, scrunching his face. 'If you know what I mean.'

I laughed.

'That's not a bad one is it? The mother-in-law must be on them. You can have that one if you want,' said Wilson.

'Thank you.'

'Consider it yours.'

I looked at the picture on the cover of the matchbook. It was a detailed pen sketch of the very bar in which we sat. I could see our stools in the picture. It was strange, to be sitting in the Grand Hotel's bar on two stools, and seeing the empty stools in miniature in your hands. I couldn't stop looking at it. Wilson went on and on in his usual fashion. He was fond of the monologue, was Wilson. But I just kept staring at the little black ink bar. There was something familiar about it.

'... so I said to him, look, mate, you either answer the questions or I run with what I've got in tomorrow's paper. Suit yourself, I said ...'

I had been to the Grand Hotel bar once or twice. That was true. There was the time when Tommy the Spoon Player gave his legendary rendition of Flight of the Bumble Bee. It's still talked about. And there was a brief visit on Wilson's bucks night, before we chained him naked to the fence of the Bavarian Steakhouse. But it was the view on the matchbook, that precise angle, that I had seen before. Before living it, sitting in it, with Wilson on this afternoon of whisky sours.

'Sure enough he crumbled,' said Wilson. 'Just like that. Another for the road?'

I got a cab back to the Parthenon later that night. I could have stayed out later. Jordan was in Brisbane at a French polish course. She wouldn't be back for hours. But I had to get home.

I went straight to the crystal Swedish bowl of matchbooks, picked it up, took it to the centre of the lounge room, and emptied its contents onto the carpet.

It took me a while, I can say that. Whisky sours always had that effect on me. In the end, though, I found it. I held it up in the air and shook it, as if in triumph. Not a joyous triumph, but one underpinned with sadness, with confusion, with hollow confirmation. I had it. A pristine matchbook from the Grand Hotel Bar.

I looked at the tiny picture again and half-expected myself to walk into the sketch, a tiny black and white Icarus, and take my seat at the stool. Of course nothing like that happened. That was silly.

It was there, on the carpet surrounded by Jordan's paper and sulphur treasures, that I knew something was definitely going on.

6

The Flamingo Lounge, and other Historical Landmarks

Every Saturday morning, at exactly 6.30, with Jordan still asleep in our king-size bed, I sat on the balcony in my boxer shorts and studied the new matchbooks that had arrived in her growing collection.

The Flamingo Lounge, to date, was my favourite. It showed a pink flamingo, drunk and stretched out on a leopard-skin lounge. Its eyes had that cartoon-like, twirly-wirly effect. A few bubbles rose out of its beak. It was shickered, that flamingo, its reedy legs crossed and relaxed. Under better circumstances, I would have laughed at the funny picture. Now it was just funny in a tragic sort of way.

There were others, too. I didn't mind the Steamboat Willie one. I'd been on the Steamboat Willie myself, the time the Texan billionaires and I got stranded on the sand bank in the middle of the Broadwater. I don't remember much of that night now, but it's supposed to be good, the Steamboat Willie, under normal circumstances. Very romantic, they say. Out on the deck when the moon is up, they say. They had a moon on the matchbook, up in the right-hand corner. A silver moon. Steamboat Willie, too, was done out in a lovely embossed silver on a ming-blue background. Very swish. The sulphur heads of the matches were the same blue.

I held the matchbook in my palm and closed my eyes and tried to imagine Jordan with the same matchbook on the table in front of her. I tried to see the meal on her plate, the placement of her hands, the little flickering candle on the table, and the man she was dining with. I squeezed the matchbook and tried to see all that. But it was a foggy recollection. It could have been any table, anywhere. Any candle. Any plate and knife and fork and bread roll. And I couldn't see the man, only his suit coat and tie. I couldn't get above his collar. It was just dark there. Nothing else. No matter how hard I tried to get into the picture on the matchbook, to board Steamboat Willie and catch her there, I couldn't.

Within a month I had dozens of new matchbooks to admire. They came from everywhere. The Apollo Ballroom, the Midnight Beat, the Golden Chopsticks Restaurant, the Regency on the Canal, the El Toreador Mexicana, the Grape and Vine, the Sportsman's Bar, the Huntingdale Club, the Royal Mangrove International Golf Course Resort. I couldn't believe she'd been to the Royal Mangrove. I'd been trying to wangle my way onto that course for months, and here was one of the exclusive matchbooks with its sweet green mangrove buds on its cover.

When I knew Jordan wouldn't be home for hours, if at all on some nights, I took out all the new matchbooks and laid them on the carpet. I sat there like a kid with my legs outstretched. I randomly placed all the pieces of the puzzle before me. Then I began to place the matchbooks in lines, in the loose chronology of what I supposed were Jordan's secret evenings. I could mix and match and change the combinations around, depending how I felt on the night. For example, in the first position I would place the Grape and Vine—a good little place to start a romantic interlude with a glass of wine. Then I would place under it the Bowler Hat Restaurant—very intimate, very expensive. That would be followed by either Le Dome Cafe, if it was to be a quiet get-together, or the Black Garter Nite

Club and then Jupiter's Casino for a more lengthy, full-on excursion.

These rows of matchbooks fanned out from me on the carpet. I invented all sorts of variations. I had Jordan in black evening dresses all over the coast. I calculated the cost of cabs between the matchbooks. The amount of alcohol consumed. The moments where intimacy may have occurred. I marked these points of intimacy with dried apricots from the pantry. It was a fairly elaborate jigsaw. It was a jigsaw of the high-life. Of fine food and wine, of snatched kisses and held hands. Sometimes I just sat there crying with my head in my hands, my chronologies stretching out like the spokes of a broken wheel.

I couldn't believe it was happening to me. My mind didn't seem to be able to catch up with the reality of it all. Naturally I began blaming myself. I analysed myself. Asked myself difficult questions. I sat across the couch from myself and pointed with an accusing finger. You're too selfish. You're not affectionate enough. You act, at times, like a child. You take people for granted. You think the world revolves around you. You don't listen to people. On and on it went. I gave myself a pretty good going over. There wasn't a lot left standing in the end.

Then I swung away from that, and began to get angry. How could she do this to me? Didn't I give her everything she wanted? And more? Didn't I love her and cherish her and take care of her and buy her tropical fish and stroke her face as she slept and honour her? Didn't I do that? Sure I did that. There are plenty of women who'd die for a guy like me. Sure there are. I'm one of the most eligible goddam catches on the Gold Coast. (I always used goddam, for some reason, when I was angry.) I was a giant goddam marlin in the goddam sea of goddam men. That's what I was. I pumped myself up with these thoughts. I huffed and puffed and rehearsed my lines of accusation. I practised pointing my finger. I prepared myself.

She would come home, though, and all my bravado fell away. I looked at her as if she had already gone from me. I looked at her beautiful eyes, her slender neck and wispy blonde hair, her fine hands, all of that, and I would cry without warning. She would ask me why I was crying and I couldn't tell her. I was living my future without her, while she was still in Penthouse One at Parthenon Place, in our bed, in our bath, in our kitchen, in our lounge, on our balcony.

I picked up my act. I put on more romantic candlelit dinners. I left little gifts all over the apartment. I dropped in to see her at the Salon De Beauty. I tried to secure, through my international contacts, some of the most exotic matchbooks on the planet. It was beginning to work, I thought. I was starting to claim her back.

Then I found the Shelley Bay Motor Inn matchbook. It had nothing much on it. It had the symbol of a knife and fork, a bed, and a man and woman side by side. It was dull. In the matchbook hierarchy of beauty, it was down the bottom end of the scale. Just the symbols—man and woman, eating, sleeping. But it was the simplicity that struck me. Food, shelter and togetherness. It was the one matchbook that brought it all home to me. Jordan was the woman on the matchbook, but I wasn't the man.

That's when I knew we were finished.

7

The Shooting Stars

It was late in August. I remember it, because that morning I'd had my first swim of the season. It was always special, that first swim. Down there in the glassy water with all the old men and women in their bathing caps and old-fashioned trunks. Early morning swimmers and beach walkers were always the friendliest people. They always nodded or stopped for a quick word about the weather or whatever. They chirped like birds. They smiled and revelled in the first light. I've never known why early morning people are always like that, but they are.

It was a Friday. No ordinary Friday, either. By 10.30 a.m. I had closed one of the biggest deals of the month. I was on top of it. I credited the swim and all those smiling faces. I found a grain of sand under one of my fingernails and I studied it in the centre of my blotter. I smiled at the grain of sand. If anyone else had seen me and not known the story of luck I had built around that tiny grain, they would have thought I'd lost it. Gone crackers. How can you explain these peculiar thoughts you sometimes get? These little superstitions you build up in an effort to explain things, to sort out the complexities that evolve around you at any time, on any given day? You can't. You don't try. You just move on.

So I took half the day off. I deserved it. There were raised eyebrows in the office. Icarus, taking half the day off? They couldn't believe it. It just wasn't me. Or how they saw me. Icarus didn't do things like that. It wasn't my 'way'.

'See you,' I said, slipping my coat over my shoulder. 'Have a good one.'

Then I did something equally as radical. For me. I had lunch on my own. This, if anyone had known, was even more shocking than the story of the grain of sand, even more out of character than the half-day off. I never, ever, had lunch on my own. Ever. I had looked at other people eating on their own in restaurants and felt an enormous pity for them. I had, on two occasions, even invited lonely diners to my table. I looked upon eating as some sort of holy ritual between human beings. It was the old breaking of the bread thing. The sharing of the wine. There was nothing sadder than a solo bread breaker and wine drinker. So I thought.

And what made me go to Grumpy's? It was, after all, my favourite restaurant on the coast. But it had also become Jordan's and my restaurant. It was our special place. The scene of our first meal together. Our inaugural bread-breaking and taking of wine. I sat at 'our' table, led by the arm by my friend Mario. I didn't need to order. Mario knew what to bring. The entrée, the mains, the dessert, the wine. That's what I liked about a restaurant. It gave you the opportunity to concentrate on other things. This time, however, I had no-one to concentrate on. Just myself. If I had seen myself across the tables of Grumpy's I would have felt some empathy. I would have wondered what brought this man to table on his own? What circumstances had delivered him to the stiff white tablecloth, the clean wine glasses, the sprig of leaves in the centre of the square table? I both knew and didn't know as I sat there looking over the Broadwater. I didn't even feel lonely, wrapped as I was in the conversation of other diners, the clatter of cutlery and the busyness of the kitchen.

I began to smile. I ordered a whisky sour (which I rarely drank before at least six p.m.) and a cigar for after the meal.

They brought the cigar, compliments of the house, with a Grumpy's matchbook. I didn't even touch the matchbook. I couldn't remember even having seen one before, although I had been to the restaurant hundreds of times. How could I have missed it? How could I have failed to notice its delicious lavender hue with a pale lemon-coloured lobster on the cover?

I sipped my drink and felt happier than I'd been in months. The food was superb. The wine impeccable. I put the cigar to my mouth, some two hours later, and reached for the matchbook, but before I could touch it, Mario had arrived with a silver lighter already aflame.

He looked at me and smiled over the flame, then through the dense cigar smoke. It wasn't his usual smile, but one much richer, much warmer, and I nodded my thanks. He just touched me lightly on the shoulder, then. The most fleeting of touches. It made me feel good, that brief touch. It made me feel secure. That everything was going to be all right. That my life would go on and that I could be happy.

I stretched back and drew on the big cigar. I had just completed the first meal I'd ever eaten on my own. I thought, Icarus, perhaps, just perhaps, you are growing up at last.

That night I sat in my favourite leather lounge chair in the dark and waited for Jordan to come home. She had been at another course in Brisbane. She would be home by ten at the latest, she said. It was past midnight. I didn't mind. I just sat there in the dark with my thoughts and the Swedish matchbook bowl in my lap.

I had stopped imagining her late-night wanderings. I had ceased putting my matchbook jigsaw together on the lounge-room floor. It didn't matter so much to me any more. I tired of the pictures and the little rows of sulphur heads. It had become boring.

At close to one I heard her keys in the door. She closed the door gently, turned the deadlock, took her shoes off in the foyer, and made her way down the long corridor to the kitchen. I heard the neon lights above the kitchen bench flicker on. I heard her tiptoeing across the tiles. She opened the fridge. She closed it. She came around through the kitchenette area and into the lounge, and turned on the small reading lamps. That's when she saw me.

'Jesus,' she said. 'Sweetheart. What are you doing? You scared the living daylights out of me.'

I didn't say anything. I just sat there, hugging the big glass bowl.

She moved across the lounge room, slowly. I looked down at her stockinged feet against the white carpet. She moved closer and closer. Then the feet stopped, and I looked up at her with a grin on my face.

Jordan gave a little laugh.

'What is this?' she said sweetly. 'What ... what are you doing, Ick?'

She looked back at the sideboard as if the bowl of matchbooks was still there. She couldn't seem to understand it out of its place. She was confused. It was as if the matchbook bowl in my lap wasn't real.

'What's happening?' she asked.

She looked a bit frightened then. Her lips were stained with lipstick. She liked really rich, red lipstick, did Jordan. It had worn off, most of it, but traces of its brilliant pigment were still there, on her generous lips.

We must have faced each other for a minute or more. She held a glass of water in her hand. The water seemed to be rocking just a tiny bit, side to side.

'Ick?' she said, almost pitifully.

MATCHBOOKS

I kept my arms around the fat bowl full of brightly coloured cardboard and sulphur. I looked her in the eyes and I didn't relinquish my gaze.

'Do you have another one tonight?' I asked her, quietly. 'For the collection.'

I smiled again and held the bowl up to her.

There wasn't much more to it. She simply turned and left. She went into the bedroom and packed a small bag and left. That was that. She didn't say a word to me. I heard the door click shut and the bell of the elevator and the rushing of the wind in its shaft and she was gone from my life.

I didn't sleep that night. Too many things were going around in my head. Everything suddenly seemed strange. I bumped into furniture that I had never bumped into before. I made a cup of coffee and forgot to put the instant coffee in the cup and sipped the hot water and milk before I knew what I had done. I walked into rooms and stood there, forgetting why I had gone into the rooms in the first place. I caught my finger in a drawer. I cut my hand on the latch of the sliding glass door out to the balcony. It was as if I had lost all my normal human skills, my faculties. I was suddenly clumsy. I couldn't understand it.

Then, at about five a.m., I took the matchbook bowl out onto the balcony and placed it gently on the tiles at my feet.

I reached into the bowl and plucked out a matchbook. I had all the lights off. I couldn't see which one I had selected, but it didn't matter.

Then, slowly, rhythmically, one by one, I lit a match at a time. I ran the sulphur head down the rough strip at the bottom and flicked each match over the edge of the balcony. It was a still night. Totally still. I did one matchbook, then another, then another, until I had lit every last one in that Swedish glass bowl.

And after a while I was so lulled by my ritual, so totally

a part of it, that I was, at once, outside of it as well. I was down on the beach, looking up to the thirtieth floor of Parthenon Place. And I saw every last match as clear as crystal. I was entranced. I was there for hours with my feet in the cold, shifting sand, watching those tiny shooting stars, those dull orange shooting stars, falling into the darkness and fading away.

Ngomo Manza
Tom Carment

A treeless slope approached in profile indicates only the easiest of gradients, and the most obvious irregularities of form. An inexperienced climber may come to a rise of smooth stone that tempts him on without fear or consideration, to a point of steepness where it is possible to ascend but not to descend, and then to a point where it is impossible to ascend further. The difference between these two points is but a few degrees. The climber cannot see above whether the slope will lessen, or offer a protuberance to grasp, and he tends to go till unable to move. If the clouds above happen to be blowing in the direction he is facing, across the summit, the victim, looking up, as he is sure to do, will experience that uneasy sensation of the mountainside slowly lifting like a ladder coming off the wall.

This was the difficulty that the white man Alex would be surprised to find himself in, for he was no amateur climber—his childhood had been spent among these kopjes. Although he was only twenty-six years old, some of the subtlety of youth had gone from his limbs: and whereas in childhood the empty mind concentrates on the task at hand, he was that day preoccupied with other problems.

An argument with his wife had precipitated his departure for a weekend alone in the hills, taking photographs. More often now she went out dancing on Friday nights to an African nightclub in the townships with the other Australian teachers. 'A place where tourists never go,' she told him. Alex always felt self-conscious dancing and he was uneasy in the all-black township crowd—he had grown up here under a different code. Jackie had originally found him enthusiastic, sporty, well-read, even chivalrous—so different to her previous sallow-faced lovers. Then gradually, her excitement had diminished and his rationality and even temper became oppressive to her. He seemed so unemotional. 'I express my love by loving deeds,' he would say. Yet as her attachment waned, his had grown into a tense and desperate obsession. He had bought her Thomas Mapfumo records and had enrolled in dance classes. There had been moments of tenderness and reconciliation— enough to give him hope—but they did not last. He coped with his frustration by indulging in what she scathingly referred to as 'Hemingway behaviour'. At the end of the last wet season he had paddled his canoe down the Zambesi, alone. His evening strolls became so long that Sampson the dog would no longer join him.

That Friday night Jackie went out as usual, and he had sat up till late at his desk. But he was unable to concentrate on his work, and then on retiring was unable to sleep. He turned on the bedside light and attempted to read a detective story, but he looked straight through the pages and listened for a car to come down the quiet street. It was not until the first birdcalls preceding dawn that he heard the familiar crunch of gravel as the Peugeot pulled in through the gate. In his pyjamas he confronted her on the drive. She stood beneath the indigo foliage and put her hands languidly on her hips. 'It was just sex,' she said. 'I'm sorry ... we dance well together.'

Later that morning he had left her sleeping on the couch. The blanket had slipped down to reveal one breast. Alex left a note—'Gone to the Vumba for the weekend, A.' The front door was about to click when he hesitated and returned to pick up the pile of her clothes, reeking of cigarettes, and put them to soak in the laundry.

The car was now just a glinting speck below. As he approached the rock face he thought about photographing a hawk drifting above it, but on looking through the viewfinder it seemed too small and insignificant. He continued on, and as it became steeper he was only partially aware of his surroundings. He climbed fast and hard in tune with the intensity of his thoughts, and before he knew it his momentum had thrown him on, past the gradient of no descent, and he was stuck there like a gecko on the wall.

The sun was 'merciless'—no, the sun was just hot, as was normal at mid-afternoon—and Alex heard the siren from the chromeworks fifteen kilometres down the valley, which signalled the change of shift. He imagined the miners in their open metal cage going down the cool shaft. He once read of a professional diver who had been checking the underside of a big cargo vessel when someone had turned on an intake pump which spreadeagled him against a grille underwater, on the side of the hull. The diver was trapped like this for half an hour, and just when his air supply was surely finished, so the story went, someone up above had switched off the pump.

Alex's attempts to move out of his absurd position were repeatedly frustrated, and his shouts for help echoed back to him unheeded. It was very painful, stretched out there, gripping at the rock with his fingers and toes. Increasingly there came to mind vistas of incidents from his life, like film clips; some forgotten and some seemingly trivial. When he tried to enjoy or extend any one of these memories, the awareness of pain cut through them like a knife and the newsreel continued. Some incidents that he would not have wished to went on longer and recurred. One especially—a hot afternoon when Alex was six years old. He was meant to be napping, but went looking through the rooms of the bungalow for his mother to ask her for a glass of water. He saw her and a man behind a mosquito net, high up on her bed; they were thrashing about like fish just caught. She did not see him but the man did, and as Alex reached the end of the corridor he heard her whisper, 'Don't stop now ... ' He had hesitated, wondering if it referred to himself. Years later he bought at auction a Japanese print of lovers behind a mosquito net and this picture was very clear to him now, in every detail. He rehearsed how Jackie would react if he died. Was she with someone else now ... ?

Shadows from slight bumps of rock in front of his face slowly lengthened, and the clothing against the small of his back and his legs became clammy with sweat. He was reminded of a time he had welched to one of the Fathers on a boy, the school bully, who had urinated in the altar wine and laid his stools across the ivory keys of the harmonium. The boy, idolised by his contemporaries, a six-foot hulk of pimples, had retaliated in assembly line by pissing down the back of his trousers.

Every muscle was challenging his will to hold on. The pain was like a cramp you get in the night, but continuous, and his rectum felt like a blockage point of extreme pressure. Even the camera seemed heavy, its strap digging into the base of his neck.

As a child Alex was very quiet and had avoided fights

and violent games. Although, one time, on reading that chameleons can change to any colour except red, he had painted the inside of a shoebox red and placed a chameleon in it to see if it would burst. But the lizard escaped before he could secure the lid.

Alex remembered how recently an emaciated dog had wandered into his garden, its hindquarters stripped of flesh, one leg hanging useless. Alex offered the dog a piece of meat but it just sat there looking bewildered. Then it rolled the meat in the dirt in an attempt to bury it. He placed the dog in a blanket to prevent it biting him and took it to a nearby vet. The vet, a hundred-kilo African, came out from his small house carrying scissors and a syringe. He had left the front door open with the television on—a soccer match. The vet told Alex to hold the dog as he snipped hairs from the foreleg, felt for the vein and jabbed in the large needle. The blood meandered like seaweed back into the syringe. The dog suddenly arched its neck around and bit Alex's forearm—the last act of its life. The vet took the body of the dead dog by one of its hind legs, laid it on his doormat and returned inside.

There was still a scar from the dog's bite on Alex's arm and he could feel the pain in it as though he had just been bitten.

It made him feel bitter and sorry for himself. Here he was, stuck on this rock, facing death, with no preamble, no warning or premonition. A stupid accident had deflected him from his course. He thought of scenery he would not see, arrivals and departures he would not witness, and the relationship he would not resolve. He saw his obsessive grasping after Jackie for what it was—a cancerous growth, non-malignant if removed early. He could see a new self—strong and easy-going, perhaps attractive ...

Right now in some parts of the city the footpaths would

be crowded with weekend amblers passing familiar shopfronts. Certainly he would know some of their faces: the long sharp face of his friend Edgar—one of the first black students at Alex's college—on his way to the Dog House Bar. And Alex remembered the time, during school holidays, when Edgar had taken him to stay with his family in the Tribal Trust Lands. It was an unusual thing for a white boy to do in those days—he had had to get special permission from the government to go to the Trust lands. He was very excited.

One evening they were sitting waiting for dinner in the smoky kitchen hut, when one of the children heard the bull break out of the kraal. They were exhausted after a long day of walking and climbing, but nonetheless rushed eagerly outside to see what had happened. For the next few hours they stumbled across fields and through the rocky bush under a quarter moon, chasing the wild bull. Every now and then in the shadows, the bull would stop completely and Alex would stop as well to catch his breath and listen for the bull's breathing. The small trees all about had large crumpled leaves which looked like wet spinach in the moonlight—everything else was dark. And he felt glad that this minor disaster had robbed him of dinner and an early night, glad that tiredness and inertia had been transformed into such intense pleasure. And then a sudden cracking of branches revealed the bull's presence in a completely unexpected direction, and the chase recommenced. When the truant was caught they tied it to a tree with a sisal rope, and in the firelight it looked shy and diffident. Alex returned to their hut, lay down on the straw mat, and without pulling a blanket over himself immediately fell asleep.

The memory of this deep pure sleep calmed Alex now. He laughed. It was so different to his sleepless waiting for

NGOMO MANZA

Jackie, and so different to those insomniac back-to-back nights together. He wondered if she would misinterpret this action as a last desperate quest for her love, rather than the accident that it was. He laughed again, and wished her well. '*Alles Güt*', the Germans say.

A breeze came up in the evening—the sort that precedes a storm. Alex heard thunder on the other side of the mountain, yet the sky he could see was still only covered in light cloud. Two hawks appeared to hover in the updraught some distance above his head, and stayed there, testing their skill, fixed in one point of space for a long period: then, flicking back their wings, they fell together in a long trajectory down to the valley floor.

Further up the valley three small African boys were taking advantage of the wind, flying their kites. One of them let go his string and raced off into the bush after it while the others laughed. It was some time before he returned.

He followed his kite for a kilometre or so up a branch of the valley till he came to a steep gorge. And it was there he saw beneath huge approaching storm clouds, a figure, unmoving up on the rock. The boy watched for a quarter of an hour to see if this figure stirred, and then decided to go after him. He realised that it would not be possible to climb right up to this man, so at the foot of the *ngomo manza* (mountain forehead) he broke off a sapling as long as a fishing rod, but thicker. This pole may have helped eventually, but it made the climbing slow and arduous, and the boy had only reached a ledge halfway up when the first lightning struck. He dared not proceed further. He tried yelling out, but the man did not hear or see him. The boy slumped on the ledge and waited for the storm to pass.

The man above had nothing to hold on to. Water running

down every part of the kopje was a lubricant beneath his grip. Soon he followed the hawks, but without as much grace. And the only sound to be heard through the rain was his camera breaking up in its fall.

The Dark Stars
Clinton Walker

In the years between about 1983 and 1986 I had more sex with more women than I've had in all the rest of my life. That was a lot of women and a lot of sex. The fact that there was also a lot of drugs involved is tied in in a way I still can't quite understand.

I had arrived in Sydney from Brisbane with my first band and my first girlfriend at the tail end of the seventies. Lurching down the New England Highway in our old Transit van, sitting on stacks of gear in the back, passing joints around and listening to the Doors and the Clash, it seemed like the only way to begin the new decade.

We were a high school band, basically, just boys from the western suburbs. We were inspired to get together in a rush of excitement at hearing the Saints and the Sex Pistols—punk rock!—and we went from there. Called ourselves the Same Again. Played around town, what few gigs there were in Brisbane at the time. Put on a few of our own dances which, predictably, were raided by the cops. Eventually we went into the studio to cut a single—by which time we figured it was high time to get out of Brisbane. So complete with boxes containing a couple of hundred copies of our single, we set off wide-eyed for Sydney.

Billie, my girlfriend, was our singer Jimmy's sister and something of a tomboy. I'd been with a couple of girls before her, but I never thought there'd girls like Billie. She was a real person, not like the girls at school, who were all just such *girls*, tizzy and giggly and coy. Billie was a bit wild, but she was no scrag. She smoked and she could match us boys drink for drink; she loved the music, and she actually seemed to enjoy sex. But she didn't like all our swearing, and she hated the violence which was not uncommon at our gigs—though she could hold her own in any argument. She always seemed to have her nose in a book. When she worked, it was as a waitress.

She would wear, like, miniskirts, but nothing over the top, or too trashy, like a lot of make-up, just simple things, which made the most of her natural features—a nice figure, bright eyes and an easy smile. Sex with her was wonderful because we were working it out together. I guess I loved her, but then, everybody loved Billie.

The Same Again failed comprehensively to achieve anything in Sydney. But Billie and I had a ball together. Sydney was a whole new world, and we shared all our discoveries, including tentative experiments with harder drugs like speed. I even started dipping into some of the books Billie left lying around. We saw all the German new-wave movies.

After about eighteen months, with the band getting nowhere, a few of the guys decided they'd had enough. They wanted to go home. That was fine by me and Jimmy, as we both felt the Same Again had become pretty-well redundant anyway. My guitar playing was improving all the time—I practised a lot—and so it was no longer enough for me just to thrash out the same three chords every song. We decided simply to break the band up (I've still got those boxes of our single somewhere). The rhythm-section went back to Brisbane, and we never heard of them again. Jimmy and I decided to give our partnership a break and see what happened; Billie and I decided to try and get the money together to go overseas.

Billie had been working for a while and so she already had a bit saved; I got a job as a short-order cook serving steaks to cops and queens in a Kings Cross pub. This saved on our food bills as I knocked off meat. We lived on speed, beer and pork chops. Good, clean fun.

We pulled a couple of Bankcard jobs. Those were the days when they'd send cards out on spec; you'd pinch them out of mailboxes, and use them up until they hit the bad list, then convert the loot into cash.

Eventually we took off for London, where everyone was going. We planned to use it as a base to see the rest of Europe from—but things didn't quite turn out that way.

Everybody in London was using smack. Small wonder—the place was a dump, there was nothing happening, and the dope was easy to procure, cheap and extremely high-quality. It was impossible not to join in on the slide.

Billie was horrified. She was always happy to take speed because it was an upper, but heroin was completely against her nature. Plus, it involved needles. This was the first real divergence in our relationship; really, the beginning of the end. I became so smitten with my new habit, needing little else other than dope, I even lost interest in sex. For Billie, that was probably the last straw.

We never travelled outside Hackney. I had this junkie's half-arsed plan to go to Berlin, the new fashionable destination, but I'd already stuck most of my money up my arm, and certainly I had no prospects of making any more. Billie announced she was going home before her return airfare expired. Feeling defeated, I didn't know what to do other than just tag along. I still loved Billie (still do).

I'll never forget that trip home. It was one of the worst experiences of my life. I had a big blast before we left Hackney for the airport, but of course, it was only a couple of hours into the flight before I needed a top-up. And there was still more than a whole day to go cooped up in that plane. Stopping over in fucking Bahrain and Singapore! I started squirming in my seat. Ordered a double gin and tonic.

Then Billie hit me with the news. She had booked a connecting flight to go on home from Sydney to Brisbane. She bit a quivering lip, held back tears. It was something about Billie I always admired, that sort of toughness, which in my limited experience was uncommon in women. I was thankful for it again now. It was bad enough as it was without a scene.

I sat rigid with shock and fear.

'So this must mean it's over?' I asked stupidly.

'Yeah.'

'Just like that?' Desperate.

'No, not just like that at all. Can't you see—that's the problem—it's been coming for ages ...'

I ordered another drink. It was over. I couldn't believe it.

In an odd way, I was almost thankful I was going cold turkey. It was like they say about cutting off a finger to cure a toothache. I was cold-sweating and starting to get stabbing pains in my gut. At least it took my mind off any other, more intangible pain.

Billie nursed her book and stared out the window.

Back in Sydney, I looked up Jimmy. He hadn't done much in the past year either, except, like myself, acquire a heroin

THE DARK STARS

habit. This was the flip-side of the so-called Roaring Eighties, an underclass that indulged itself every bit as completely as the era's fabled yuppies. The only difference was the drug of choice.

Jimmy and I got a place together, a flat right near the Cross in Womerah Lane, Darlinghurst. Darlinghurst Heights, we liked to call it, since it perched on the other side of the hill to what we called The Dustbowl, East Sydney. Womerah Lane was a funny little sort of ghetto world all of its own. A lane onto which backed rows of identical upstairs/downstairs flats with sundecks, garages, banana trees and clotheslines all wrestling for space. It was populated by junkies, art students, musicians, gays, hookers and even the odd old-timer, yet it had a strange sense of community about it.

Our flat was downstairs at Number 17. They all had the same shotgun layout. A path ran along the outside, past the small end rooms, a bedroom, the bathroom and the kitchen, to enter at a middle room, the dining room. Beyond that were two larger rooms, divided by French doors, the end one being the best in the place as it had windows. That was my bedroom. The room next to it was the lounge. In the dining room Jimmy set up a Portastudio. He threw a mattress on the floor in the tiny end bedroom. He didn't care; all he ever did in there was sleep (alone), between the hours of about five or six a.m. and two in the afternoon.

Jim's routine quickly became apparent. As soon as he got up, he'd start looking to score, and then he'd stay up all night mucking around recording. The next day do the same thing, and so on and so on.

We never even discussed getting a band together. It just seemed given that Jim wanted to do what he was doing. He never played anyone, me included, his tapes. But whenever our paths crossed he was pleasant, unless he was strung out, and his sardonic sense of humour never deserted him. We ran our respective habits quite independently, like a lot of junkies that live together do. You just had to watch your stash.

Dope, to me, was no big deal, inasmuch as it was generally so easy to get. All you had to do was find the cash to keep yourself on. And I could always get work as a roadie to supplement the dole.

I was getting into a pleasant enough routine of my own. I'd met Sandy, the woman who lived by herself upstairs next door, and she and her flat became something of a refuge for me. Sandy was a bit of a mystery, at first. She was older than me, her flat was full of Asian curios and artefacts, and she just seemed to have a calm about her.

I'd go up there, and the hash pipe was always on the ready. We'd sit around and get stoned and talk, and though I was never one to really open up, it was comforting just to talk to someone, especially a woman. Women, after all, had always seemed to me to be at the centre of things. My mother, despite a propensity for hysteria and liking for a drink, had held our family together; my father I was deeply ambivalent about, if only because I hardly knew him. He just never seemed *there*. And then he left.

Sandy and I slept together, for which I was thankful, strangely, more than anything else. The sex wasn't so passionate as it was warm and satisfying. Sandy knew what she was doing and took the lead in doing it; I was rapt and she seemed happy enough herself, so who could complain?

Sometimes other guys would come knocking on the door, and they'd come in, and they'd hang around just like me. When another bloke showed up, it was a case of the last man left standing would go to bed with her. Sandy gave the impression that either/or was fine by her. Later, I figured she probably would have been quite happy taking more than one man to bed, but I wouldn't have cared for that; me and two women, sure, but another bloke, no way.

I was still really quite naive. I mean, at first, I couldn't understand how Sandy could afford to live in the style she did, and how come she had this bleeper which would go off at all hours, prompting her to make a phone call and then shoo me away saying she had to go to work. I eventually figured she was a call girl, which made no difference to me one way or the other.

I was still smarting from the break-up with Billie.

'She's always been so fuckin' moralistic,' Jim said, rightly or wrongly perceiving that only the drugs had split us. 'I mean, when we were kids, you know, and we'd get into trouble, she'd always cave in and tell Mum, you know.' But even then, Jim couldn't hold back an affectionate chuckle.

Jim himself had always been a wild man, the sort of guy who couldn't resist a dare, who'd hang out the window of a moving train just for fun. (That's why being the front-man in an explosive punk band had been so perfect for him—at least until that became predictable in itself.) And so maybe, I thought, Billie being Billie was just trying to protect her brother from himself. But I tried not to think too much about Billie at all.

I set myself an overriding new objective. I had to get into a new band. Somehow, it all fell beautifully into place. A guy called Eric Snow was back on the scene. He was a bit of a legend, having been in outlaw bands in the seventies, but he'd disappeared from view—been in jail, as it turned out—and was only now trying to get something going again. He'd found a couple of young guys who played bass and drums, and he was looking for a guitarist. We met at a gig, and clicked. I was in.

To me, this was perfect. The rhythm-section guys were shit-hot, and Eric was great too. He was no fool; he'd gone inside for dealing, but he took it as a sign. Did his time smart. Got clean and got fit. Took to pumping iron. And studied, Philosophy and Communications. So he'd become kind of like an intellectual Iggy Pop except he was about seven feet tall—and that only made him more imposing.

The Dark Stars, as Eric named us, started coming together in the rehearsal room, so we went with it. The Snowman, as we called him, told me I was a fool for using, but I was too good a guitarist for him to let go.

The band made its debut at a pub called the Southern Cross in Surry Hills, and it went fantastically.

There was a real scene blossoming at the Southern Cross. It was an exciting time. The charts might have been full of foppy haircut/synthesiser bands, but at the same time, there were lots of new rock'n'roll bands around which constituted the roots of today's alternative music. The Southern Cross was always packed. Plenty of girls. This was, again, before rock'n'roll became an almost exclusively male domain, when it still even had a measure of radical/intellectual chic. The Southern Cross, then, was full of all sorts of arty wannabe's as well as straight rock'n'roll animals. And us Stars were its new darlings.

On the weekends, the nearby Trade Union Club would have bigger bands on, and a bar that stayed open till dawn. The last band would finish around two a.m.; you then repaired to the bar on the first floor. It was brightly lit and the incessant jangling was not only of poker machines but also the band just finished still ringing in your ears, and the buzzing of your own flesh under the influence of whatever sort of stimulant it was you were on. Everybody was on something, mostly speed, though I stuck to my steady heroin habit. The popular image of junkies on the nod is accurate to an extent, but equally, because it dulls all pain, heroin can also keep you up and going. Which it did me.

It became apparent that there were women and sex for the taking here. They say guys get into bands to get laid, and while that's true to an extent too, it doesn't tell the whole story. All the musicians I knew back then at least fantasised that they could make a career out of music—not that they would have used the word 'career'—but if 'girl control', as we called it, also came along the way, well, you'd be mad not to take advantage of it, wouldn't you?

I had my rock star pose down. I'd read a couple of books which added an intellectual dimension, and even for all the self-loathing that drug-addiction implies, I suspected I couldn't be that bad a guy. So, I had the look, I bathed regularly, and I was considered witty and charming. Plus, at twenty-five, I now knew how to do it, or at least I thought I did. If I was stoned, well, that not only made me at ease with myself, more confident, but also added an edge of danger which—long before AIDS put a stop to abandon generally—seemed to make me even more attractive.

I didn't want to get involved, just get laid. I'd never really done a lot of one-night-standing, but it came easy. (Went just as easy too.)

And so you'd stumble out of the Trade into the grey dawn of Saturday or Sunday with a pretty young thing, only somewhat worse for wear, on your arm, and you felt like you'd live forever.

The cab ride back to my place was mercifully short, as the both of us champed at the bit to get at each other. Fumbling through the side door, we excused ourselves as we tiptoed, giggling, past Jim, who'd be nodding off with an acoustic guitar cradled in his lap, and we'd close the doors on my room and go from there.

So who can remember who did what to whom? Nobody got hurt, and everybody had fun.

All this time, I'd been writing to Billie, telling her that she was the one I really wanted, and eventually she agreed to come down for a visit. She wanted to see Jim anyway. I should have known it would turn out the way it did—that Billie had planned the whole trip just to tell me what's past was past—but of course, I was blind. That I made a pathetic effort to hide my habit only heightened Billie's disgust. She'd obviously hoped to let me down gently, but I made it impossible for her. Jim, for his part, was just so stoned the whole time he could hardly even talk. I don't know what upset Billie most. She left after two days and three nights. I couldn't understand why she wouldn't sleep with me just for old times' sake. After she left, I put my fist through a wall, which was a pretty silly thing for a guitarist to do.

But I soon got over it, superficially at least. The band was really starting to happen now, and so I had plenty to occupy me.

They say men reach their sexual peak at eighteen. Don't believe it. In my mid-twenties, life was like a sexual smorgasbord, and I wanted to try every dish on offer at least once. So I helped myself. This was where sex became like drugs, it all became mere consumerism. The twelve-step goose-steppers might say they were both the same addiction. I don't know about that, but I do know that the more you have, the more you get, the more you want.

It wasn't just fucking groupies either. Indeed, it was considered quite *declassé* among us budding rock-gods to be seen with one of *them*. No, since this was a scene frequented by actresses and artists and women who seemed only a step away from full yuppiedom—professionals like journalists and doctors—*they* were the prizes. With an actress, say, you could bask in the reflected glow—or vice versa—and maybe you'd get your photo together in *TV Week*. With a professional woman, well, they had money, and for her, a dangerous rock star always added some colour and cachet to a lifestyle which was otherwise populated by suits. We can all be whores sometimes.

I had a lair of my own. I could close off the rest of the flat so all that filtered through into the lounge and my bedroom, which opened onto each other, was the occasional low murmur and clunking of Jim's all-night recording sessions. We had the TV, gas fire and a bed—all you could need. I'd occasionally duck out to the bathroom with my works to have a quick taste and then my mojo would really be working. It's another myth that junkies can't get it up. Junkies can get it up, all right, if they want to, it's just a question of whether or not they can come.

You could hole up for days like that.

I developed a new pattern, rapidly turning-over 'girl-friends'. I would acquire them and then when the sex lost its novelty or a new option, or challenge presented itself, I'd discard them.

Certainly, I had a hair-trigger. A girl once said to me, Nice tie (it was a silk fifties job). I took it as a sign. We ended up spending a couple of wild weeks together. And that was that. Fast, and clean.

The women I wanted, I got. It was a power I was fully aware I had, and I flaunted it.

The world of sex was something to explore. It wasn't so much that it was a Kama Sutra-like parade of peversions, but rather that even as it kept returning to a couple of basics, themes upon which the variations were only ever slight, every experience was still totally different. Sight, sound, smell, touch, taste, every sensation in every woman making different demands. Some girls go up, some go down, others will, others won't. There was no picking 'em. (Emotionally too I suppose, but then, I tried not to get too involved on that level.)

I was still occasionally popping up to see Sandy, although I'd stopped sleeping with her. We still talked, and Sandy, I suspect, was suss enough to see what was happening to me—if not herself. I told her how I'd been asked out by a woman I knew and liked but didn't really desire, as such, and how we'd gone nightclubbing and tooted coke till dawn, which was noteworthy because, believe it or not, I disliked tooting cocaine. Mandy was a budding and politicised film-maker, and definitely a spunk. But I didn't want to sleep with her, just because she didn't have that effect on me. I would have been happy just staying friends. Sandy asked did I sleep with her, then?

'Well, yeah,' I shrugged, 'I had to, she ...'

Sandy cut me off: 'Typically male,' she sneered. Even though I didn't know exactly what she meant, the remark disturbed me.

I was starting to resent Sandy, even if I didn't like myself for it. It was as if she spread herself so thin, she was unable to actually give much of herself at all. And even I gave something, I thought, however erratically. But more than that, although I didn't want to admit it at the time, was the fact that Sandy was challenging me, forcing me to look at myself.

That all this disturbed me even more than the abortion I'd recently caused another woman to have is perhaps indicative of the depth of my self-absorption.

I was nonetheless beginning to wonder if I was on the wrong track.

At the same time, the band was racing away—we had released an EP and we were so hot we were on the cover of *RAM*, and on Double-Jay and *Countdown*. At the ABC studios in Melbourne, Molly swanned around with a Scotch in one hand and a boy on the other. The little girls in the audience couldn't have been less interested in a hardcore rock'n'roll band like us—they wanted Boy George—but Molly gee'd them up anyway.

We were touring a lot. And of course, as they say in showbusiness, What goes on the road, stays on the road ... We had, in fact, just got an offer to tour America on the back of the success of our EP there, and so we all felt like our shit couldn't possibly stink.

But then something happened that would dig its claws into me. One night I was at my local having a quiet drink alone when a girl I knew a little and actually disliked came in and offered to buy me a beer. Naturally, I accepted. She was taunting and teasing me, which I suppose was her nature—and why I wasn't fond of her. At any rate, for whatever reason, we ended up going back to my place. Sleeping with this girl was the last thing I ever thought I'd do, and so maybe because I resented the fact that here I was now doing just that—that I had lost control—I took it out on her. I wasn't violent in the slightest—violence towards women appals me—but certainly, I was brusque in a way I'd never before been in bed. I guess I felt as if I was saying, Well, fuck you, you wanted it, you'll take what you're given, and this is all you're getting. Without even so much as the semblance of care or tenderness, and I'd always tried to muster that. Maybe that's what she wanted, what she liked—she didn't seem put-out—but the incident worried me. It was as if I'd stepped over a line.

Then, I took up with a girl called Karen. She was the singer in a cool new country band around town called the Wooden Spoons. She dressed like a rockabilly chick, wearing a ponytail, Western shirts, gingham frocks and cowboy boots, and in bed I'd say, Baby, leave the boots on! She was a nice girl and I liked her, and I even had the idea that if things worked out, I might try and stick with the relationship, make a go of it.

By this time, our American tour had been organised. Karen offered her flat down at Bondi Beach as the venue for a going-away party. She couldn't have done anything worse. The party was a disaster. I myself usually planned ahead and carried enough dope to cover contingencies, but someone, most likely Jim, who'd actually come out for once, had rung The Man. The Man arrived and half a dozen of us sequestered ourselves in a room and started shooting up.

Karen tolerated my habit, but this was going too far. Just as she was about to launch into a fully justified tirade, however, Jim dropped in a heap on the floor. OD'd. Typical. He'd by now acquired the nickname Jimmy OD.

This was perhaps the only predictable thing Jim ever did. He was burnt out, his wild streak exhausted, everything he'd been consumed by his habit, not so much out of self-loathing as the power of the drug itself and the junkie's insatiable appetite for more, to go deeper into that abyss. Jim accepted this self-destruction just as he had wilfully tempted fate so many times as a kid.

The sight of Jim turning a hideous shade of blue-grey on the floor jolted Karen into speechlessness. A friend led her out of the room in horror, and she collapsed in tears.

We picked Jim up and walked him around the room, but he wasn't responding. We decided to haul him down to the beach and throw him in the surf. That worked. We dragged him out of the water coughing and spluttering. But then he passed out again on the sand. We dragged him back down to the water, and left him rolling around in the wash. He soon came to, and we all straggled back to the party. When we got there we were asked to leave.

The others did so. I stayed. The party had been cruelled. Karen wouldn't speak to me. She went to bed, and I crashed on the couch.

THE DARK STARS

The next morning I couldn't have been more contrite. I wasn't leaving until the following day, so I had time to talk my way out of trouble. To be honest, I was astonished by, not to mention grateful for Karen's capacity for forgiveness. I don't deserve this, I remember thinking to myself.

I'd already moved what valuables I did have down to Karen's so Jim couldn't hock them, and I left her the next day sure that we'd pick up where we were leaving off when I returned in five weeks' time.

The American tour wasn't bad. It wasn't great, but it wasn't bad. What it did do was make us aware just how enormous the task of merely gaining a foothold in America would be. Better that, though, than being big fish in a small pond at home.

After a while on the road, you can tend to get into a cocoon. It's easy to lose touch, especially when money's tight and ISD calls are expensive. I finally called Karen from LAX just as we were about to board the flight home, just to say I was on my way. She seemed distant, which was understandable, but there was something else. She had something important to tell me, she said. Jim had died. Just the other day.

I was mute. Even when you might be expecting something like this, you can never be quite prepared for it. I felt as if all the air had rushed out of me. Sandy had found him, Karen told me, with a spike still stuck in his arm.

Karen started to try and say something else. 'Look,' she stuttered, 'there's another thing ...,' but I'd already drifted off in my mind. And my plane was boarding.

'I'll see you tomorrow,' I whispered and hung up.

After clearing the usual shakedown Australian Customs imposes on incoming rock bands, I made my way straight to Womerah Lane.

Pulling up in the cab, jetlagged, generally fazed and in the very early morning light, the old place had an eerie tranquillity about it. I stuck my head in the flat, just to eyeball it. It had a sulphurous smell about it. Then I went up to Sandy's. Some things never change. But as much as Sandy remained her sympathetic yet realistic self, if there were any signs in all this I could see them for myself, or at least thought I could, and I didn't need Sandy to point them out to me. Not that I didn't appreciate her concern, but really, I just didn't want to know.

She told me Billie had flown down from Brisbane to take Jim's body back up there to be buried by his parents. She gave me the number where Billie was staying, and I kept moving.

I went back down to the flat, gave it the once-over. I still can't bear to think I was half-hoping to find Jim's stash. He didn't have any possessions to speak of, other than an acoustic guitar and a pile of used and re-used cassettes. In the corner of his room was a box of Same Again singles. He'd hocked the Portastudio.

I got Billie on the phone, and arranged to go around and see her before she left for the airport. She was staying at a motel in Surry Hills. I didn't know how I felt about seeing her this way.

I quickly called Karen. There was a surprise in store for me there too. In my absence, she'd hooked up with someone new. I might have known. I guess I knew I was a scumbag, and I was only now getting my just deserts. 'Fuckin Jesus!' I barked when I hung up the phone. I grabbed a couple of things, locked the flat, and kept moving.

The Chron Lodge was an incongruously sixties-modern motel on an otherwise Victorian Crown Street. Billie opened the door to let me in. Her eyes were red. Wordlessly, she watched me flop on the end of the bed, then sat at the dressing table, looking anywhere but in the mirror.

I felt guilty and ashamed.

'Fuck this,' Billie whimpered. 'You bastards.'

I stared at the floor, the thin brown carpet.

'Just so fucking selfish. You mightn't care if you kill yourself, but other people do. God knows why.'

I felt something turn in the pit of my empty stomach.

'I hate the pair of you. I hate Jim because he's dead, and I hate you because you're alive.'

But Billie was bigger than that. She raised her head out of her hands and took a deep breath, brushed the hair out of her eyes, and appealed to me, 'Can't you see, it's just such a waste ...'

I loved her then as much as I ever had. I also knew we could neither of us go back.

'Look, I've got to go,' Billie said.

I helped her into a cab, then ran to escape the blazing light of day in the darkened lounge bar of the first pub I saw. I passed the afternoon in a torpor of dark spirits. Somewhat revived, I went round to Karen's to collect my things, but I suppose holding some faint hope she would come around. If nothing else, I desperately needed to get laid. Sex was scarce on the road in America for an unknown Australian wannabe. But Karen virtually laughed in my face as she shoved my ghetto blaster and acoustic guitar in my arms.

I trudged down along the beach wondering what the hell to do. Staring out to sea, I saw nothing, no answers. I jumped on a 389 bus to the Cross, where I checked into the Hampton Court Hotel. Got a nice front room overlooking Bayswater Rd: The Mansions Hotel where I'd done that cooking job all those years ago; the brothel next door that boasted 'The Biggest Bed In The World!'

On impulse, I did something I'd never done before. I knew plenty of hookers and call girls, but I'd never before paid for it myself. I picked up the phone book, found a likely-looking local agency, and ordered a girl.

She was at the door in minutes. I let her in. She was wearing a trenchcoat, which she took off to reveal a teddy. She was okay.

'What do you want?' she asked.

'I just wanna fuck,' I sighed.

She laughed. 'Gee, I haven't heard that for a while.'

When she left exactly an hour later, services duly performed, I felt curiously unsatisfied, maybe even more desperate. My empty stomach was turning bilious.

I phoned The Man. He would take longer than minutes to arrive. I paced the room, swilling bourbon. Already, it seemed like the girl hadn't even been around.

Nothing was the same any more. Jim was dead. Like most of our contemporaries, the Dark Stars had set their sights on America, and both the Trade and the Southern Cross were already winding down. I had nowhere to go.

Worst of all, everyone was all of a sudden talking about this new disease called AIDS. It just seemed like a conspiracy to deny me all the sex and drugs I needed.

The Man finally arrived. I couldn't get the stuff into me quick enough.

When I came to it was an hour or so later. I must have OD'd. I'd OD'd before, of course, but this, again, was different. I was alone, for starters.

I lay on the hotel bed smoking, all my nerve-ends frayed. It wasn't that I was thinking I was lucky to be alive, or that there were any warning signs in everything that had happened in the past two days. All I could think was that whatever it was I was looking for, I'd come to the end of the line, and I hadn't found anything.

Maybe I was on the wrong track. Tired of living from moment to moment, without even realising that drugs were

illusory and that sex was not an end in itself but a means—
I can articulate it now—by which I sought connection, and
continuity. Because a life without that is a life without
impact, or resonance, and that's almost no life at all.

Nowhere along the line, after all, had love come into it.

Without even knowing what I was doing, I eased gradually, instinctively out of it.

Maybe I just realised I was all alone in the world and feared I'd stay that way.

The enforced demise of the band was in a way the best thing that could have happened. With a big recording deal signed, we cut our first album, and then we went back to America to tour in support of its release there. But something got to Eric. He went off the rails again and got back on the gear. As a result, the band collapsed. A few fans and critics mourned a great potential nipped in the bud.

I was more or less forced to get my shit together. I embarked, as they say, on a solo career. Through everything, my passion for music—the guitar—had never abated, and with re-adjusted, more worldly-wise personal ambitions, coupled with playing the odd session and a little teaching, it still serves me well enough.

Eventually I met a woman I loved, and we made that choice to commit ourselves to a life together. So far it's working, not least of all, I think, because I now understand the need to give as well as take, and that that giving comes back to you several fold.

It helps too that a woman understands a man.

On this day, I don't want to stray from the hearth.

Whisper It
Jonathan Griffiths

It's like the gods were against me from beginning to end, like I was being tested. Am I in love or aren't I? Is it worth it or isn't it?

I took off in the afternoon. I packed my bags and I had all her stuff to carry down because she was going straight from uni. So I loaded up and headed down to the bank. I went in to get my pay out because I still owed $700 on the ring—and my pay wasn't there. It must be going in at four o'clock, sometimes that's what happens.

So I went down to the main branch in the city, which is open till five—and it's near the jeweller. I got there at half-past four, lugging all these bags—and my pay still wasn't there. What the fuck am I going to do?

I said, 'My pay is there, check it out.' So they checked with my branch and said, 'Yeah, it's gone in but they put it in under tomorrow's date. Sorry, we've made a mistake but we can't help you until tomorrow.' And I was like, going to explode. I walked out of the bank and I was just numb, I didn't know what to do. So I went to the jeweller's, asked them if they'd take a cheque—and they said they wouldn't. They'd love to help me but they couldn't.

I walked out of there and if I'd had a machine gun I would have gone on a killing spree. I was furious. So I thought, right—I'm going back to that bank and I'm getting my fucking money. They didn't want to give it to me but I pushed and I pushed and I pushed—and I walked out of there with an $800 advance on my pay.

I was so relieved. I headed back to the jeweller's, got there just as they were closing—and got the ring. I ran out, jumped into a taxi, went round to a florist's, picked up a rose and headed down to Central Station. Then the taxi driver couldn't change a $50 note. He had the shits with me and I wanted to smash his face in. I was fuming. Everything had gone wrong—like, it worked out okay in the end but I was just so wound up, so angry and so fucking miserable because the whole world was against me. And I was lugging all these bags around, that had been getting heavier and heavier and I was just sort of dragging this rose along the ground.

Then she walked up, all bright and sparkly—she didn't know anything had gone wrong. She had no idea why we were really going away, and that it almost hadn't happened. She was really happy to see me, 'Hi, how are you? Is that for me?' And all I could do was poke it at her. And I made up all these stories about why I was so shitty—and she was even happier that I'd gone to get her a rose when I was so cranky. She said it proved my love even more.

Anyway, we jumped on the train, relaxed, and headed up to Leura. By the time we got there I'd calmed down and was almost happy. This was where it was all going to happen. We got off the train and it was freezing—this icy arctic wind slicing right through us. We battled our way through the elements and fell into the restaurant. It was perfect: subdued lighting, a crackling open fire and the scent of burning eucalyptus in the air.

The waitress led us to our table, right beside the open fire. I put my bag beside me and positioned the ring so I could reach for it at the right moment. All the way through the entree I kept thinking, I'll ask her now, I'll ask her now. And as soon as I thought that I'd reach for the ring, I'd seize up, I'd feel sick, I'd just freeze up so I couldn't say anything. So I'd think, okay, I'll do it later.

The waitress brought the main course and the same thing happened—every time I'd reach for the ring I'd freeze. I had the duck, she had trout. We held hands and ate forkfuls of each other's food. If ever there was a moment to ask this was it—but I didn't know what to say. I looked deep into the fire, searching for inspiration, for just the right words. We finished the duck, the trout, the vegies, the sauce, the sprig of parsley—and I still hadn't found the words. When the dessert arrived I thought, right, this is it. I've got to ask her now—I've got to. So I reached into my bag and I got the ring and hid it in my lap, in my clenched fist. And then somehow the talk got around to marriage and I thought, now! Now's the time. Ask her! Ask her!

Then she grabbed my hand, the hand with the ring in it. She put it in her lap, she wanted my hand in her lap, on her knee, stroking her leg. And I held my fist tight. And she said, 'Open your hand,' and I said no.

She said, 'What's going on? Open your hand!'

I said, 'No—I can't.' But finally I did—and there was the ring. She looked at it, then looked at me and she flung her head sideways and tears arced out of her eyes and her hair swung around.

She looked at the ring again then looked at me and said,

'Aren't you supposed to ask me something?' I didn't respond, I couldn't.

'Ask me,' she said. I shook my head. 'Ask me,' she repeated. I shook my head again, I couldn't say anything.

She leant over and said, 'Whisper it.'

So I said, _{'Marry me.'}

And she said, 'Yes.'

Neighbours
Tim Winton

When they first moved in, the young couple were wary of the neighbourhood. The street was full of European migrants. It made the newly-weds feel like sojourners in a foreign land. Next door on the left lived a Macedonian family. On the right, a widower from Poland.

The newly-weds' house was small, but its high ceilings and paned windows gave it the feel of an elegant cottage. From his study window, the young man could see out over the rooftops and used-car yards the Moreton Bay figs in the park where they walked their dog. The neighbours seemed cautious about the dog, a docile, moulting collie.

The young man and woman had lived all their lives in the expansive outer suburbs where good neighbours were seldom seen and never heard. The sounds of spitting and washing and daybreak watering came as a shock. The Macedonian family shouted, ranted, screamed. It took six months for the newcomers to comprehend the fact that their neighbours were not murdering each other, merely talking.

The old Polish man spent most of his day hammering nails into wood only to pull them out again. His yard was stacked with salvaged lumber. He added to it, but he did not build with it.

Relations were uncomfortable for many months. The Macedonians raised eyebrows at the late hour at which the newcomers rose in the mornings. The young man sensed their disapproval at his staying home to write his thesis while his wife worked. He watched in disgust as the little boy next door urinated in the street. He once saw him spraying the cat from the back step. The child's head was shaved regularly, he assumed, in order to make his hair grow thick. The little boy stood at the fence with only his cobalt eyes showing; it made the young man nervous.

In the autumn, the young couple cleared rubbish from their back yard and turned and manured the soil under the open and measured gaze of the neighbours. They planted leeks, onions, cabbage, brussels spouts and broad beans and this caused the neighbours to come to the fence and offer advice about spacing, hilling, mulching. The young man resented the interference, but he took careful note of what was said. His wife was bold enough to run a hand over the child's stubble and the big woman with black eyes and butcher's arms gave her a bagful of garlic cloves to plant.

Not long after, the young man and woman built a henhouse. The neighbours watched it fall down. The Polish widower slid through the fence uninvited and rebuilt it for them. They could not understand a word he said.

As autumn merged into winter and the vermilion sunsets were followed by sudden, dark dusks touched with the smell of woodsmoke and the sound of roosters crowing day's end, the young couple found themselves smiling back at the neighbours. They offered heads of cabbage and took gifts of grappa and firewood. The young man worked steadily at his thesis on the development of the twentieth century novel. He cooked dinners for his wife and listened to her stories of eccentric patients and hospital incompetence. In the street they no longer walked with their eyes lowered. They felt superior and proud when their parents came to visit and to cast shocked glances across the fence.

In the winter they kept ducks, big, silent muscovies that stood about in the rain growing fat. In the spring the Macedonian family showed them how to slaughter and to pluck and to dress. They all sat around on blocks and upturned buckets and told barely-understood stories—the men butchering, the women plucking, as was demanded. In the haze of down and steam and fractured dialogue, the young man and woman felt intoxicated. The cat toyed with severed heads. The child pulled the cat's tail. The newcomers found themselves shouting.

But they had not planned on a pregnancy. It stunned them to be made parents so early. Their friends did not have children until several years after being married—if at all. The young woman arranged for maternity leave. The young man ploughed on with his thesis on the twentieth century novel.

The Polish widower began to build. In the late spring dawns, he sank posts and poured cement and began to use his wood. The young couple turned in their bed, cursed him behind his back. The young husband, at times, suspected that the widower was deliberately antagonising them. The young wife threw up in the mornings. Hay fever began to wear him down.

Before long the young couple realised that the whole neighbourhood knew of the pregnancy. People smiled tirelessly at them. The man in the deli gave her small presents of chocolates and him packets of cigarettes that he stored at home, not being a smoker. In the summer, Italian women began to offer names. Greek women stopped the young woman in the street, pulled her skirt up and felt her belly, telling her it was bound to be a boy. By late summer the woman next door had knitted the baby a suit, complete with booties and beanie. The young woman felt flattered, claustrophobic, grateful, peeved.

By late summer, the Polish widower next door had almost finished his two-car garage. The young man could not believe that a man without a car would do such a thing, and one evening as he was considering making a complaint about the noise, the Polish man came over with barrowfuls of woodscraps for their fire.

Labour came abruptly. The young man abandoned the twentieth century novel for the telephone. His wife began to black the stove. The midwife came and helped her finish the job while he ran about making statements that sounded like queries. His wife hoisted her belly about the house, supervising his movements. Going outside for more wood, he saw, in the last light of the day, the faces at each fence. He counted twelve faces. The Macedonian family waved and called out what sounded like their best wishes.

As the night deepened, the young woman dozed between contractions, sometimes walking, sometimes shouting. She had a hot bath and began to eat ice and demand liverwurst. Her belly rose, uterus flexing downward. Her sweat sparkled, the gossamer highlit by movement and firelight. The night grew older. The midwife crooned. The young man rubbed his wife's back, fed her ice and rubbed her lips with oil.

And then came the pushing. He caressed and stared and tried not to shout. The floor trembled as the young woman bore down in a squat. He felt the power of her, the sophistication of her. She strained. Her face mottled. She kept at it, push after push, assaulting some unseen barrier, until suddenly it was smashed and she was through. It took his wind away to see the look on the baby's face as it was suddenly passed up to the breast. It had one eye on him. It found the nipple. It trailed cord and vernix smears and its mother's own sweat. She gasped and covered the tiny buttocks with a hand. A boy, she said. For a second, the child lost the nipple and began to cry. The young man heard shouting outside. He went to the back door. On the Macedonian side of the fence, a small queue of bleary faces looked up, cheering, and the young man began to weep. The twentieth century novel had not prepared him for this.

And Then a Funny Thing Happened
John Stapleton

At 9.15 a.m. already running late, everything looked tawdry, the colours just plain wrong. A Qantas 747 was taking off half a kilometre away. They watched it climb in the winter wash. Red kangaroos in industrial skies, poetry out of chaos, promises never fulfilled. The din was unbelievable. Assured by the Federal Airports Commission that things would improve for their long-neglected suburb when the new runway went in, at a mere cost of $320 million, things had instead got decidedly worse. The children cowered in the park. Conversations stopped. Television shows were viewed in gaps made by thunder. I wish I was on it right now, Anna whinged for the umpteenth time, putting his own discontent into words for him to reject. He just wanted to get to work. Being late every morning of his life made him conspicuous, which was the last thing he needed right now.

Mornings were not Anna's best time, and this morning was no exception. She was going to India the next day, having scammed a trip he couldn't afford for himself, forcing him to be the bigger person. By all means go, have a good time, I've been there several times, I'll look after the kids. Enjoy yourself. After all, you were pregnant for two years in a row, he said, co-opting her argument. Take the opportunity. We can't hold each other back just because we had children.

The truth was, he had forgotten what it was like to be on his own and wanted to remember, to think his own thoughts. There were floods of affection, of feeling wanted, settling into an identity. Becoming a man, a husband, a father. And now the anger.

'Won't you miss me?' she whined, screwing out some indication of affection from him. His thoughts were getting ruder by the day. Shut your fucking face, for Christ's sake, just shut the fuck up. 'Of course I will,' he said, his mind skating. Who was bringing who down here?

An old woman in black watched them from the other side of the road, holding her grand-daughter, fiddling with the hose, preparing, despite the worst drought in living memory and repeated warnings on the news, to wash down the concrete in front of their house. Most of the neighbourhood women completed the same ritual each morning, just as their ancestors had done in the remote white-washed villages of their birth. He didn't know her name. She was Tony's mother, recently arrived from her village on the other side of the world. She didn't speak a word of English. Tony, tubby, plain, trapped by an even plainer wife, driving an old, once flashy, metal tank of a car, was his favourite neighbour. He was the only one who would lend him money when things got bad.

Bound by an industrial estate, an airport, a highway and the most polluted river in the country, this part of Tempe was a pocket of late nineteenth-century working cottages whose charm had been totally desecrated by the Macedonian and Yugoslav emigres squeezed there by property prices. Brick cladding and concrete drives were symbols of success in a new country. He and Anna had bought what they regarded as the best house in Tempe, an 1880s wooden farm house. They had sanded the floors, added a verandah, planted dozens of trees all round. His neighbours came to commiserate. They had been young once, and hadn't been able to afford cladding either.

'Stop complaining', he snapped, fumbling as he tried to strap in the kids, even more annoyed than usual at the useless seatbelts.

It had been a long winter, his lungs hurt and the rank smell of unleaded petrol enveloped the house.

After a lifetime of being out, of travel and adventure, just going to work, battling through the traffic and the days just to spend the evenings at home, felt very commonplace. He had become a cliché, the journalist who wanted to write. The cardpack of dreams had vanished at the same time as his life had become full with the love and complexity of a woman and the endless demands of children. There was no question now of giving up his job. There were financial worries, distractions, nights when he went to bed too early and could barely remember the man who didn't like to go to bed at all. For the first time in his life there was responsibility for the lives of others. With a one- and two-year-old crawling over him constantly, adoring ever-demanding worms—my daddy's a good boy, Sammy would shout loudly—it began to seem as if reading was for childless people. He was becoming illiterate. He had been reared in a magical realm, taught by books that there were greater, loftier ideals than daily work rituals and keeping a roof over his head.

Anna looked weary. 'I'll be so glad to be going, to get

away from you all,' she shouted over the noise of the plane. She would say anything to wound. Meeting him, having Sammy and Henrietta, were the worst things that had ever happened to her. She was determined to let him know what a colossal failure he was. It was his fault they weren't rich, living like the people in her favourite magazine, *Vanity Fair*. You'd think, the way Anna went on, she'd been living on the Champs Elysées being courted by fabulously rich, wonderfully entertaining, beautiful European playboys rather than in a flat above a rock band in Surry Hills, Sydney, Australia. 'I lost my youth when I met you,' she said; and when he failed to respond: 'I can't stand the way you just stand there.' He bowed his head under the tirade and counted the hours. Go, by all means go!

It wasn't just his own hypocrisies, the stabs of passion and memory—the sexual trace elements, guilty, pornographic images—or the uncertainties that he felt over his love for her that bothered him, but the hypocrisies of everyone. He was sick to death of Sydney. The too-bright harbour, the soulless business heart, the idiot tourists gawking in the Cross, the rotten little junkies, the wasted displays, the North Shore middle class, their truly horrid wealth and self-possession, he was sick of the whole damn lot.

It hadn't always been so.

The past was one of surviving on the street as young men have always survived, of never having sex without a gain, usually material, shifting through endless relationships and casting himself loose in gay bars. Sydney had acted as a spectacular backdrop to his own wild adventures, the dazzling light of the bays and the beaches silhouetting his own enthusiasms. He emerged before the moustachioed clones and the claims of pride. In those whispering, furtive times it had been like entering a secret, underground society.

AND THEN A FUNNY THING HAPPENED

There was a sense of adventure, of singularness, a belonging in their outrageousness among the crowds he met. But so many of the figures that cut a swathe through those bars and late-night coffee shops were doomed. Happy endings were few. Successful couples unknown. Love, which he did not seek, was chaotic, dark. His was an age-old curse. Limp wrists and perversion, a lingering self-hatred. Gay men weren't strutting the sidewalks and sweating it out in the gyms, but perched on bar stools, convinced they were aberrant, not true men. They swallowed the lie, the beliefs of their taunters. Their faces did not glow with health or confidence. They reached deep inside, and waved in everyone's face their own deviance. Michael passed among them, seeking experience, in love with all their personal demons.

To be a queen became for them an honourable title, a badge to be worn with inverse pride. When he first began there was no Mardi Gras, no gay pride, no Oxford Street. There weren't gay saunas or bookshops or coffee houses, newspapers or magazines. Instead he entered a wonderful, subterranean world, where a drag queen trailed a finger across his cheek and told him how beautiful he would look in a dress, a world where he was instantly popular, a million miles from the soulless suburb where he grew up. It didn't take long for the poison to arrive. Through the dream, the discovery which went on for years, person after person flung themselves at him, declaring undying love. Their deaths or their threatened suicides became the ultimate emotional blackmail. Yet another he had spurned died the day after, drinking a bottle of scotch before noon and collapsing right in the middle of Sydney's most famous gay bar. For months afterwards the boy's friends screamed at him out of car windows, blaming him. It was easy to believe that he was inherently evil, that to love him was to court bleak disaster.

He had always been wanted. He never had to worry

about where the next drink was coming from. There was always someone who wanted to make love to him. Adopt him. From the first time, in a back alley of the motor show when he had wandered away from his father and his brother, lonely and upset and bewildered by the chaos of pubescence. A man had been kind, interested, listened to him. Had led him away from the crowd, up a back alley. Had kissed him. He had been completely astonished when the man's face had disappeared to below his belt. Desperate to lose his virginity, he nonetheless had no idea what was happening. He'd never heard of oral sex. While he had looked up homosexuality in the *Britannica*, he had no idea what the act involved. He tucked the man's telephone number into his school trousers, and rang it a fortnight later, at the beginning of the school holidays.

While men were readily available, the opposite sex remained a mystery. None of the girls at school would go out with him, though he screwed up courage several times and asked. In a beachside suburb he was the ultimate weirdo—he read books. He watched the other boys in the showers after Physical Education, intoxicated, frightened, curious. His classmates sent him up, taunted him, picked fights. Hit me with your handbag, hit me with your handbag. He could hear the chant in the roar of the surf, high in the pine trees. Hit me ... Hit me ... Later he found out his worst tormentor was simply jealous and had only discovered his predilections because he was getting off after school with the same man.

Around the Cross all the boys pretended they were straight and only on the game for the money. He could never admit his attraction for his friends. They would all pretend there was a girl waiting for them round the corner. He played the part too, or got very coy when his own sex life was discussed. Try as he might, he still hadn't managed to lose his heterosexual virginity. Still, there was no shortage of men. There was always a sugar daddy dangling. He went from one to the next, worshipping at the knees of corrupt saints. He wanted to be looked after. The hostility of his father, the belt snaking out towards him, the endless brutal anger, the absolute lack of affection, was replaced by an ancient kindness. He lapped it up. He was always so pissed by the time he ended up in bed he couldn't have cared less who or what was gobbling him off, as long as he had a bed for the night. They would buy him cars, rent apartments, take him out to dinner, listen as he told them, drunk and excited, of all the things he was going to do in life. Old men, young boys, it was a time-honoured relationship. He learnt a lot from them. Some did their best by him, encouraged him to go back to school, to read books, listen to music. Took him to concerts, restaurants. Paid his school fees and later university expenses. It wasn't just sex they wanted, though they always wanted that. Their physical repulsiveness was overstepped by emotional intricacies. They all wanted to be loved, and the preposterousness of expecting love in return from a sixteen-year-old boy never struck them.

As he grew older things changed. Once the serial subject of unrequited love, now it was his turn to experience the agony of wanting someone who didn't want him. Desperately in love with a painter who didn't want to know about him, he made a complete, desperate fool of himself. Shattered self-esteem led him to weepy, melancholic dawns across the white terraced houses and the flowering frangipani of Paddington. At the same time the experience of being gay in Sydney was changing, becoming less singular as a gay culture and identity developed. No longer unique but communal, he longed for love, a relationship, a type of marriage. He wanted desperately to have a boyfriend, to be part of a couple. He didn't want to be single any more. He mooned though a succession of bumbled affairs, young men standing awkwardly in the back yard, waiting for him to make the move ... I was thinking of making a pass at you ... Were you now?

Then, one of his regular sweeps through Adelaide, where he went probably twice a year to hang around with old friends and where, to his great amusement, he accessed a different class of art queens, it finally happened. He met someone fresh, new to the scene, ripe for love. They lasted together nine years. Other people always remembered them arguing. But there were good times as well, sticky intimacy, fun, exploration. With his continuing lack of professional success, he thought of the relationship with Martin, his love, their togetherness, their coupledom, as one of his greatest achievements. He wanted it to be ideal, to go on forever, to rise above the physical, the material. With a certain megalomania, for these were still very much uncharted waters, there being no rules for gay relationships at a time when everything was up for discussion, theirs was to be one of the great, historic loves. Though what he went through seemed utterly singular, it followed a pattern, the seven stages of gay relationships: attraction, sexual fascination, intimacy, familiarity, habituation, disillusionment, break-up. At first everything was gripped with meaning, the world and his place in it, as a rush of new love tingled through him and they seemed forever to be running towards each other. They went for long walks through his favourite place in the Adelaide Hills, a huge old ruined nursery where fields of jonquils and daffodils had gone wild. There followed years of living together. Travelling in a great arc across the world, when they couldn't have been closer. Living in London. Becoming as one. To the final chaotic days when Martin always had an interest that wasn't him, some bit of fluff on

AND THEN A FUNNY THING HAPPENED

Saturday night, a blond hairdresser to while away the afternoons, constant, ghastly triangles. When he slammed doors and broke furniture and threw books out windows. Smashed Martin's windscreen and tried to run him over. When he could finally take it no longer, in a staggering series of months where he left for India without telling him beforehand and came back because he missed him. Finally they broke up for the last time. He felt utterly destroyed, truly believed it was the worst thing that had ever happened to him.

And then he had been alone.

It was the days of the Mardi Gras now, when gay pride was everywhere. At the same time his peers started to die of AIDS. He felt trapped by the new definitions. He was from a different time zone. The new politics only reached so far in the confused babble. Somewhere, during his long bouts of heavy drinking, he had adopted the earlier beliefs of his old drinking buddies, to be gay was somehow to be corrupt, his sex a sickness. Crowds of old friends were dying, and the darkness of those sad days, with so many talented people ending in the most miserable of ways, echoed with his own irredeemable past. There was someone evil, vicious and camp inside. He found himself, deeply drunk on black bourbon and cokes, laughing inside a fat, corrupt body, lisping inappropriately. His mannerisms went limp-wristed, his eyes took on an understanding, worldly-wise look.

And then a very funny thing happened.

Bewildered, drunk, taking too many drugs and swilling too much bourbon through the small hours, he started to fall apart. He ended up in detox. Twice.

When he got out the world was a different place. For the first time in his life he was lonely. He was older. No longer could he just sit on a bar stool and wait for someone to buy him a drink. His idea of picking someone up, getting completely wasted and seeing whom he woke up with in the morning, didn't work any more. He didn't have to barely look sideways to pick someone up. He hung around with recovering alcoholics and addicts in coffee shops, briefly intrigued by the new scene. Most of the men were younger than him, boasting energetically of their adventures with women.

He started looking at girls.

And just as he did Anna showed up.

They'd been sitting in a coffee shop with a group of people; someone had been going on and on about twelve-step programs, born again. The wonders of self-improvement, taking control of your own life. They exchanged glances. And the thought occurred to him immediately. I could sleep with her.

She was pretty and had a nice smile and they slept together on their first date. They had sat up on the balcony of his apartment at three a.m., one of the best views of Sydney laid out beneath them. It had been time to go home or to go to bed. And she had shown no inclination to leave.

He'd been so nervous.

The greatest surprise was that it had been so enjoyable. Much to his relief, things worked in bed the way they were meant to. He found her erotic. He wanted to fuck her.

It was news to him that he could conduct a successful relationship with a woman, but the romance had blossomed. It wasn't love like the first love, but he was happy in a way he hadn't been for a long time. She was good fun. He was proud to be going out with her, enjoyed being with her.

One Sunday afternoon, luxuriating in a well-earned day off—he normally worked Sundays—they sat drinking lemon squash on his balcony, high in his eyrie above the view he loved so much: the huddle of Woolloomooloo terraces below leading out to the peeling Finger Wharf, the ferries picking their way through the white sails of the yachts, the distant thunder of the trains as they crossed the famous coat hanger of the Bridge, Kirribilli and the northern suburbs behind.

I'd like to have children some day, he said, making it casual.

She looked surprised, said nothing.

It was true, in an abstract sense. It had been true for years. Something missing. A fundamental instinct. He wasn't brave enough to say, I would like to have children with you.

She believed in monogamy. He had grown up in the seventies, when envy and ownership were the greatest sins, but there had always been part of him that was instinctively monogamous. He felt far more comfortable going to bed with someone he was relaxed and familiar with, the exact opposite to the prevailing bar ethos. The thought of abandoning what he regarded as his fundamental right to sleep with whomever he liked whenever he liked, to deny himself the need, even the requirement of his chosen art to experience all, especially the intimacy of others, struck him at first as profoundly odd. Martin had certainly been no believer in monogamy. He had always argued for an open relationship, sexual friendships. In their travels together Martin had always regarded sex with the locals as an essential part of the experience of foreign places. What did it matter, as long as the core was secure. The trouble was, the core was never secure. Although it sometimes worked well, all too often he felt like the long-suffering, deeply humiliated, homely wife, turning her head away, ignoring the affairs of her husband. Putting up with it because the other option was to be entirely alone.

In the end monogamy was a deep relief. He didn't have

to put up with the humiliation of living with someone with a constantly wandering eye, the insecurity of endless triangular relationships. His ability to love her without worrying about who was round the corner was part of his growing confidence. He no longer had to go to parties with his partner, and wonder if they would be leaving together, publicly shamed once more. The introductions. This is my boyfriend, though whether he desires me as much as you, whether he will be sleeping with me tonight, is a moot point. He had had a gutful of so-called open relationships.

Days rolled into months. He didn't want to be trapped by the past, chained by definition. He didn't see any reason to mention another life. Whenever he and Anna talked of the past he was very vague. Omission didn't seem dishonest.

Then some kind soul, one of his flatmates in fact, blurted it out to her, But I thought he was gay!

Anna had gone white with shock. She had no idea. It wasn't the era to be sleeping with bisexuals, certainly not without a condom. His HIV had been negative and he assumed he had been safe because he didn't like being fucked and had had a steady boyfriend through the periods of high transmission. But she wasn't to know that.

We've got to talk, she said, in one of those tones which have driven fear into men's hearts since time immemorial, there's something about your past that I know and you don't think I know.

In the future there would be gnawing jealousies and uncertainties, but at the time she was a model of how someone should behave in such a situation. I just want you to know that who you're with at the moment is who you're with, and the rest doesn't matter, she said. With someone else the revelation could have destroyed the relationship. With her it didn't.

They moved in together.

Within hours of moving in she told him: I'm pregnant, again.

She'd already had one miscarriage, falling pregnant within weeks of his first declaration that children were an option. Within days of telling him she miscarried, which solved the dilemma of trying to work out what to do. In any normal sense they simply hadn't known each other long enough. He got very pissed and cried in the pub. He had wanted the baby, no matter what. She sat up in bed with tears in her eyes. Someone was missing, someone had gone. There was a strangely intense passion in their lovemaking in the days after she recovered, as if she was deliberately trying to get pregnant again. There was nothing rational about it. They had barely known each other three months. Later, they were always puzzled how it had come about, how they had landed so solidly together, in such a way that they couldn't imagine life without each other. They would never advise anyone to do what they had done. It was only luck that things had worked out as well as they had. He had never even met her family before she fell pregnant with Sammy.

It was around then that he truly began to love her, caught in some sort of destiny bigger than them both. He did not feel in control. He tried to downplay what was happening. After the disaster of Martin, he didn't want to get hurt. He was still getting used to the idea of a heterosexual relationship. He enjoyed the sex as much as or more than he had had with anyone in his life. It was so nice, felt so gratifyingly normal, to have a straightforward fuck. His sexuality had frozen on a few old images, and now it was moving again.

The only thing he missed was the excitement of intimacy with strangers and the tumult of the bars. Though sexual partners weren't exactly plentiful, and picking people up for a bit of abandoned, casual sex hadn't been his forte, he had assumed he would miss sex with men. He didn't.

Four months after giving birth to Sammy, Anna was pregnant again. He talked her out of having an abortion.

Before they knew it, they had two kids and their lives had changed utterly and irrevocably.

They settled for the full suburban nightmare, the car, the mortgage, the endless bills. He abandoned the past, keeping few friends through the change. He bunged on the normal bloke routine, wore working boots, swaggered when he could have minced, worked hard in his own introverted, torturedly honest way as a reporter on the paper, achieving a certain recognition, readability linked elegantly with the landscape or the nature of the event, the strings of facts. But in the past few months he couldn't face his own life any more. His internal contradictions were reaching some kind of impasse ... 'Couldn't you help me with this fucking seatbelt,' he shouted accusingly.

She glared at him hatefully. 'Oh god, I just can't wait to go!'

He roared off without looking back. Things were going bad between them and he felt he was getting the raw end of the deal. He looked after the kids in the morning, put them to bed at night, worked all day. She'd hang around the house, gossiping to girlfriends on the phone, ignoring her university work, acting like a member of the oppressed if she had to pick up a broom. With the kids in childcare her load wasn't exactly heavy.

A semitrailer belched smoke in front of them. The window was broken and there was nothing he could do to avoid the fumes. His eyes watered as he coughed, and behind him in his car seat little Sammy, normally bright and eager and happy, also coughed, his asthma getting worse. Arguments disturbed him. He liked everything to be in place. He loved his DaddyMike and AnnaMum.

'Daddy, I don't believe anybody any more,' he said, his two-year-old face serious, upset.

'That's a funny thing to say, Sammy.'

'I don't believe anybody any more,' he repeated.

'Why do you say that?'

'I just do.'

The following day everything happened at once.

Anna left, the plan being that when he and the kids came home she would no longer be there. Discreet, almost accidental, they were trying to make the departure as undramatic as possible. On the same day Henrietta and Sammy were starting at a new childcare centre, away from the Lebanese woman who had been caring for them while Anna went to university.

On top of everything, it somehow didn't surprise him somehow that this was the day he got a pep talk from the vicious little closet queen who paraded as a news editor, the first pep talk he'd ever had in his life.

'It's a long time since you've surprised us,' he said. Yeah, it's a long time since I've been surprised, he thought, you fucking little creep. You have no idea what it's like to write to daily deadlines, year in, year out.

Alone at last, and despite being saddled with children, he looked for ways to exploit his freedom. Though not a sexual thing, he missed some of the dizzy drunken madness of the gay scene. Preparations for Mardi Gras were well underway. Although it was decidedly easier being heterosexual, just in the way people treated him as a normal person and not a performing clown, it was if, nothing else, odd not to have that gay identity any more. It was so much a part of you, how could you turn your back on it all, Martin had asked. Easily, he thought. He hadn't twisted his sexuality into politically correct shapes, hadn't come to it through a bourgeois desire for experimentation, difference.

For him sex with men had never been a statement of rejection of middle-class norms, it had been born of emotional chaos.

He couldn't quite see how he could go to the Mardi Gras with the two young ones, but he would have liked the almost therapeutic abandonment of the occasion. Perhaps the mother-in-law could mind the kids. He roped his friend Stephen into helping him with them on some of the after-work cruise arounds to openings and launches in the month-long Mardi Gras arts festival leading up to the parade. They were certainly the only children at most of the events, a statement which appealed to Stephen. Whereas in the past these events would have been just the beginning of a long night out, they always had to leave early as he headed home to get the kids to bed. Stephen was one of his few old gay friends who had accepted his shift in sexuality. Most of them thought he was no longer being true to himself. If a married man left his wife and took up on the scene, he was applauded. If you moved the other way, you were a betrayer, of yourself, of the community. 'I've got two kids now,' he'd told an old friend proudly one night, shortly after Henrietta's birth. 'I don't know you any more,' the friend said, and walked away.

He went with Stephen and the kids to the opening of the Mardi Gras art show. Martin, still the ultimate culture vulture, was there, soaking it all up. Courage in the face of AIDS. Our growing identity. Our tragedy. Death in brotherhood.

They nodded at each other, said nothing. The brutal, devastating times hovered unspoken between them, the days when all his hopes, everything he had wanted, had centred in the other person, and had disintegrated entirely. He had always thought that if he ever saw Martin again he'd fucking kill him. But it wasn't like that. It was almost therapeutic.

There were paintings about love and death and sex all around them. It was hot and hard finding a beer in a sea of champagne. They sensed each other but didn't say a word. There was too much between them to be forgiven. The sense of betrayal was too deep. For a long time he had never thought it would reach this stage, thought they would be friends if not lovers for life.

What had passed between them, was passing between them, was trivial in this world where there were deeper themes. Grief, the human spirit, enormous courage, the saddest of deaths of men far too young to die. Friends and acquaintances had gone by the dozen, a whole stratum of Sydney life. They weren't ready to go.

It was only a month since Bruce had died. Headboy, as he had been known, was a big handsome strapping lad who hadn't been ready to go. Much of the inner city was plastered with Headboy graffiti. His ultimate dream had been to be in a rock band. Headboy got in a few gigs before he got too sick to perform any more. He, Michael, would go round and visit him, sit in his public housing flat, feel the silence lap around them. It was so difficult to know what to say. *How you feeling? Cheer up, things will get better.* Things patently were only going to get worse. Angry at everything, Headboy made no effort to make his visitors feel comfortable. He was dying and didn't like one fucking thing about it. In and out of hospital for months, he could only envy the health of others. On his last day Michael went to see him in hospital. As he walked down the corridor towards the ward some of Headboy's friends were walking the other way. 'It's too late,' they said, tears in their eyes.

Sometimes he sat in the pub and heard stories of the different people he used to know. Matthew, a wild boy round the place, loved a joint, loved a drink, hated work, had said, twisting his thumb and forefinger together, a bitchy little fucker when he wanted to be, you know what this is mate, the smallest joint in the world, and it's rolled just for you. They always got plastered. Sometimes they grew close, in conversation, in alcohol. He bounced from pillar to post. Lived the life. Then he was skeletal, very sick. Inexorably, it came time to go. He gathered his three remaining friends at his flat, said his goodbyes. It was the cruellest of things. Drunk, he shot $400 worth of smack. In the end they had to smother him with a cushion.

In the crowd the kids clung close. Unlike the old days, he didn't know many people to talk to. It grew crowded and claustrophobic. He caught glimpses. It had seemed like love at the time. Now all he felt was anger at the wasted years. And relief it was over. Who'd want that life anyway? Leaving was the best thing he'd ever done, and he could never imagine being so demeaned ever again.

He talked to someone he'd once known quite well, now a writer of reputation with a new book out, *The Comfort of Men*. The carnival of bodies, the tribal eroticism, all seemed such a long way away, a long time ago.

'What have you been doing?' Dennis asked.

'Breeding,' Michael said, gesturing, both arms full with children.

'I was trying not to act surprised,' Dennis said.

'It's nice to have their mother away; I needed the space,' he said, a little pissed from the champagne. Buttering up to the boys who always like to hear stories about how badly any relationship with a woman was going. 'Now I've got the mother-in-law.'

The gathering reached a point where no more champagne could be got, the kids grew grizzlier and grizzlier, and he had to go. Stephen helped him get the kids into the car, and he knew he did not go unnoticed—he saw Martin standing glass in hand on the pavement chatting to

Dennis. He struggled the kids into the old bomb he'd outgrown but couldn't afford to replace. Martin, pretending not to watch, watched every move, taking in the cool air, his head at that particular, arrogant angle he had learnt to dislike so much.

He dropped Stephen off at the house in Erskineville he shared with his boyfriend, dropped the kids off with the mother-in-law and went out. He had every intention of getting completely pissed. The babble of the bars, the deep darkness of bourbon and cokes, could always be guaranteed to distract him. In losing himself, he found himself, perched on bar stools, gossiping to new acquaintances or old.

I dreamt of you, out there on the front, David, an old drinking buddy, said, referring to the Gulf War which had fascinated them both. I dreamt we made love, right there on the battlefield. There were guns going off all around, tracers in the sky. There were soldiers, hunky, in all the trenches, and you, with your reporter's pad, and I was fantastically pleased to see you. He laughed and tried to shrug him off; David was always so embarrassing the way he gushed at him. For no particular reason he had always avoided sleeping with him.

David was always propped on a bar stool somewhere, an artist of sorts, sympathetic but useless. It was hard to turn away from someone who was telling you what a fabulous person you were, even if he was drunk and tiresome.

You had ash on your face, and grease, and the sky was turning white from a Scud missile, and you were just fabulous, you loved me so much.

He tried to look away, embarrassed, and David grabbed his face in his hands and said, 'Don't be like that with me, I'm just telling you how I feel.'

A few more drinks and he escaped. It was nice to go home, to sleep alone.

The night of the Mardi Gras came. He was covering it for the paper. He didn't bother to meet up with the photographer. The night had become so vast it no longer mattered whether words matched pictures. Pad in hand, a couple of drinks under his belt, he wandered down to the beginning of the parade. He picked out old people and those with children, asked them why they were there. They all glowed with enthusiasm. This one event had done more to alter the attitude towards gays and lesbians than anything else.

Then he started interviewing people in the parade itself as they stood waiting for it to begin. There were the North Coast fairies, out to have the time of their life, fluorescent, tight, crotch accentuating board shorts, brown bodies finely muscled, the drugs already beginning to work. There were the political groups. The AID support groups. The suburban groups. The Bi-sexual Network. The leather queens in cages. Then they were off. Armed with his press pass, he walked with them, through the long cheering corridor of people. He remained detached, but it was impossible not to be carried away by the wild exuberance of it all, the eccentric and the wonderful, the Diesel Dykes, the Fruits on Loops, the girls in the pink Chevrolet. Work it, girls, work it, a loudspeaker admonished. A fat hairy drag queen beamed with exhaustion and excitement at the crowd. A drunken caricature of a builder, the weight of a hammer pulling his working shorts down below his crack, fell over in front of him, staggered to his feet and lurched on. The crowd couldn't contain themselves. Parts of the night, of the visual spectacle, took him to another plane, his own quiet life left far behind.

Too soon it was over. Those with tickets went on to the post-parade party. This was the main event. Everything else was a prelude. Sleeping was for the living vegetables, the truly duller than the dull. This was the centre. The entrants in the parade disappeared into the great maw of the Showground, into their personal nights of promise, pinnacles of high times, abandonment, hours of non-stop dancing, the promise of sex everywhere. Truly the best of times. Not even his position as the man covering the event for the city's most prestigious paper had done anything to help procure a ticket.

He went to the post-parade press conference, drank a free beer, took notes as the chairwoman proclaimed it, as he or she did each year, the most successful and problem-free Mardi Gras ever.

Shortly after he was standing in the middle of Taylor Square, watching the crowds scatter, the clean-up crews go into action, when he found himself standing next to Louis. They'd met more than twenty years before when they were both impoverished adolescents in London with nowhere to live. They'd spent one long night riding the tubes, catching trains just to stay warm.

He had not expected to see Louis ever again, was surprised to run across him back in Australia several years after their first stray encounter. He never bothered to make anything more out of the acquaintance but had continued to run into him every few years, one of the stray filaments of encounter which made up his life.

He compared notes on the evening, at the same time watching the crowds still dispersing. The pubs were deliberately shut, waiting for the potentially trouble-causing straights from the suburbs to return to their breeding grounds, the heterosexual heartlands. The street was carpeted with beer cans and trash. The lights of the sweeping machines turned the street yellow, adding malice, turning the crowd into looming giants. Men in white overalls were already in action. It would take hours to find a taxi. There was no point in even trying to go home now. If he did he would be walking.

'I've got some free vouchers for the Love Art shop,' Louis ventured after a while. 'You want to come and check it out?'

'Anything special goes on there?' he asked.

'There are booths and a live sex show. Every now and then a bit of straight trade gets there, really spunky guys. Football players. They're gorgeous. So naive. So randy. They just love having their dicks sucked, their girlfriends won't do it for them. I've had some good times there, it's the luck of the draw.'

So they walked on down to Love Art.

Although in one brief incarnation he had worked as a sex shop attendant, his typewriter perched on the glass cabinet of dildos, such places always made him feel uncomfortable. He was immediately embarrassed to be there, hated to think that he would appear as one of the desperates, genuinely seeking orgasm amidst the grime, rather than possessing the comfort of an observer. So much for the abandonment of Mardi Gras. Already there were quite a number of men milling about, the ticketless. Most of them were middle-aged, none was attractive. Louis knew the attendants, chatted on. He was obviously a regular.

After five minutes they were upstairs. It was pretty tacky. Men stood around in the corridors outside booths. They were all waiting for something, the heat to start working, lurid passion in dark corners, voyeurs and participants, the magic of hormones and muffled gasps. Again Louis knew people, and introduced him to a few. Then Louis dolled out some of his discount tokens, explaining that the live show would be starting soon and he needed the tokens to be able to watch it. A series of booths circled what he soon discovered was a stage.

It's started, Louis said, pointing him into a booth and then disappearing.

AND THEN A FUNNY THING HAPPENED

He went in. The booth enclosed him, in front a blank screen. He had never been in this situation before, didn't know what to do. He put in a coin. The screen lit up. There was a young man on the stage, in underpants, dancing, a pile of porn books in the corner to encourage his erection. He kept looking down as he danced, a small cassette radio on the floor. He was Mediterranean in appearance, wearing sweaty grey underpants. He was wanking as he danced, only half-aroused, invisible eyes watching, assessing. It must be damn hard keeping it up, he thought, more than enough to make me shrivel, discerning, demanding eyes scraping the skin off your cock and your ass. With a clank the screen went blank. He put in more tokens. The performance was continuing. He didn't know how to behave. There was enough of a voyeur in him to find it vaguely erotic, or at least interesting, but he also felt very uncomfortable and out of place. He'd rather be in bed with someone he loved, despite the hard times, not lined up with the desperates, their orgasms devoid of affection.

The screen went blank again and he put in another token. The performance was getting hotter, slowly. The boy was at least a little more aroused. He seemed to be paying particular attention to him, pulling down the screen that connected the booth to the stage so that he didn't have to keep putting in tokens. Giving him a freebie. He knew even less what to do. He watched the guy dancing, flirting, pulling down his jocks and letting them back up, revealing what there was to reveal. There were cubicles all around him, the uglies watching.

He felt a sudden wave of claustrophobia, didn't want to be there any more. He had lost track of where Louis was. Bewildered by his own lack of interest, he took one last look and exited the cubicle. There were still men standing around. Dark. Red paint. Dust. Underground eroticism. He didn't feel any sense of gay pride. He fled down the stairs, into the street, giving away the remainder of his tokens to someone as he left. He couldn't get out of there fast enough. There wasn't any question of saying goodbye to Louis. He didn't know where he had vanished to.

The street hit him in a wave of disoriented light. The crowds were still dissipating, groups wandering around looking for action. He had emerged from something secret, intimate, furtive, far from the glorification of gay sexuality which had been so much a part of the formal part of the night. In back rooms, saunas and back alleys the grumblings and grunts, encounters to be savoured and boasted about, would go on till dawn. At least for a while the loneliness would be ripped away. He didn't care. He'd had too many rapid encounters, met too many bastards who just wanted to unload. He felt no personal sense of belonging. The days were gone when he would emerge blinking, tripping, part of the grand adventure, the great random congress of the night. He kept on walking, away from the Mardi Gras, the triumphs of the night, other people's triumphs. The centre of things was somewhere else.

Anna came home several days later, a week earlier than scheduled. Though he had not been physically unfaithful, mentally he had had his spree. His desires to escape the confines of married life had been fulfilled. The kids were overwhelmingly excited to see their mother, rushing into her arms. After weeks of no physical contact it was a pleasure to wrap his arms around someone, to be caught up in an embrace, the kids hugging them at the same time. Inside, something had broken. He accepted now that he was in love, a couple, that this was his path. That there weren't alternatives, other loves just waiting for him to change his mind.

That night they made love like they hadn't done for a very long time, if ever. It felt completely right. There was a renewed passion in everything he did. He'd forgotten how wonderful it could feel. 'I love you,' he whispered, lying back, spent, kissing her again, her hair damp. He didn't want anything else any more.

He listened to her stories of Calcutta, New Delhi, Jaipur. She unloaded bags of Indian cloth. Hung a brightly coloured Punjabi wedding tent under the ceiling of the verandah. All the nastiness, the bitterness as they turned in on each other, had gone. 'I really missed you, missed the kids,' she said, after having been so keen to get away. She, too, now seemed to accept that the cards they had been dealt—their relationship, the children, the house—weren't a mistake after all. The kids were delighted to have their mother back, running up and down the hallway screaming with excitement. The house took on a semblance of order again. They were a family once more. He couldn't make love often enough, couldn't get enough of her. All the troubles of the past vanished. He felt happier than he had ever been.

Life settled back to normal. The following Monday, at 9.15 a.m., already running late, everything looked tawdry, the colours just plain wrong. The drum of the planes taxiing to their hangars came through the open windows. 'I could really do with a hand with the kids,' he said through the bedroom door. 'You can go back to bed for the rest of the day, for all I care.' 'Can't you deal with them for Christ's sake,' she moaned. 'I do everything else.' 'Oh, sure. Come on', he said, completely exasperated, 'it's not much to ask.' 'I'll get up in a minute,' she said, and he knew she wouldn't. He pulled on the kids' pants, searched desperately for a pair of matching shoes, the clock ticking away. The news editor, balding head, white pressed shirt, had been on his back more than ever the past week. He herded Sammy and Henrietta into the car, went through the usual drama trying to find the car keys. There was another life, there had been another life, and it wasn't his any longer. He found the keys and stamped down the hallway. 'Thanks for your help,' he shouted as he slammed the door. It was then he discovered he had a flat tyre. Unfortunately that had been his fabricated excuse for being late just the other day. They'd never buy it, not twice in a row. A Thai Airways 747 was climbing into the sky a kilometre away. Family or no family, he wished he was on it.

Where the Mine Was
John Dale

It grew dark early that afternoon. He was at the back of the house stacking firewood and saw the huge black clouds muscling in over the town and out along the crooked sealed road to where the mine was. He worked harder, piling armfuls of logs hard up against the back porch. From the edge of the bush two black currawongs eyed him suspiciously. He went inside and washed his hands in the kitchen sink as rain began to spit at the windows.

The stew pot was bubbling on the stove. He lifted the lid and stirred thick bits of sweet potato and kangaroo meat around with a long wooden spoon. 'Dinner's ready!' he called and his wife came through in her bluey and faded work jeans, clutching her green helmet in one hand. 'How is she?' she said.

'Fine, Ray. Sleeping like a baby.'

'Good.' He ladled her dinner into a deep bowl and broke out some bread. They talked of what was happening at the mine while she ate. Two more days to go before he was due back on shift. A Valiant growled past the house and pulled up at the end of the street. AC/DC was pouring from the open doorway opposite and half a dozen four-wheel drives and utes were parked with their wheels up on the footpath.

Ray took a Boags draught from the fridge and went over to the window. The curtains were wide open and he could see men from B shift drinking out on the front lawn of that new primary teacher's house.

'You filled my thermos, honey?' Tanita asked.

Ray nodded. 'In your crib bag.' He breathed on the windowpane and rubbed it clear with his sleeve. Rain was coming down hard now and he watched the men from B shift scatter like starlings back onto the teacher's porch. Lights flicked on in all the front windows and Bon Scott's voice got drowned out by the rain. 'I wonder if she knows what she's doing,' he said. 'Inviting those bastards over.'

Tanita squatted down beside the open fire and attacked the log with a big iron poker. Sparks leapt up onto her bluey and she brushed them off. 'Well, she's over twenty-one, otherwise they wouldn't've sent her up here.' She glanced at him as she stood up, winding a strand of her wiry black hair between her fingers.

'How come they gave her a house in the married quarters, that's what I can't figure. You remember how long we had to wait for a place?' He dragged the curtains roughly across the window. 'Tomorrow I'd like us to take a run up the coast if this weather breaks. Get some steaks, some decent coffee in. I sure get sick of that shit they sell up the store.'

Tanita picked up her green lid and her pack of twenty-fives. She swung the crib bag over her shoulder.

'It's pissing down out there,' Ray said quickly. 'You want me to ring in sick for you?' He paused. 'We could do it up on the couch the old way.'

She took her orange raincoat off the hook beside the front door and shook it out. 'You know what C shift are like. It's not worth the hassle. They got this thing at the moment 'bout women drivers taking sickies and having babies ...'

'Maybe I'll wait up for you,' he said, smiling. He followed her out to the carport and watched her pull on a pair of the company's yellow gumboots. She was a big strong woman with deep brown eyes and thick lips that looked like they were meant for kissing. Ray put his hands on her shoulders and fitted his own mouth tight against hers. 'Take care near the crusher, hon, it's going to be as slippery as hell on the road.'

'You know me, Ray. I'm a cautious woman.' She slid into the Falcon and revved the engine. Water shot out from under the tyres as she backed down the drive. The headlights arced across the roofs of the mineworkers' houses and then she was gone into the night.

For a while Ray stayed out on the doorstep, sucking on the end of a cigarette and watching the rain angle across the drive. A couple of B shift mill rats were arm-wrestling on the hood of a Landcruiser across the street. Ray flicked his butt onto the lawn and went back inside. He stuck his feet up on the round coffee table and trolled the dial on the set. *Escape from Alcatraz* was on, but he'd seen that when he was about five. He wondered if there was any channel in the world that showed decent television on Saturday night. Not out here anyway. He kicked the off-button and sat there in front of the fire listening to the rain sweep across the roof and staring into the flames.

The phone shook him awake. He sat up in the chair like a setter, blinked and then rushed down the hall to answer it. 'Ray,' a male voice said into his ear, 'that you, Raymond?'

He could hear bottles clinking and rowdy voices in the background. Janis Joplin was singing 'I need a man to love.'

'Come over and have a drink Ray.'

'Who is this? That you, Henderson?'

'There's someone here who wants to talk to you, Raymond.'

'Why don't you bastards grow up,' he said.

The voice laughed. 'What's the matter? Your wife's out on the trucks. Come and have a drink, you cunt.'

Ray jammed the phone down and stood there in the dark, his fingers resting on the receiver, his breath coming in short sharp bursts. What had she said, the bitch! He could feel his heart thumping against his ribcage. He waited for the anger to pass and then tiptoed down the hall to the second bedroom, poked his head in around the door. A nightlight glowed dimly from the far corner of the room where a dark-skinned girl of fourteen was sleeping. One of her arms dangled over the side of the pine bed and two of the fingers on her other hand were pressed against her mouth. Ray listened to the wheezing sound coming from her chest. Christ it was stuffy in here! Her nightie had pulled down over her shoulder to reveal the full curve of one small breast. Ray stared at it, fighting back the thoughts. He tried to think of the car. Of the rust in the rear panels that needed to be cut out. Anything except the sight of his stepdaughter lying there. Images rushed at him and he saw himself throwing off his clothes, taking two long strides towards the bed. He stood in the doorway imagining it all, waiting for it to pass. He knew it would. It had before. You just gave it time.

The girl stirred under the doona, 'Daddy,' she called in a sleepy voice.

It still sounded weird when she called him that. He swallowed hard, shifting his weight in the doorway. 'Yeah, hon,

Ray's here. Your chest sounds bad. Want me to get your inhaler or anything?'

'Can you bring me some water. Please.'

He went out to the kitchen and came back with a glass full. Held it up to her lips, let her drink from it like a little bird. He touched her kinked black hair with his fingers. She looked so much like her mother sometimes.

'Thanks, Ray.' Smiling up at him with open child's eyes, her small brown breast gone back now inside the nightie.

'Sleep well, Chrissie, okay.' Her asthma had grown worse since they'd moved up here to the west coast. He shut the door behind him, went down the hall and through the kitchen. He opened the back door and stepped out into the rain. Let it rain. Let it run down his hair and into his face, let it stain his pants. Standing there in the darkness cooling down. When the feelings about her had first come he'd made himself a promise. Morals weren't his big suit, but he'd sworn then that he would never touch her. Not that it stopped the feelings, but they were something you could never talk about anyway. Not with Tanita. Not with his shift mates. Sometimes he was sure that Chrissie knew, that she was wanting him to be more than just a second daddy. Four days ago he was going down to the toilet and she'd called out to him from her bedroom, called out in this grown-up voice: 'Ray, come here, Ray!' She was wearing a short tight skirt he'd never seen before, fishnet stockings. 'What do you think,' she said, turning in a circle, 'do you like it?' Of course he didn't tell her what he thought. And she'd just stood there at the edge of her unmade bed, smiling up at him like she could read his mind.

He shook the water off his hair like a dog and stepped back onto the porch. He bent down and picked up an armful of firewood. Something hairy brushed across the back of his hand and ran up his arm. Ray shuddered as a large female tarantula leapt from his shoulder into the doorway and crawled laboriously across the kitchen floor. He followed the spider inside and dropped the logs down onto the hearth in the living room. Christ, he needed a drink! Having a drink right now was the main priority. In the kitchen he yanked the fridge door open and checked the racks. Nothing. They were right out of bullets. The tarantula eyed him from above the stove as if he was the intruder. And maybe he was. Maybe they all were out here. In five years' time this whole town would just be bush again; that was a condition of the mining lease. He lit a cigarette and stood in front of the fire, his lungs kicking with the nicotine. Rain clattered on the roof and gurgled down the drainpipe. He ran his hand through his damp hair, stuck the screen up against the fire, took his sheepskin-lined coat off the rack beside the front door and left the house.

Music was playing across the road, people were laughing and the front door to her place was wide open. For half a second he toyed with the idea of crossing the road, going straight in and telling her she was crazy. There was a saying in this town that B shift would rather fight than fuck. And trouble here was just too easy to get into and too hard to climb out of. Drawing his head down into his warm fleecy collar, Ray walked up to the only hotel in town. Some of the older miners were knocking balls round the worn pool tables and nursing their small beers. They nodded at him and he returned their enthusiasm. He wondered if there was anything more lonely than a public bar on a Saturday night. He ordered a slab of Boags Bitter and two packs of Camels unfiltered. Irene, the bargranny, slapped the box down on the counter like it was nothing. 'Tanita working tonight, love?' She rang up the total in the till and turned back to the TV. *Escape from Alcatraz* was still on. Irene was going

WHERE THE MINE WAS

deaf and she had the sound turned up so loud that you could hear Clint out in the car park.

Ray walked along the side of the main road in the pissing rain, past the blackwoods and the Tassie blue gums. Way off in the distance, between two hills, he could see the lights from the mine burning yellow. Twenty-four hours a day, 365 days a year those lights burned while men, women and machines blasted, trucked and crushed the ore, then fed it down the pipe to the giant Japanese freighters waiting offshore. Sometimes when you were out walking you could feel the earth trembling under your feet.

At home he got out the bread knife, sliced the carton into four and stacked the door of the fridge with cold ones. He popped a can and sat in the dark, listening to the cars coming and going across the street. Amara Nicholls, that was her. The first time he'd laid eyes on her was at the Asian Cooking night that some of the Filipina wives had put on at the school. Ten dollars a head—all the spring rolls, chicken and fried rice you could eat. Most of the married men had gone along. She'd told him a joke that night about single men. Bears with furniture is what she'd called them. And when she'd laughed he'd looked right into her mouth. In the whole town there were maybe twenty single women compared to three hundred bears with not too much furniture. It was odd how so many of the single women gravitated towards the married guys. As if they preferred their men already house-trained. That night they talked about the mine and Windermere—a suburb down in Hobart they both knew well. He'd hardly even noticed her scarred lip then. It was funny how that never bothered him.

He reached a hand up behind his head and felt for the underwear drying on the back of the armchair. Casually he picked up a pair of Tanita's black panties and held the soft lacy cotton to his cheek, smelled the warmth from the fire.

These were new; he'd never seen these on her before. His eyes scanned the label. Tens. Tanita didn't wear tens, she wore sixteens. Ray threw the panties onto the vinyl sofa and stood up quickly. He drained his beer and went out to the fridge. Across the street he could hear the twang of a steel guitar and pounding of drums. His fingers gripped the cold metal handle, then he wrenched the door open, plucked four cans from the box and tucked them under his arm.

Out in the carport, he told himself he wouldn't stay long. Go over there, show his face for five minutes, find out what was happening. He went down the drive and crossed the road, the rain running down his forehead and off his broken nose. A miner in a blue and white checked jacket on the front lawn was holding onto the trunk of a tree, steam rising from between his legs. Ray stopped at the gate, glanced at the line of mud-streaked cars jammed in her driveway and a big shiny Harley he'd never seen before. He took a swig of Boags and went uneasily up the steps and in through the door.

An old black voice on the stereo was growling to a loud bluesy beat: 'You done me wrong.' Miners leaned against the cement-sheet walls drinking in bunches of fours and fives. Ray threaded his way between them, holding his can out in front of him so it wouldn't spill. The air was thick and blue with cigarette smoke. A pair of young miners lay face down on the floorboards, but most of B shift were standing in a tight circle, drinking, scratching and staring at something happening in the centre of the room. Ray elbowed his way through the checked jackets and peered over a broad set of shoulders at seven women dancing cheek to cheek with their partners while thirty or more single men looked on in silence. Barefoot and slender, Amara Nicholls had one arm around the waist of a large red-haired man wearing a cut-off Levi's jacket and a dirty bandanna tied around his forehead. Her eyes were half-shut and her mouth was open just a little. She rolled her head softly from side to side and clicked her thumb and finger to the beat. Ray watched as she took a big fat joint from the red-haired biker, its end glistening, and sucked the smoke deep into her lungs. The sweet smell of dope drifted overhead and a voice growled from the speaker right next to Ray's ear, 'I'm in the mood for some of your love ... ' He lifted his can to his lips, edged nearer the window, wishing now he'd stayed at home. Empty bottles and overflowing ashtrays littered the food table. The cheese platter and the bowls of chilli chips had all been pawed through. A cigarette filter poked up out of the remains of the onion dip. Ray stood there staring at Amara, her hips swaying to the music and most of the miners' eyes in that room fixed on the tight backside of her jeans.

'Ray!' she yelled suddenly. 'Raymond!'

Heads turned as she broke free of the red-haired biker's grasp and weaved through a ring of drunken miners towards him. She pressed her mouth up against his cheek and he felt the ridge of scar tissue on her top lip.

'I didn't think you were coming,' she said. She slipped a small warm hand inside his sheepskin jacket. 'I've missed you, Ray.'

'We gotta talk. Can we go somewhere?' He could sense the miners on either side of him tuning in to their conversation. 'The bears,' he whispered. 'How come you invited all the bears?'

She laughed and grabbed his elbow. 'Come on,' she said. 'I need to take a piss.' From across the room the red-haired biker watched them, thumbs hooked under the big chrome buckle on his belt. Ray glanced at the man's black riding boots. He had a bad feeling about tonight. He followed Amara down the hallway, stopped outside the bathroom door while someone inside coughed and flushed and then a drunken young mill rat staggered out doing up his zip.

Inside the bathroom Amara closed the door and flicked the catch. Hair clips, tubes of gel and different coloured fish-shaped soap lined the edge of the plastic bath. She looked at him expectantly, one eyebrow raised.

'Henderson rung me,' Ray said. He could hear the rain beating on the iron roof, a bass guitar vibrating noisily through the thin walls. He watched her unzip her Levi's 501s and peel them down as far as her knees. 'I think he's twigged to us.'

'So?' She squatted on the seat. 'It's finished, Ray. All over. It was your decision.'

'But the whole town's going to find out now,' he said. 'They'll be talking about us in the crib room.'

Amara tore off a strip of toilet paper, folded it in her fingers and wiped herself. She dropped the paper into the bowl. 'You know when I first came to this town all I used to drink was a glass of wine with a meal sometimes. Now it's a bottle every night.' She stood up. 'Three more months and I'm out of here.'

Ray stared at her thick dark bush. He was thinking of all the places they had done it. In the rainforest, down behind the primary school and best of all—out in the button grass. Anywhere that was dangerous, anywhere they ran the risk of being seen.

He said, 'I want you, Amara, I want you bad.'

She hitched up her jeans. 'What about your wife, Ray, what about all that stuff you said?' She took a step towards him and hooked her arms around his shoulders. Up close she smelled of dope and gin, and something much sweeter than both. He liked the smell of her body. That was what had attracted him from the start. He could feel his desire for her growing, the blood squeezing through his veins.

'Kiss me, Raymond.'

He pressed his lips tight up against hers, felt her tongue probe round the back of his teeth. Her zipper was open and he slipped a pair of fingers inside, worked them down under the elastic.

A fist rapped on the bathroom door. 'Hey,' a voice yelled. 'There's people busting for a leak out here!'

Amara drew his hand out slowly. Her eyes were big and green and he could see the light bulb reflected in both of them. She turned and flushed the toilet.

'We just going to walk out there together?'

'There's always the window, Ray, if you're so freaked.'

Above the showerhead a small rusted louvre window looked down onto the backyard. No way could he fit through there. He grabbed a face cloth off the rail, ran it under the cold tap. 'Okay,' he said. 'You first.'

Amara slipped the catch. A big-gutted miner clutching a bottle of stout by the neck was standing outside the door, shifting his weight from boot to boot. He took a handrolled cigarette out of the corner of his mouth and stared at the face cloth Ray had pressed over one eye.

Stepping past him, Ray said, 'I think you got most of it out.' He followed Amara down the hall, head tipped back.

In the kitchen she laughed. 'You're a bastard, Ray. I think that's why I like you.'

Ray tossed the wet face towel onto the sink. John Lee Hooker was tapping his foot slowly to the boogie and a group of older miners were huddled in the corner talking about their future. Ray looked out through a cracked glass pane at the rain coming down in sheets. He could smell her on his hand.

Amara waved an arm in the air. 'Ray, there's someone I want you to meet.'

The red-haired biker with the dirty bandanna was cutting a path through the miners towards them, his big knotted fists swinging at his sides. Ray felt the muscles in his gut tighten.

'Ray, this is Eddy. Eddy—Ray.'

Ray came up with his hand fast, thinking if the biker refused it he'd turn and walk away, but Eddy took it, gripped it hard. Deep acne scars peppered the skin underneath the man's jaw.

'You a miner?'

'Ray's a shovel-operator,' Amara said. 'He loads up the big trucks.'

'What, them fifty tonners?'

'Yeah.' Ray nodded. 'You looking for work?'

'Eddy works with me, Ray.' Amara said. 'He started last week.'

Ray blinked. 'You're a teacher?'

'We've had some problems at school. Eddy's been fantastic with the grade fives.'

'Never let the little monkeys get the drop on you.' Eddy winked. 'Wanna beer?'

Ray refocused on Eddy, getting a totally different picture of the guy. 'No, I'll get 'em.' He went over to the fridge and worked two stubbies out of someone else's pack. A voice behind him said,

'Well, well, if it ain't the A shift ladies' man.'

Ray turned. A heavily-built miner with a thick black moustache was staring at him.

'Listen, I wanna word with you, Henderson.'

Henderson grinned, displaying two missing front teeth. 'Mate, I'm all ears.'

'You're all bullshit,' Ray said. 'Don't you go ringing my house again at night. I've got a sick daughter there—'

'Better watch that kid, mate. She's gonna break a few

hearts in this town. I seen her walking up the street the other day in this tight little skirt—'

'Shut your mouth,' Ray said.

Henderson whistled, leaned his shoulders back. 'Mate, looks like I struck a nerve.'

'What are you saying?'

'Saying nothing, Raymond. You're doing all the talking.'

Ray slammed two stubbies down on the sink; glass cracked and beer dribbled down his wrist. The kitchen went quiet. Ray's heart was hammering in his chest and he felt the hairs on the back of his neck sticking up. He said, 'I want you to apologise.' The moment the words left his lips he knew they sounded ridiculous, but he was boxed into this now.

Henderson grinned at his two offsiders; the B shift pit boss never went anywhere alone. Ray could sense the older miners in the corner holding their cans still, cigarettes burning quietly off the edge of their lips.

'Mate,' Henderson said, 'Mate, all I'm doing is filling you in.'

Ray saw the smirk on his face and grabbed him by his bluey, shoved him hard backwards as a female voice called out for them to break it up. Henderson got to his feet, but he was not smiling now. A black lick of hair dangled over his dark eyes. He charged at Ray, head tucked low like a ram. Ray sidestepped and smacked an elbow in Henderson's face. It was crazy, a thirty-nine-year-old man acting like this, but deep down Ray wanted to really hurt him. They tumbled out the back door into the rain as the miners crowded around, eager for excitement. Ray could smell tobacco on Henderson's coat. His fist struck bone and he swore; Henderson came at him again, driving Ray off the path into the mud. The other men cheered as they slipped and Ray landed hard with his knees in Henderson's kidney, rolled him over like a big winded sheep and fixed both his hands around his throat.

Amara pushed her way through the crowd. 'Stop it, Ray! Stop it!'

Henderson's tongue was flapping out the corner of his mouth when a siren pierced the rain.

Ray stopped squeezing, lifted his hands in the air. Miners turned their heads towards the faint lights of the mine and everyone went quiet. The siren wailed and wailed in the distance. Ray climbed up off Henderson, who lay there clutching at his windpipe with thick muddied fingers. Ray wiped the blood off his nose; his boots squelched with water as he walked. His heart was still speeding and he stood for a moment in the back yard, listening to the siren.

Men and women were already heading for their cars. Ray grabbed Amara's arm. 'I need a lift out there quick.'

'Ray,' she said, 'oh my God, Raymond.' She was pulling at her lip.

'What is it?' Eddy said, 'What's going on?'

'That your Hog out front?'

Eddy nodded.

'I'll tell you on the way,' Ray said. 'Let's go.'

Miners were starting up their utes and four-wheel drives out in the street. Lights came on in all the houses and men and women opened their doors and stood out under the carports in pyjamas and robes looking through the rain towards the mine. The siren kept wailing. Ray jumped onto the pillion seat of the customised Softail as Eddy started it first kick. They shot off down the drive and out into the street before most of the cars had even got their lights on. Down past the tailings dam they flew, Eddy crouching low over the tank and Ray leaning the wrong way into corners, down past the singlemen's quarters where the lights burned and men were rushing half-dressed out of their cabins, Ray holding onto Eddy's thick belt, his eyes shut tight in the rain, murmuring under his breath the same words over and over, Don't let it be her please, please not her! Whatever he had done wrong it didn't deserve to come back on Tanita.

'They got a fire out there?' Eddy yelled over his shoulder.

'That's the emergency siren,' Ray shouted back into the rain. 'They only sound it when there's been an accident. My wife's down there now.'

'You're not with Amara?'

'No, I'm not.' He felt Eddy nod. The Harley gripped gravel as they climbed towards the yellow lights of the mine, the siren growing louder and louder the closer they got. He clung to Eddy's waist so tightly that Eddy had to yell for him to ease off. All around them tall dark eucalypts and sassafras dripped with rain. Ferns, moss and lichen covered the dense rainforest floor and the hills on either side were shrouded in mist. They swept around a sharp bend and there at the end of the road, lit up in the rain, was the mine.

Eddy whistled. 'That is some fucking hole you got here!'

The top had been sheared off a mountain and millions of tonnes of rock scooped out from inside. A wire fence ringed the approach to an enormous open-cut mine that stretched back across the landscape for kilometres. Steep gravelled roads led down deep into the bowels of the earth. Cranes stood guard over huge piles of crushed ore as fine as dust. Ray could see white hats and State Emergency Service Volunteers conferring outside the mill beside two fire trucks and a Landcruiser Sahara with its motor running. He jumped off the Harley before Eddy had even stopped, ran over to the main gate where a huge yellow sign said:

WELCOME TO SOUTHERN MINES

DAYS SINCE LAST ACCIDENT:
85

OUR BEST PREVIOUS RECORD:
87

MINING OPERATIONS:

SAFETY IS PART OF EVERYBODY'S JOB

Ray burst into the guard's box, water dripping off his hair. 'Who is it, Phil?'

The old security guard puffed anxiously on a cigarette, his face webbed with wrinkles. 'A CAT's flipped over near Crusher Gully.'

Ray just stood there. 'Not Tanita's?'

'All I know, Ray, is we got one truck gone over and a driver trapped down there.'

'Call them up!'

'Can't do that, Raymond. You know the procedure. Radio's only for emergency crews.'

'I'm going down then,' Ray said.

'You're not rostered on. King's out there. He won't let unauthorised personnel through.'

'What's he gunna do, Phil? Shoot me?' Ray slipped out of the guard's box and under the boom gate. The noise from the siren was so loud it set his teeth on edge. He made his way quickly across the yard towards the fire trucks. The SES volunteers and white hats seemed to be waiting on some signal. The mine boss was talking rapidly into a cellular phone. When he spotted Ray, he stared at him through his bottle-thick glasses and barked at one of the engineers, 'Get that man a helmet!'

Someone slipped Ray a white hat and he stuck it on as the boom gate kicked up and the town's ambulance tore in straight past them. Everyone jumped onto the fire trucks and the mine boss and five white hats piled into the Toyota Turbo. With sirens screaming they tailed the ambulance down the gravelled incline towards Crusher Gully, Ray gripping the shiny handrail of the truck and praying under his breath it wasn't her. Not now. Not when everything was coming good. An SES volunteer squeezed Ray's arm, but didn't say a word. None of the men was talking and Ray was too busy trying to stop the worst thoughts creeping into his mind.

Coming out of the mist he saw them, moving slowly across the floor of the mine like enormous four-legged beasts, a convoy of graders, dozers and big yellow trucks. Towers of emergency lights lit up the pit and the granite-hard core of the mountain was exposed to the rain and the noise of sirens and the whirr of heavy machinery. Two of the dozers, a grader and the breakdown truck carefully winched something up from the edge of the gully. Even from this distance Ray could make out the shattered windscreen and the caved-in cabin of a fifty-tonne CAT. Slowly, the truck was dragged up by its front axle over the edge of the dump and Ray felt a stab of happiness. The number painted on the side wasn't hers. It wasn't her bloody truck! He bit down hard on his lip to stop himself crying out with joy as the ambulance pulled up ahead and the SES crew jumped off the fire trucks uncoiling hoses and passing down welding gear. Ray stared at the skidmarks dug into the gravel right on the very edge of Crusher Gully where the driver had locked the anchors on. His eyes shifted to the other miners standing out in the rain with bowed heads and he felt something dark slip past them, like a thin quick shadow across a wall.

Shivering with cold, Ray climbed down off the fire truck

and pushed his way through the white hats and the men and women of C shift, seeking her among the grey overalls and blue coats and green lids. At the edge of a line of parked yellow trucks she spotted him and ran towards him and threw her strong arms around his neck and he lifted her off the ground, held his big black woman in the air for a second. Her skin and coat smelled of the damp earth and he bounced her up and down gabbling into her right ear, 'Christ, Jesus fucking Christ, Tanita!'

'I saw it, Ray.' She shook her head and blinked rapidly. 'I saw him go over.'

He lowered her back onto the ground.

'Gary Peard,' the words rushed out of her. 'It's Gary Peard—he was backing up with a full load on and then his wheels just clipped the edge. He went over so fast, like something had a hold of his truck.'

Her big brown eyes looked straight at him.

In all the time they had lived together he had never once seen her cry. He worked a hand up inside the buttons of her bluey, under her woollen shirt and touched her stomach with his fingers. 'You all right?'

Nodding, she sniffed and wiped her nose on the back of her hand.

'I thought I'd lost you, hon,' he whispered, holding her belly.

The siren quit wailing then and except for the shuddering from the engines of two large CATs, a heavy silence descended over the pit. The mine boss took off his glasses and rubbed at the bridge of his nose. Miners were standing in a tight circle around the smashed-in truck and Ray and Tanita pressed forward, peering over the shoulders of the men and women from C shift.

They'd cut Gary Peard out of his cabin and lowered him onto a stretcher. His crushed helmet lay in front of the giant

WHERE THE MINE WAS

black wheel of the truck and the town's only doctor, wearing a clean white shirt with the sleeves rolled up to his elbows, was kneeling in the mud probing with his fingers at the top of Gary Peard's head. When the doctor pulled away Ray saw what was hanging from the front of his shirt.

Tanita dug her nails into Ray's palm and Ray stared as Gary Peard was lifted into the air and then slid neatly into the back of the ambulance. The driver didn't even bother with the siren. Silently the ambulance climbed the hill, its red light blinking through the mist. For a while Ray stood there with his arms tight around his wife and the light, silvery rain streaking the sky. As they walked back to her truck, men and women from C shift came up and touched Tanita's arm or brushed their rough hands against her wrist. Truckies, dozer-drivers and engineers—everyone began to reach out a hand or press the tips of their fingers against a workmate's coat. Even the mine boss was going around gripping men and women by the elbow and the miners were nodding to each other in a curt sort of way as if they'd just come on shift, but no-one said a word.

Tanita climbed up into the cabin of her big yellow rig and Ray squeezed in beside her, perched on the edge of the heater. Steam hissed from the legs of his trousers; his boots were caked in mud. She started the engine and one by one the big trucks rolled out. When the convoy had reached the top of the road, Ray turned and glanced back down at the mine, at the bands of iron ore buried so deep in the heart of that mountain they had to be blasted out with explosives. The emergency lights had been switched off and the rain was falling softly on Crusher Gully, falling, too, across the main pit and the abandoned craters and steep gravelled roads. Falling from one end of that huge black mine right out to the dark misted hills in the distance. And Ray wondered who would have to tell old Mrs Peard it was her son.

Outside the concentrating mill the trucks pulled up in a row and cut their engines and the mill rats came out, taking off their red helmets and walking directly for the gates. Men, women and children, some still wearing pyjama pants and dressing gowns under their orange-striped raincoats, had their faces pressed up against the wire fence waiting. The car park was packed with families from all four shifts and shopkeepers from the town handing out pies and foam cups of coffee. A young sandy-haired woman was crying at the gate, her fingers entwined in the wire mesh. Ray knew there would be no work at the mine tomorrow. He scanned the faces at the fence and caught Amara and Eddy watching him as he walked through the crowd with his arm wrapped around Tanita's shoulders.

'You drive,' his wife said.

'I want to tell you something, hon—'

'Just get me home, Ray, please.' She threw him the keys and he opened the door of the ute and adjusted the seat back. She slid in beside him, unbuttoned her bluey and the top stud on her jeans, sat with her legs wide apart, sweat beading the corners of her lips.

'You all right, Neet?'

She was hanging onto the doorstrap, but she didn't answer, just waved at him to get going. Her chest was wheezing as if she had one of her old attacks coming on and she wound down the window and gulped in the air. Wet black trees hissed past on either side, the road cutting through the forest like a part in a man's hair, Ray driving fast now, changing gears quickly, glancing at his wife out of the corner of his eye and thinking how strong this woman was. He took a hand off the wheel, reached up under Tanita's shirt and laid it gently over her sweating belly. Held his hand there as they drove home through the rainforest sure that he could feel the tiny heart beating.

Room 311
Lex Marinos

The man let the door close behind him. Weighted perfectly it sighed and then clicked despite its bulk. There was enough city light to see clearly. The man slid the key card, arrow down, into the slot on the wall. A recessed light above him lit up the short hallway, further down a bedside lamp, brass with a black shade.

If there was anything different about the room the man was unaware of it. There was just the familiarity. Not in a comfortable way. The sort that breeds contempt. Wardrobe, fridge and coffee-making to the right. Bathroom to the left. Half a dozen steps and into the main room. The man dumped his bag on the small bag-dumping stand. Took his tobacco out and threw it on the bed, took his jacket off and threw it over the desk chair. Kicked off his slip-ons, reefed off his socks. Rolled a smoke and went into his routine, also familiar.

Got rid of the rest of his clothes and took a bathrobe from the wardrobe. Wondered how many other words there were ending in robe. Couldn't think of any, let it slide. Dipped into his bag and pulled out his shaving kit. Dipped into his shaving kit and pulled out his dope. Rolled a joint, but didn't light it. Not yet.

The man opened up the TV cabinet, rolled out the TV, took the remote back to the bed and began flicking. Past the movie preview channel, get to that later, onto some current affairs. Jeff Kennett pretending to be a talking turd. Leave it on for the sound.

The bathroom white and chrome like a surgery. Halogen lights. Trendy. On a dimmer switch. Very trendy. The bath was actually a small spa. Forgivably trendy. Put the plug in and started the taps. Found the complimentary bottle of bath gel. Along with the shampoo, conditioner, moisturiser, sewing kit, toothbrush, razor, emery board, cotton buds and soap roses. All laid out on a flat piece of what looked like coral. Ecologically unsound. Must mention that if ever he filled out the confidential questionnaire designed to help the managing director make the hotel's service even more perfect.

Kennett had been replaced by someone from East Timor. The man found the room service menu and began scanning. He lifted the phone and pushed 4. Hello-room-service-Jason-speaking-how-can-we-help?

A-club-burger-with-chips-and-salad-and-some-chilli-sauce-please.

Certainly-sir-anything-to-drink?

No.

That-will-be-twenty-minutes.

Thanks.

The spa was half-full and the bath gel suds were going mad like some B-grade science movie from the sixties. The man slowed the taps down and went back into the room. He stopped at the fridge and checked the contents. For about 120 dollars he could drink the minibar including the macadamia nuts and the Toblerone. There was a time. He took out a green can of beer and popped it.

From the window he could see down into Flinders Lane. Nothing much going on. Further out were the Jolimont railway yards, the Tennis Centre (last time he was there he saw Prince), the MCG (last time he was there he saw Carlton beat North under lights). The window wound out about ten centimetres. Suicide-proof. To throw yourself out you'd have to be so anorexic you'd probably float. Still it was air. The man lit the joint and exhaled into the night. He wondered whether he should put a towel across the bottom of the door. There was a time. A moment of indecision. Whether to suck on the beer or the joint first. The beer.

He wondered whether he should call someone. It would mean going through all that crap. How are you? Long time. I was just down here for the night so I thought I'd give you a call in case you weren't doing anything. Last time I saw you you were doing something. Have you seen him or her or them? How's work? How's life? Hows? Whats? Whys? Too hard. Too old. Too tired.

It was easier years ago. How are you? I was just down here for the night, do you want to get together? I'll be right over.

The man held the joint against the cold can until it fizzed out. Save some for later. East Timor had turned into tomorrow's synoptic chart. Time for the spa before room service arrived.

The water was just right. Not hot, not cold. Sometimes you fluke it. Suds everywhere as the water jets turned the spa into Rotorua. Nice on the kidneys, ticklish on the feet. As the dope started to roll the man realised he couldn't hear the TV over the spa. That meant he probably wouldn't hear the room service knock either. Maybe they had already been. Had he been in there too long. Turn the spa off and just soak. They'll come back or ring. He drained the can of beer. Felt the need for a piss. Would have liked a block and tackle to help himself out of the bath, but managed anyway. Briefly thought about Archimedes. Kicked the bathmat over to the toilet and smiled to himself that he'd remembered to lift the seat.

Dripping and pissing when the doorbell went. Timing. He smile moronically at himself in the mirror. HANG ON. The piss showed no sign of abating. Be patient he thought. Maybe he said it out loud. Finally. Down to spurts now. Finally. A few shakes. That seemed to be it. The man flushed the toilet, put on the bathrobe. Latrobe he said. That's another one. Weak. There must be something better. He opened the door.

Jason's colleague was Amelia carrying a tray that could have carried her. Beautiful in the delicate sort of way that only Asian women can be. Amelia put the tray on the table. Malaysian, Vietnamese, Filipino, he wondered. Before he could ask her she had produced the wallet with the receipt and a pen. As he signed it he thought of a Chinese girl that he had slept with years ago. Behave yourself.

Enjoy-your-meal-sir and she was gone. They'd only slept together a couple of times but he remembered her well. Skin the colour of coffee with condensed milk. Smooth and small all over. Passive. She lay there and let him do things to her, closing her eyes as he took her nipple between his teeth. She wouldn't let him go down on her. Where was she now? Maybe she was Amelia's mother.

The man unwrapped the cutlery from the serviette, lifted the hot stainless steel thing off the plate and stared at the food. He started eating chips in his fingers. Suddenly the size of the burger and the thought of dead animal seemed impossible. He rolled another smoke and took another beer from the fridge. A red can this time. He found the remote and started flicking. The movies he had either seen or didn't want to see. The adult movies were on channels 14, 15 and 19. He found the program guide, read it three times before he could understand the instructions, checked the digital clock beside the bed and figured the movie on Channel 15 had either started five minutes ago or finished twenty-five minutes before.

The man punched up Channel 15. $10.95 flashed on the right-hand top corner of the screen. If you want to buy this movie press the green button. The man did as he was told. The picture hiccupped before coming to rest on a woman on a bed talking on the phone. Miniskirt and a lot of leg. Miniblouse and a lot of tit. Intercut with a guy sitting at a desk. Suit minus the jacket. Evidently there had been a mix-up at the laundromat. They each had the other's washing. He was holding a pair of her panties. She started playing with her tits. The talk became breathier. His hand went inside his trousers. Her hand went underneath her dress. She started squirming. They agreed to meet each other later on at a club. Recognise each other by wearing something red. No mention of exchanging laundry.

The man remembered a girl in a red blouse. He found the remainder of the joint and relit it. Sucked deep. Back when he was a student. She shared a house with some friends of his. One night he had called over and she was the only one there. They had shared some flagon wine and a pipe. Also it seemed some telepathy. Soon their hands were all over one another. He remembered she was wearing a blouse with what seemed to be a thousand small buttons. He had started to fumble a few of them open when she smiled and stepped back and just pulled the blouse up over her head. They had great sex that night and for months after. Until he went overseas for a year. When he came back she had moved. Into a unit in a block of flats with a sauna. They did it in there once. Fill me up she used to say. Gradually lost touch. Despite getting a dose of NSU he remembered her well.

More beer. More smoke. The man's attention returned to the video. He was distracted by the reflection of the bed lamp in the screen. He turned around to turn it off. Above the bed was one of those pastel flora and fauna moonlit paintings that grace hotel walls and nowhere else. Was there a gallery somewhere that specialised in this style? Hotel art. There was another one above the desk. Same artist if that scrawl was a signature. Who would put their name to it? Both paintings screwed to the wall. Presumably to prevent guests who were so overwhelmed by their beauty from just ripping them off the wall and stashing them in their luggage. He switched off the light.

The man picked up a chocolate that had been placed on the pillow. A nice touch. He wondered how that had originated. Did some smart young executive in the hospitality trade in America or Japan come up with the idea. Why don't we sneak into the guests' rooms while they're out, turn down the bed and leave a chocolate on their pillow for when they return. That might be a nice touch. Presumably the idea caught on because everyone likes to eat chocolate before they go to sleep.

The man ate the chocolate although sleep didn't seem that close. He remembered another woman. The dope had kicked in again. They met at a radio station when he was doing some freelancing. Had dinner at his suggestion. Went back to her place at her suggestion. She was recently divorced, no kids and wore a G-string. They got into it pretty quickly. While they were getting carpet burns on the loungeroom floor, he had taken a chocolate from a bowl on the table and held it in his mouth as he went down on her. Soft centre to soft centre.

Spinning now. The chocolate or the memory had made him hungry. He dipped a couple of cold chips into the chilli sauce and scoffed them. Took a messy bite out of the club burger. This would require serious chewing. Washed it down with the last of the red can. Back to the fridge. Green or red? As if it made a difference. Eeeny meeny. The greenie. Halfway back to the bed he stopped returned to the minibar and poured a miniature Johnnie Walker red into a glass. Let the beer chase that. Now where were we.

Another toke. The video had moved on to the club. The sound track was a repetitious electronic rhythm track with a not quite funky bass and a not quite raunchy sax. The man was sure he had heard it before. He wondered if all pornos used the same track. The heroes were looking around the room but didn't see one another. Instead she homed in on a Latin stud in a red satin shirt. The guy hit upon Miss Platinum wearing red gloves. Oh no. First mistaken laundry. Now mistaken identity. What a plot. What permutations. She dragged the pleasantly surprised Latin stud into the ladies' toilet. Cut back to the guy ogling Miss Platinum's silicone.

The man flopped back on the bed. Careful not to spill his drinks he pushed his way up to the pillows. Rested the glass on the bedside table beside the hotel notepad and the hotel pen as he arranged the pillows behind his neck. He muttered something but couldn't quite make it out. With some effort he refocused on the TV. Back in the ladies' toilet the woman was gripping the architrave of the cubicle door as the Latin stud jackhammered her from behind. Mouth open, eyes wanton looking straight down the lens. It's a job, what the hell do you do that's any better? Bass and sax. The man couldn't hold her gaze. Slugged the scotch. Sent the beer straight in to douse the flames. Closed his eyes. Let the empty glass rest on the bed. Maybe it would get some sleep.

The toilet reminded him of his wife. Well the toilet didn't. That's incorrect. The scene in the toilet reminded him of an occasion with his wife. That's better. Just before or after they were married. A party at a friend of a friend of a friend's. A humid evening. He followed her into the bathroom and they did it standing up as the party went on without them. *Heart of Glass* thumping away.

Really spinning now the man remembered women from over the years, years ago. Faces legs breasts stretches of flesh hair eyes lips. Some without names. He remembered them well. Different then. Was it more free or just young? If you can't be with the one you love etc. His wife again. The hotel rooms they'd shared. Like this some of them. But not like this, Singapore, Philippines, Indonesia, Vietnam, Malta, Greece, Italy, France, Spain, Egypt, Turkey, and other places. The man became aware of his heartbeat.

The man forced himself to sit up and take some deep breaths. Back on the screen the guy was standing halfway up a spiral staircase. Naked. Miss also naked Platinum was a spiral below him, sucking him off between the iron lacework. Bass and sax. The man groped for the remote and hit the mute button. The man steadied himself. Reached for the phone and deliberately pressed the buttons. Careful not to hit a wrong one. Not until the phone was ringing did he think to check the time. Late. Should he hang up. Too late.

Hello.

It's me. I just ...

... take your call right now, but if you'd like to leave a message we'll get back to you as soon as we can.

The man was momentarily confused hearing his own

voice coming back at him. Why was the machine on? He always hated it. Where was she?

Beep.

It's me. I just ...

Too hard to synchronise mind and mouth so he replaced the receiver, awkwardly misjudging the distance to the dial pad.

The man flopped back on the bed. His head kept descending after his body stopped.

The remote again. Careful to hit the right button.

Bass and sax.

Grunts and moans.

The man's hand went down inside his bathrobe.

Ex-Wife Re-Wed
Frank Moorhouse

She did not tell him herself, Louise told him with that status of voice used for gossip of profound content—'Did you hear about Robyn?'

He noticd that Louise did not use their usual expression 'ex-wife'. Robyn had not been known as anything else but 'ex-wife' since they divorced—Jesus Christ, was it really fifteen years ago—and she remarried. She had become again the person 'Robyn' not just the 'ex-wife' character in Louise's and his conversation.

'Well? Tell me.'

How would Louise have heard anything of Robyn, who now lived in Portugal and who moved in a different world?

'It's the Big C.'

The Big C. Louise's voice was enlivened by her role as the bearer of grim news, by being able to dance death into their lives.

Louise was one of the few of his current friends who had known the 'marriage'.

'How did you hear?' He wanted to know how she knew and he did not—given that neither of them was any longer in contact with Robyn.

'Purely by chance,' Louise said. 'I was in Lyon at a trade exhibition when I met her.'

'Does she say I gave her the cancer?' It was a joking toughness to block the shock and the pity which were reaching him. 'She blamed me for everything else.' Louise managed a small laugh, it was their style of humour not Robyn's style of humour. 'How bad is it, Louise?'

'Bad. Irreversible.'

Next day there was an uninformative overseas call from Robyn on his answering machine. The first contact for years. He did not telephone but wrote a letter which told her he knew about her illness and which like all other exchanges since they'd broken was another effort to discharge the guilt he felt about their time together. A fading guilt, and an unfairly borne guilt, given that they'd married as teenagers. At times of low spirit, though, he still felt it was he who'd failed, who'd broken the vows. Of course it wasn't like that, but at these low times he felt he should have stayed with the marriage despite the incompatibility which had shown up early. Would he have been any the worse off? Maybe he would have been anchored enough to become a writer when he'd mistakenly thought he would need to be unanchored. He was still plagued by how she'd crashed their bright red car on the third day they'd had it and he'd yelled at her, failed to comfort her. It was their first significant possession, a materialisation of their relationship. He should have comforted her; instead, he yelled at her. Or was she unconsciously crashing their relationship? As a callow husband he'd attacked her for feeling premenstrual tension. He had read to her from a book which said it was 'all in the mind'. He had forced her to admit that

EX-WIFE RE-WED

it was 'all in the mind' and to pretend she suffered nothing.

His letter to her was short, he said he'd heard she was ill and he was willing her recovery and rooting for her with all his spirit, which he was. Rooting was an odd word for him to have settled on, in their country-town school days it had been fucking. He pondered this and then left the word in the letter.

He said that for his part he remembered good times and rich moments from when they'd been young kids going into life together. He said he still suffered too from things he'd handled badly. He mentioned their 'farcical reunion' a few years earlier.

She wrote back saying how affected she was to get a letter and that she too certainly carried good memories in her heart and had since laughed about their 'farcical reunion'.

Their daughter whom he'd never known was now at university in the States.

She said she was returning to Australia and hoped he'd be in the country and able to see her and that it would not be a second 'farcical' reunion.

After a boozy night with old friends at the Journalists' Club he drove her back to their home town which was no longer a town so much as a suburb of a city.

'We should call it "the suburb" I suppose, not the "old town",' she said.

'I guess we still see the *town*.'

'I can still feel the town.'

She had lost much weight but still seemed agile and he still saw in her the movements of the girlish hockey player. She gave off what he saw as a strained cheeriness and he had not mentioned her cancer and neither had she. He didn't feel he should raise it, sensing it to be perhaps antitherapeutic to acknowledge it or that cancer was something best handled with hauteur rather than candour.

'The old school is really now the *old* school,' he said, 'as old as anything ever gets in this ever-renewing country.'

'Let's go to the school. I'd like to see the old school again.'

He felt the unspoken part of her sentence.

'Remember planting those trees in the new school when we were prefects?' she said, as they sat in the car looking at the row of eucalyptus trees which they'd planted, now well grown—twenty-five-years old. The summer wind gave them a green-silver light and the leaves seemed to shake, frustratedly, against the unmoving solidity of the trunk and limbs. The trees took him back to before high school, to the primary school and hot endless days when she and he had been children in the playground, hot and breathless, aware of each other but unable to express or understand this uncomfortable awareness, only able to express it finally by chasing, hair-pulling, tickling.

'A penny for them.'

They had been going so well and now she'd come out with one of those detestable phrases which he remembered once made up so much of her conversation. Her intelligent ordinariness had enraged him back then. During adolescence he'd fought against what he'd seen then as the tyranny of ordinariness and the tyranny of convention. He'd used excessive behaviour, flamboyance borrowed from literature, self-dramatisation, rule-breaking, bohemian posing, all as resistance to, and inoculation against, the ordinariness of his country-town life. He'd laid down rules for his friends' conversation at high school—no clichés, no wishing people good luck, no salutations, no greetings. And now, even near her death he couldn't let her get away with it, out it came.

'I don't know what I was thinking but I'm now thinking

about how we tried to ban those sorts of expressions when we were here at school.'

'What sorts of expressions?!'

'Oh, sayings like, "a penny for them".' He felt foolish for having made the point.

'Oh God, so you did.'

He was trying to be light but somewhere there in him was the adolescent trying to remake the world, to impose his own minor tyrannies. He hoped she didn't sense it. Back then she'd always been praised for her 'common sense', for being 'down to earth'. He'd been striving for an 'uncommon sense'. His models then were artists, revolutionaries, dreamers—none of which he'd become, becoming instead a servant of an international agency, practising mundane idealism, circumscribed dreaming, deferred dreaming, the illusions of a negotiated revolution. He turned again to her, recalling that along with the down-to-earthness she had also believed in some non-rational things, the meaning in coincidence, the usefulness of astrology. He then wondered fleetingly if she really did have cancer or whether this was a mid-life panic, had she really been diagnosed or was it some sort of intuitive self-diagnosis? She was capable of that.

'Yes,' she said, 'you didn't want people to say hello or goodbye, it wasted time, we were to speak only if we had something to say worth saying or truly felt. Yes. And everything had to be "original".' She snorted.

'I was a bit of a zealot.'

'You sure were.'

This hurt, he didn't want her to confirm that, he didn't think he'd been a zealot. 'Did you really all think I was a zealot?'

'Oh yes. There was lots of talk about you. You were always trying to make the school—or our year—into some sort of branch of the Communist Party or a commune or whatever it was you were reading at the time. *Walden*. Maybe not a zealot but a very, very serious boy. Maybe that's why I married you.'

He remembered that it was back then that he'd had to confront his first sad misconception about the world. He'd wanted to believe that his friends at school were true students, his teachers true scholars, all concerned only with inquiry. That all adults respected truth and the weight of evidence.

This misconception still caught him out, still took root in his mental garden and, of course, was still the fallacy he had to work by.

'You were pretty queer,' she said, 'but impressive in your own way.' She pushed his arm playfully. 'Don't look so worried—we didn't think you were a loony. We were more worried that you would think we were dumb. Did you think I was dumb back then?'

'I married you. You got a better pass than I did.'

'We know that examinations don't count in the long run. Did you think I wasn't an intellectual? And anyhow men marry women dumber than themselves for security.'

'I was sometimes driven up the wall by your common sense. You saw through all the bullshit.'

But she was never sure what was really bullshit and she had neither insight nor vision.

He laughed. 'I miss it now and then. We need you in Vienna.' He didn't believe that.

She asked about schoolfriends, Carl, Sylvia, Friedman. 'Do you ever hear from them?'

'Not at all really. Sylvia's with the Schools Commission. She's always being written up in those articles on successful feminist women.'

'Sounds just like her.'

Sounds just like her.

'Let's go into the school.'

They got out of the car. It was vacation. The school was empty. Nothing as empty as a vacant school.

'Let's go to Room 14. The Prefects' Room.'

He was thinking of another room, where they had almost made love for the first time, Room 17?

'Why not Room 17?'

She turned to him smiling, almost a blushing smile. 'Of course, I'd almost forgotten that. Oh yes.'

They walked along the corridors, the smell of chalk, always oranges? or fruit-cake? Or were these smells in his mind?

They stopped and looked into Room 17, the art room. She took his hand and squeezed it.

'We came very close,' she said.

'The Gestetner's been replaced by offset.'

They went on to Room 14 where the flirtings, the brushings, the illicit hand-holding, the supercharged touchings of pre-courtship, had begun.

The room was crowded with superseded household appliances, jugs, toasters, heaters, snack-makers.

'They have more electrical gadgets than we had.'

'We had a jug—for instant coffee—they've got a restaurant-style dripolator.'

She leaned into him affectionately. 'You wrote a story for the school magazine about nuclear war beginning the day you got your examination results—remember? And you end up being involved in all that even now.'

'Not quite "all that", but yes, that's where I ended up.'

'Though now you're for using nuclear power aren't you?'

'Only because it's inescapable for the time being.'

'But you were aware of the threat before other people.'

'Not really.'

'Before *we* were at school. You were a peace movement before there were peace movements.'

'What it shows twenty-five years later is that I was politically wrong—the bomb hasn't dropped—maybe it stopped war.'

He realised he was slightly disturbed by her holding his hand; it was, he realised, irritation with himself, a fear of contact with her. Because she had cancer. He was angry with himself and took her other hand against this stupid gut reaction.

'I think I was using it metaphorically—the bomb.'

This idea seemed to be unacceptable to her. 'How? Why?'

'I think I was really writing about the bomb of puberty dropping on the peace of my childhood.'

'I don't think you were. I don't think you were that clever.' She laughed to avoid any offence.

He let go of her hands and went to the window to look across at the playing field. She came up behind him and embraced him from behind, her cheek coming against his. Again he felt a resistance to her but suppressed it.

'You haven't mentioned my cancer,' she said. She tried to say it in a comic voice but it threw a shadow of effort. 'For godsake, mention my cancer,' she laughed, and going to the window, opened it and shouted, 'Cancer!' and then closed it. 'There, it's mentioned. People won't mention it. I didn't think it would happen with you and me but it has. People won't say the word. But I *have* to talk about it.'

The effort at lightness was so colossal and so transparent and courageous he felt tearful.

'You look so well—it hadn't crossed my mind,' he said, holding his voice normal, 'but OK—how's the cancer going?'

His voice came out far from normal.

She made physical contact with him again, leaning into him. 'Oh I have my winning days and my losing days. It's incredible that I can really say at the end of a day—I'm winning or I'm losing. But I'm not strong enough to count the winning days against the losing days. That's where I'm a sook. But I'm not a defeatist.'

She had never been a defeatist. But the word sounded too close to being crushingly, inescapably upon her. She stumbled over saying it.

'Does it hurt a lot?'

'Hellishly in the lower pelvis sometimes.'

'I've heard that chemotherapy is rough.'

'Oh I've given that up. I didn't believe that anything that makes you feel that bad could be good for you.'

'Louise said you were having Cobalt 60 inter-cavity irradiation.'

'I gave it up.'

'But why, Robyn, why?'

She squeezed his hand. 'Don't feel offended because your magic is being refused.'

It wasn't *his* magic—nor was it 'magic'.

'I changed therapies,' she said, 'as Susan Sontag said, all the medical therapies are like warfare—they bombard, they attack, they search out and destroy.'

'For godsake, Robyn, they *work*.'

'Calm down, calm down. So does my way.'

Her way.

'I'm meditating and I have a vegan diet which is all I feel like eating anyhow—now hold on—don't be so quick to make a mock of it. It works too, you know. I'm doing imagery therapy—the Simonton technique.'

'The what!'

'Calm down. I imagine the white cells eating the cancer,

as simple as that. I believe in the power of the imagination. But I don't see it as a violent act—I imagine it as peaceful. The imagination is a much under-used power.'

She looked very tired from having had to put it into words against her sense of his opposition. She had stated it as a testament of faith. Oh he was still so zealous with her. He angered again against himself. He wanted to take both her hands and kiss them as a supportive gesture and as a way of dissenting from those negative responses his personality was giving to her. But still he could not bring himself to do it.

'You're not looking like an invalid,' he forced himself to say, 'so something's working, maybe.' He tried to bite back the word 'maybe'. 'I'm sorry I mocked you—you know me, always the schoolboy rationalist.'

'But a rationalist who was sophisticated would accept that there are these grey areas in medicine and especially in cancer healing. Strange things do happen.'

'Yes. I'm for anything that works for you,' he said, feeling happier with that form of words, 'but why don't you try everything at once? The Cobalt 60, the alternative therapies, the lot.'

'But don't you see that if you try the medical things you're being passive—you're putting yourself in the hands of other people and saying "cure me". With the other therapies you are active—it's me working for my own cure.'

But there was nothing in the book that said you shouldn't put yourself in the hands of others when ill. Trusting, or involving others, might be part of being committed to your life. He didn't want to argue with her. He was afraid of upsetting the balance of her will, in so far as he was granting validity to willpower cures. He suspected, though, that do-it-yourself cures might be a diseased reaction to disease. We could not depend upon the beneficence of the unconscious. He wouldn't rely on his.

'Remember that last party we had here at the end of fifth year,' she said, 'no, of course, you were already in Sydney. We had my old gramophone here,' she went over and stood where the gramophone had been, 'we drank soft drinks and ate cakes which the girls had baked.' She stood in reverie. 'Gee ... ' She became tearful.

He wanted to go to her but the resistance was still there.

They traced their school lives slowly as they wandered about the empty school.

'I was truly deeply shocked that day in Room 17. I mean, I hadn't actually seen a man's ... a penis before.'

'It took you more than a year before you would look again.'

'You're lucky I *ever* looked again.'

They stood in the grassy fields where twenty-three years earlier they'd made tentative pre-intercourse love. If his mother or her mother were not at home they would sometimes go there and pet more until they ached and were almost sick from arousal without release.

As they stood there in the long grass, she said, 'I sometimes wonder what gave me the cancer, was it—this is silly I know but I have to say it—could it have been men's penises not being clean enough?'

He tried to joke. 'I don't think so—British women would all have cervical cancer.' It was a typical idea for her to have, and, who knows, maybe right.

'I don't mean you,' she touched him, 'you were a good middle-class boy and clean, but well, others ... ' She gave a small guarding smile as if he might even now be upset by mention of other men, 'others after you weren't always good middle-class boys.

'Did a doctor suggest this?' 'It's a private theory, I have

lots of private theories these days. Being ill in a serious way gives you a special sense of knowing your body.'

They left the school. 'I always remember the Head saying something that was very important to me,' she said, 'remember him saying that school wasn't preparation for life—it was real life, real living. It's true, and school is an important part of living.'

In the car she suggested she'd like to go to the church where they'd been married.

Outside the church he said how normal their lives had looked then—church, fellowship, Sunday School, confirmation, débutantes, engagements, balls, marriages, births.

'I missed out on confirmation,' he said to her, 'that was one of my protests.'

'But you *were* confirmed,' she said, 'I was the one who refused to be confirmed and caused all the ruckus.'

'No,' he said, feeling determinedly sure, 'I was the one who refused to be confirmed.'

'No, sorry I was the one who held out, you were forced into it by your mother but you were certainly confirmed.'

He flushed, she was right, he'd been rewriting his history. Why? When had he started that legend—lie—and then forgotten to correct it?

'You talked about doing it,' she said, 'you talked of rebellion but your mother put great pressure on you. My mother oddly enough was a bit against it for some reason. Low church—found it too popish.'

He was embarrassed, he must have made up the story when he was a teenager in Sydney as part of the picture of rebellious adolescence in a country town.

'Are you honestly confused?' she asked.

'What does it matter now,' he said, 'yes, you were the one.'

They went into the dim church and walked up the aisle where they'd walked as nineteen-year-old bride and groom. 'Is this the altar?' he asked her. 'I never quite knew where the altar began.'

'Yes, but Rev. Benson called it the communion table.'

'The altar was where they once sacrificed animals.'

'Not in this old town,' she said, 'here we sacrificed kids. Kids like us.'

She turned to him then with tears and came to him. 'Hold me.'

She held on to him.

'It's OK,' he said, 'you're OK, Robyn.'

'I'm dying,' she said, 'I know it.'

'You're fighting it—you'll win, you were always a winner.'

'We will at least know all the answers then,' she said.

Towards what end?

She looked up at him hopelessly. 'Marry me again—just for today—let's marry for the day. We may never see each other again anyhow, whatever happens.'

He strove to get her meaning.

By 'marry' he assumed she meant they should pledge to each other some vow of affection.

'We were little children together,' she said, 'and we went through all that stuff of adolescence, and we were each other's first love, and I did bear your child—even if you never claimed her.'

He had lived as if this child did not exist. He had decided years back that he could not be a father for the child because of the circumstances, his alienation from Robyn, his emotional deficiency. But he'd also made the decision to protect himself from the pain of being held away from the child. If he had once permitted his fatherly feelings free rein they would have tormented him forever. He had still to keep them unreleased. He had explained this to Robyn on a number of occasions but she had never accepted it. He wouldn't try again.

He knew then for the first time, or faced for the first time, the fact that parenthood had passed him by.

He'd passed through another of the doorways.

He felt no deep affection for her. He felt a sympathetic bond of, probably, a unique kind. He didn't feel caught up in a rush of new affection or restored affections. Perhaps he felt sentimental. What he felt most was recoil from her disease. This continued to make him angry with himself.

'You do still feel something for me?' she asked.

'A great deal.'

'Do you feel some love for me?' she asked.

'Of course I do,' he lied, searching for validation of this statement—he did feel a type of love. In some fudged and twisted way, yes, there was a love, she had a unique place in his personal being. 'You have a special place in my heart.'

Yet why not lie? He found he was frightened of lying for fear she would detect it and be hurt more.

She took his hands and turned both of them towards the altar.

The western light was coming in from behind them at the back of the church but was still faintly reaching the windows above the altar.

She turned to him.

' "Do you take me",' she whispered, ' "as your spiritual wife for this day" ' —she faltered—and then added, ' "and for all the days until we die, from this day forth?" '

He looked at her and saw her frailty and fear. Yet all he could react to was her extension of the made-up vows from 'this day' to 'all the days until we die'. He sensed that she was taking theatrical pleasure from the pseudo-ecclesiastical wording of it, the church, the light.

'Yes,' he decided to say.

'Say it,' she said with insistence, 'say it to me, say the words.'

He felt the saying of it to be an act of serious import. He found he could not take it lightly or fraudulently. He searched inside himself for the validation, for the authority to say it. Somewhere inside himself he found a permission.

'"I take you as my spiritual wife for this day".' He tried to stop it there.

'"... and for all days until I die, from this day forth",' she instructed.

He noted that she changed the wording and emphasis to refer to her death, but if he said 'until I die' it would refer to his death. 'And for all the days until I die, from this day forth.'

'You may say,' she said softly, bravely, poignantly, '"until you die"—meaning until I, Robyn, die. I don't want it to be meaningless. I don't want you to swear to something you cannot hold to.'

They had been children together and then adolescents together. They had gone forward into life together. He remembered telling her once that D. H. Lawrence, or someone, had said that first love remained with you forever, was an irrevocable bond.

He shook his head. He tightened his hold on her hands. '"Until I die".'

'Thank you, Ian.'

They held hands silently for a few seconds at the altar in the afternoon light, in the country town church of their childhood.

He then became uncomfortable, worried that someone might come into the church but realised then, that they had some right to be at the altar. This was their town, their church.

'Come on,' she said, urging him. 'Do it for me.'

' "Do you take me as your spiritual husband for this day and for all days until you die, until this day forth".'

He feared he had the wording wrong.

'Yes yes, "I take you, Ian, as my spiritual husband for this day and for all days until I die, from this day forth",' she said, with a forceful sincerity. 'You may now kiss the bride,' she said, smiling.

He moved to kiss her and, as he did, was ashamed that he could not give himself to the kiss with a wholehearted spirit, instead he made the kiss a brotherly kiss, hoping that it was also intimate enough for her to believe it to be the kiss she sought.

Maybe if he'd been able to give her that kiss passionately without withholding, maybe if he had been able to make love to her on that visit to the home town—or at least give her physical embraces of a wholehearted kind—she would have stayed alive. Maybe with her method those gestures by him would have been enough to tip the balance. Maybe she died because of people like him in the world. Maybe he was a negative cell. Or maybe this was egocentric thinking and placed him unrealistically large and unrealistically close in her personal galaxy.

He was in the bar at the UN City in Vienna, drinking alone, when he heard of her death from Mark Madden, an American chemist with the NEA who had been her lover at some time after the marriage.

Madden and he also had been close for a few months when he'd come to Australia as a young student drop-out. They'd re-met on the IAEA circuit at times. Despite these close links and their respective distances from their homelands, he and Madden now usually avoided each other in the bar. This night Madden had come across to him and said, 'Robyn died this morning, I thought you mightn't have heard.'

Why would Madden think that? But yes, Madden was right, he hadn't heard.

'God,' he said, 'that's rotten.'

He felt a real sadness and a regret for her now permanent absence from his life, or to be precise, the 'absent presence' she'd been in his life since they'd separated.

'She was a sweet, sweet person, a very special sort of human being,' Madden said, as they had a drink together. That sort of talk, he thought, was why he didn't drink with Madden.

'I knew her as a giggling hockey-playing schoolgirl,' he said to Madden, 'that is my enduring memory.' It was a way of asserting the superiority of his knowing of her over Madden's knowing of her. Two male egos still clashing like stags over her dead body.

'She was essentially a poetic person.'

'Poetic? I never saw her as poetic. I didn't see that side of her.' Nor did he believe it.

'It wasn't a "side of her" it was the whole damned person.'

'I'm not doubting you Mark, just that I knew a much different Robyn. How do you mean poetic anyhow?'

'I mean, man, that she wrote poetry.'

He and Madden had once been really close and now it was nearly all animal antipathy.

'Robyn wrote poetry?'

'She had poems in magazines. Yes.'

He was surprised by this and resented Madden knowing and his not knowing.

Privately he still felt his relationship to Robyn to be

superior to whatever she'd had with Madden, but he was finding it impossibly disorienting to believe that this self-important, unnaturally fit, tomato-juice-drinking chemist in the tartan check trousers and black jacket could have been a lover of a girl he had once been married to and shared innocence with. He noted alcoholically his secret vow to her in the home-town church. Not that the vow had carried any obligations but it had from time to time invaded his consciousness in an ill-defined way, suggesting obligations which he could not discover.

Nor could he match this guy Madden with the guitar-playing gentle American youth he'd known in those years before. It seemed wasteful of nature to have put all that growing into that guitar-playing youth only for it to come out as the self-important NEA chemist, Madden.

'When was it that you had an affair with her?' He thought he might as well drop niceties and delve into matters he'd always left unexamined. Or maybe it was information he'd once had and which his mind had not held.

'Robyn and I did not have an "affair".'

'I didn't mean to demean it.'

He did wish to demean it.

'As you know, it was after you two had split. I had two periods of loving Robyn—in New York years ago, in the old peace movement days with SANE and then again much later in Lisbon, when she was stringing for the *Herald-Tribune*. We were very close then in Lisbon.'

We-were-very-close-then-in-Lisbon.

'And I became very fond of your daughter Chris.'

'She hardly qualifies as my daughter.'

'Hell man—face up to yourself—she's your daughter. She's living with some guy old enough to be her father—if you're in anyways interested—out in the mid-west somewhere.'

'Robyn said she was OK.' He didn't want to know about the child. People shouldn't tell him about the child. He could not afford to know about the child.

'Hell she is.'

They sat there in their own silences.

He tried to remain sociable. He had no bond with his biological daughter. They'd had nothing to do with each other since her birth. He maybe would come to regret this but now he felt nothing for her state, no inclination to try to make a bond with her. Impossible. Would she come seeking her 'real' father one day and go away bewildered and disappointed that he was not a mythical father but simply a crumbling, solitary international civil servant who'd failed to become a writer, who drank too much? A man of too little feeling. That wasn't true. He wept nearly every week. But for what did he weep? He was perhaps, though, someone who did not know how to live properly, he would tell her.

'I told her to try everything—she said she'd given up chemotherapy. I told her to have conventional therapy and alternative therapy at the same time.'

'That was bad advice, friend. She wanted faith not smart-arsed advice. The last thing she needed was to be steered back to invasive therapy.'

He should have known that Madden would be that sort of person. He did hope though that he had strengthened Robyn's will. Or was that wrong? Should he have instead argued more strongly against the hocus-pocus? Maybe that was his true offence against her. Not challenging her irrationality stongly enough.

Madden went on. 'She had to go for it, health and disease, the whole caboodle. Wasn't it Mann who said that disease is simply love transformed? She had to turn the disease back into love.'

'I thought that maybe self-help was the disease disguised. Disease disguised as therapy. Neurosis pretending to be the doctor.'

'She was trying self-love—I don't see that as disease.'

'Well we know now she was either on the wrong therapy or she didn't have enough self-love.'

'Or she began too late after being screwed about with Cobalt 60.'

'I thought you were a man of science.'

'I am a scientist and that's why I'm open to new strategies. I know we don't know it all, Sean.'

Madden was one of the few in his life who still called him Sean. A leftover part of their former intimacy. Madden had forgotten that Sean was not the name he went by.

'Did you encourage her to try the other therapies?'

'Yes, I did. I put her on to the Simonton technique.'

'You filled her full of crap, in other words.'

'Don't call it crap when you know fuck-all about it.'

'It is crap and she's dead to prove it.'

Alcohol was making him reckless.'

'I take strong exception to that remark.'

'Do what you bloody well like with it.'

Again they lapsed into their own silences, but both with increased pulse rates and broken breathing.

He then recalled something from his marriage and felt sickened by the recall. He had not thought about it since that time. It had not come to him during their reunion in the home town.

It was in the collapsing days of the marriage, or just before when they had been trying to restore its zest. Or maybe he'd really given up and hadn't cared what happened. He'd intimidated or inveigled her into sexual games, including an episode with a whip. Now that he looked back on it, knowing also more about himself, he had wanted to be the whipped one but had in fact whipped her. She'd gone along with it all and responded to it as sex play, but it hadn't helped the relationship. Probably because they'd got it back to front—that is, if she really had any such inclinations residing in her personality and had wanted to whip him. She was happier though with things closer to the orthodox. He wasn't sure how much the games had been created out of frustration, rage, about their blocked and dulled relationship. But the thought which pushed itself into his mind now there in the UN bar in Vienna was a remark she'd made after one of those nights. She'd said apologetically that she wished she were 'better at it', but that she'd been frightened of being whipped on the breasts because she feared that it could give her cancer. He'd denied this possibility—on no knowledge whatsoever. He now knew that a blow can cause cancer. Not that they'd been exchanging 'blows' or really striking each other with any force. At the time he'd laughed at her for equating sexual deviance with sickness and cancer as the punishment for dabbling in evil. He wished he'd sought her forgiveness about this before she died.

'God I loved that woman,' Madden said, with an even more emphatic American sincerity, fuelled probably by the tequila that he was now drinking, having switched from tomato juice. Having drunk down the tequila and ordered another immediately, as if the speed of his drinking publicly proved his grief. Then he said, 'And she was damned bright—one of the brightest women I've met.' This was said in an affirmative way, as if Madden was 'pulling' himself up out of the grief.

He wished Madden would piss off and leave him free to dwell on her death in his own maudlin way. And he didn't want to be in the UN bar. It was too brightly lit, too much a bar of publicly acceptable behaviour, a bar to be in after work not after after-work. Madden was the wrong person to be with.

'Oh come on, Madden, she was many good things but she wasn't bright in that sense. She was a very good journalist but she was not intellectual. At times I found her painfully banal.'

'You callous bastard—I ought to sock you.'

Sock you. High school language.

Sock you.

He wouldn't mind a fist fight with Madden there in the 'school' bar. Turbulence and disorder would discharge his frustrated urge to be maudlin.

But no, the institutionalised setting had them both in its command.

He stood up, grunted a goodbye to Madden, put down a pocketful of schillings and left to go back into Vienna. To an old bar. To the grand bar of the Imperial where he might be grandly maudlin. As he walked out in the night air to the train station he said to Robyn out there in the cosmos, 'You were a bright burning flame of a girl Robyn, and you were for a time my passion, but oh why did you go with guys like Madden?'

Or guys like him. But she hadn't gone with him when he was a 'guy', she had gone with him when he was a boy.

The train took him across the Danube.

He had another thought: 'She went with guys like Madden therefore I am a guy like Madden.'

Ah, the time of self-laceration. If he couldn't be maudlin he could be self-lacerating.

No, she would have not been involved with him if she'd met him as an adult. Or would she? What was the difference between Madden and him—both solitary men adrift in an international community? Community?

He'd had great personal power as a youth in that small town, a student prince in his imitation of flamboyance, his curious, neurotic energy. Now he was something of a drunk, a failed writer, a 'co-ordinator' of reports.

At the first drink in the Imperial he observed that he was not a 'guy like Madden'. He was a guy who could perceive the possibility that he was guy like Madden and fear it. He was therefore not a guy like Madden. Madden was not sitting in the UN bar fearing that he was like him. Madden had no doubts about his nature.

He went back to bed wishing that he had never known his ex-wife, only his wife. No. He wished he'd known only the hockey-playing girl who was to become his wife.

Upstream
Ian Beck

Coming over the crest of the hill with the town below and the line of hills in the distance, I could see how little had changed. There had been talk once of bringing the rail line in from the coast, but the project had been dropped in favour of rural subsidies and Brilga had survived without ever prospering. Now, after ten years, it was still the same.

The river flanked the town on three sides. It was big enough for seasonal flooding, and the roads that crossed it were lined with markers that showed the depth of water in winter. Between the river crossings an avenue of poplars screened the town from the highway. All the buildings in the main street were single storied, and the shadow of the grain silo in the Farmers' and Graziers' Co-operative stretched across their roofs and moved like a sundial around the town.

I drove past an abandoned petrol station and onto a wooden bridge. I could see the river below. It swirled around the pylons and sparkled in the open places downstream. Crossing the bridge brought it all back. That was where we had swum in the summer. On days when the air was dusty white and the sunlight lay like a weight on your shoulders, I had swum there after school with Darryl Burney and Michael Hospers and a boy whose name I have forgotten. The river was wider then, and the irrigation systems had not drained its tributaries; but below the bridge it was still the same and driving across it I felt my heart lift, as though someone I had once loved had just passed by in a crowd.

I turned onto a gravel road beside the river and drove through the shade of the trees. Flooding had changed the look of the country, but the willows had kept the banks intact. I remembered swimming downstream on the current, and the sudden chill when you entered the shade of the banks. The water there was cold and, diving through the roots of the willows, you could see the colour of the water change as the bottom dropped away. The roots were tangled and filled with the driftwood the floods had left. After a season underwater the wood was silky smooth and so rotten it crumbled like stale chocolate. At night we had burned the dry wood and fished by the light of the fires. I remembered fishing there with my father when I was still young enough to be troubled by the darkness and the way the worms moved on the hook. Dad had fished with my uncle and two of his friends from the war. They had all been in the army and, listening to their stories, I had got the impression that the war had been an enjoyable and often highly amusing business. The friends were cheerful and athletic and made jokes about Dad's hand whenever he lost a fish. I tried to remember their names but they were gone now. What stayed was the glow of the firelight on the water and the steady pull of the current on the lines and the sudden feeling of the night when the others had moved downstream.

The willows at night could be a disturbing place. It had not been pleasant catching the river carp when there was no-one to take them off the hook. They had the slick maggot-whiteness of things that lived away from the light, and did not struggle when they were landed. It was different when we fished upstream. The fish were smaller there, but catching them in the bright fast-flowing water with the sun in your eyes and the spray drifting down from the rapids you did not get the same feeling as fishing the willows.

On the far side of the town's only high ground the river moved through open fields and around islands of brush and pine. There were billboards beside the road and a signpost pointing out tourist attractions. The falls above the rapids were not indicated on the sign. I would go back there one day. It would be a good spot to take the children if I could manage to get them for the weekend. We could camp under the gum trees that grew on the rocks beside the river and fish the places I had fished as a boy. There was a road into that part of the river now, but in the days when I had known it the country was still untouched. To get to the river then you walked through a valley and down a slope with granite outcrops between the trees. The river flowed through the rubble at the base of the slope and over a terrace of water-smoothed stone to the rapids. Walking through the valley with your knapsack on your shoulders and the heat rising from the bush, you could hear the rapids ahead—fresh and cool-sounding in the stillness—and see spray above the trees.

Sometimes on weekends I had camped there with Michael and Darryl and a boy named Billy Oates. Michael fished for carp with a trout rod and a line so light it disappeared in the palm of his hand. He worked the river like a trout fisherman and threw back most of the fish he caught.

He was dedicated and knowledgeable and fished in competition with Billy. We worked different parts of the river and camped overnight on a spit of pebbles below the rapids. Lying in the lean-to at night you could hear the sound of the rapids and the breeze moving through the trees. There was all of summer in those sounds and a feeling of things renewed that you did not get in town. That was a long time ago, when I was young and the change of seasons was exciting.

I glanced at the clock on the dashboard and wondered if there was time to visit the town. The traffic would be heavy on the coast road, and the boys' mother was certain to have made plans for the day. I could visit the town another time. There was a house there where my father had died and a street where I knew the names of most of the families, but Brilga was like a vast and well-loved country, and I would need more than an afternoon to see it all. It was something to keep in reserve if the trip to the rapids fell through. Arrangements like that required the same degree of preparation and skill as a courtroom summation. I had learnt the ritual by now, but until the boys' mother had accepted me as a stranger there would always be that element of point-scoring.

A line of cattle was moving up from the river and crossing the road ahead, and I slowed and watched some children on pushbikes weave in and out of the herd. The cattle were sleek and sluggish and their bellies dripped moisture. Watching them brought back mornings on a farm near the river, walking cows to the milking shed with Owen Forbes in the cold light after dawn. The farm was on the fringes of the snow country, and on winter mornings the cold steamed the breath of the cattle and froze the discarded milk in the drains around the dairy. The milk was never pasteurised and when the polished steel pails were brought back to the house Mrs Forbes would skim off the top layer of cream and spoon it onto our breakfast cereal. Sitting at the table with a plate of bacon rashers and inch-thick toast and eggs the colour of the rising sun, I had not minded being woken so early, nor the feeling of homesickness that came sometimes in the night.

On Owen's farm I had realised for the first time the difference between living in a country town and living in the country itself. It was something you realised when you saw rabbits bloated with myxomatosis or fox skins stretched on a fence to dry, or when you showered in the cloudy bore water that irrigated the farm. I saw it, too, in the summer, when the dust blew in from the fields and made everything feel powdery and the river changed to pools of rust-coloured water between the boulders.

On summer evenings we would go downstream to a place where tree trunks had dammed a tributary and sit in the stagnant water until dusk brought the illusion of coolness. I remembered lying in the green water with the stars out and a warm breeze in the reeds, listening to Owen and his father sing 'The Pub With No Beer' and 'The Cat Came Back' and 'The Queensland Drover', and trying to keep my eyes from the cleavage of Mrs Forbes's swimsuit. Mrs Forbes was young then and when she stepped out of the water her swimsuit clung to her and made me dream at night of girls who looked like the Pepsi Cola girl and came to my bed for reasons I did not fully understand.

All that had gone when Owen died. He was an only child, and afterwards everything changed; but for a long time I had been part of two families and certain love was the cheapest currency around.

The cattle had gone and the road stretched straight and flat through the fields. I followed it to the main highway and turned onto the coast road. The river had disappeared behind fields of yellow wheat and a windbreak of poplars. Their branches striped the road and flickered on the windscreen.

I watched the shadow of a cloud move over the wheat and thought about the people I had known in my childhood. With the exception of Michael I had not kept in touch with any of them.

The last I heard, Darryl Burney had joined the army and gone to Cyprus with the United Nations Peacekeeping Force. At the end of his enlistment he was coming back to town to run his father's electrical shop. Billy Oates had thrown in his job at the Farmers' and Graziers' Co-operative and disappeared in an undergraduate ghetto somewhere. Owen Forbes had been killed in an accident on the Calga road when he was twelve years old; and Michael Hospers lived now on the coast with my ex-wife, at a place where the river emptied into the sea.

He Found Her In Late Summer
Peter Carey

1.

He found her in the later summer when the river ran two inches deep across glistening gravel beds and lay resting in black pools in which big old trout lay quietly in the cool water away from the heat of the sun. Occasionally a young rainbow might break the surface in the middle of the day, but the old fish did no such thing, either being too well fed and sleepy or, as the fisherman would believe, too old and wise to venture out at such a time.

Silky oaks grew along the banks and blackberries, dense and tangled, their fruit long gone into Dermott's pies, claimed by birds, or simply rotted into the soil, vigorously reclaimed the well-trodden path which wound beside fallen logs, large rocks, and through fecund gullies where tree ferns sent out tender new fronds as soft and vulnerable as the underbellies of exotic moths.

In one such gully a fallen tree had revealed a cave inside

a rocky bank. It was by no means an ideal cave. A spring ran continually along its floor. Great fistfuls of red clay fell frequently and in the heat of the day mosquitoes sheltered there in their swarming thousands.

Three stalks of bracken outside its dirty mouth had been broken and the sign of this intrusion made him lower his hessian bag of hissing crayfish and quietly peer inside.

It was there he found her, wild and mud-caked, her hair tangled, her fair skin scratched and festered and spotted with infected insect bites. She was no more than twenty years old.

For a long time they regarded each other quietly. He squatted on his heels and slapped at the mosquitoes that settled on his long, wiry brown legs. She, her eyes swollen, fed them without complaint.

He rolled down the sleeves of his plaid shirt and adjusted his worn grey hat. He pulled up his odd grey socks and shifted his weight.

She tugged at her dress.

At last he held out his hand in the way that one holds out a hand to a shy child, a gentle invitation that may be accepted or rejected.

Only when the hand was lowered did she hold hers out. It was small and white, a city hand with the last vestiges of red nail polish still in evidence. He took the hand and pulled her gently to her feet, but before a moment had passed she had collapsed limply onto the muddy floor.

Dermott adjusted his hat.

'I'm going to have to pick you up,' he said. It was, in a way, a question, and he waited for a moment before doing as he'd said. Then, in one grunting movement, he put her on his shoulders. He picked up the bag of crayfish and set off down the river, wading carefully, choosing this way home to save his passenger from the blackberry thorns which guarded the path along the banks.

Neither spoke to the other, but occasionally the girl clenched his shoulder tightly when they came to a rapid or when a snake, sleeping lightly on a hot rock, slipped silkily into the water as they approached.

Dermott carried his burden with pleasure yet he did not dwell on the reason for her presence in the cave nor attempt to invent theories for her being so many hundred miles from a town. For all of these things would be dealt with later and to speculate on them would have seemed to him a waste of time.

As he waded the river and skirted the shallow edges of the pools he enjoyed his familiarity with it, and remembered the time twenty years ago when it was as strange to him as it must be to his silent guest. Then, with the old inspector, he had done his apprenticeship as his mother had wished him to, read books, learned to identify two hundred different dragonflies, studied the life cycle of the trout, and most particularly the habits of the old black crayfish which were to be his alone to collect. It was an intensive education for such a simple job, and he often reflected in later years that it may not have been, in an official sense, compulsory, but rather a private whim of the old inspector who had loved this river with a fierce protectiveness.

The examination had been a casual affair, a day trek in late spring from where the old Chinese diggings lay in soft mossy neglect to the big falls five miles up river, yet at the end of it he had successfully identified some two hundred trees, thirty insects, three snakes, and described to the old inspector's satisfaction the ancient history of the rocks in the high cliffs that towered above them.

It was only much later, after a child had died, a wife had left and floods had carried away most of his past, that he realised exactly what the old man had given him: riches more precious than he could ever have dreamed of. He had been taught to know the river with the quiet confident joy of a lover who knows every inch of his beloved's skin, every hair, every look, whether it denoted the extremes of rage and passion or the quieter more subtle moods that lie between.

Which is not to suggest that he was never lonely or that the isolation did not oppress him at times, but there were few days in which he did not extract some joy from life, whether the joys be as light as the clear web of a dragonfly or as turbulent as the sun on the fast water below Three Day Falls.

The winters were the hardest times, for the river was brown and swollen then and crayfish were not to be had. Then he occupied himself with a little tin mining and with building in stone. His house, as the years progressed, developed a unique and eccentric character, its grey walls jutting out from the hillside, dropping down, spiralling up. And if few walls were quite vertical, few steps exactly level, it caused him no concern. Winter after winter he added more rooms, not from any need for extra space, but simply because he enjoyed doing it. Had ten visitors descended on him there would have been a room for each one, but there were few visitors and the rooms gave shelter to spiders and the occasional snake which feasted on mice before departing.

Once a gypsy had stayed during a period of illness and repaid his host with a moth-eaten rug of Asiatic origin. Other items of furniture were also gifts. An armchair with its stuffing hanging out had been left by a dour fisheries inspector who had carried it eighty miles on top of his Land Rover, knowing no other way to express his affection for this man on the river with his long silences and simple ways.

Books also were in evidence, and there was an odd

assortment. Amongst them was a book on the nature of vampires, the complete works of Dickens, a manual for a motor car that now lay rusting in a ravine, and a science fiction novel entitled *Venus in a Half-Shell*. He had not, as yet, read any of them although he occasionally picked one up and looked at it, thinking that one day he would feast on the knowledge contained within. It would never have occurred to him that the contents of these books might reflect different levels of truth or reality.

'Nearly home,' he said. They had left the river and passed through the high bracken of Stockman's Flat. He trudged in squelching boots along the rutted jeep track that led to the house. He was hot now, and tired. 'Soon be there,' he said, and in a moment he had carried her through the thick walls of his house and gently lowered her down into the old armchair.

She huddled into the armchair while he filled a big saucepan with water and opened the draught on the stained yellow wood stove.

'Now,' he said, 'we'll fix you up.'

From the armchair the girl heard the words and was not frightened.

2.
There was about him a sense of pain long past, a slight limp of the emotions. His grey eyes had the bitter sweet quality of a man who has grasped sorrow and carries it with him, neither indignant at its weight nor ignorant of its value. So if his long body was hard and sinewy, if his hair was cut brutally short, there was also a ministering gentleness that the girl saw easily and understood.

He brought warm water in a big bowl to her chair and with it two towels that might once, long ago, have been white.

'Now,' he said, 'one of us is going to wash you.'

He had large drooping eyelids and a shy smile. He shifted awkwardly from one water-logged boot to the other. When she didn't move he put the towels on the arm of the chair and the bowl of water on the flagstone floor. 'Don't worry about getting water on the floor,' he said.

She heard him squelch out of the room and, in a moment, imagined she heard a floor being swept elsewhere in the house. Outside the odd collection of windows she could see the tops of trees and below, somewhere, she heard the sound of the river.

She picked up a grey towel and went to sleep.

3.

The tin roof was supported by the trunks of felled trees. The stone walls were painted white, veiled here and there by the webs of spiders and dotted with the bodies of dead flies. In one corner was a bed made from rough logs, its lumpy mattress supported by three thicknesses of hessian. A tree brushed its flowers against the window and left its red petals, as fine and delicate as spider legs, caught in the webs that adorned the glass.

She lay naked on the bed and let him wash her.

Only when he came in embarrassed indecision to the vulva did she gently push his hand away.

When the washing was over he took a pair of tweezers, strangely precise and surgical, and removed what thorns and splinters he found in her fair skin. He bathed her cuts in very hot water, clearing away the yellow centres of red infections, and dressed each one with a black ointment from a small white jar which bore the legend, 'For Man or Beast'.

He denied himself any pleasure he might have felt in touching her naked body, for that would have seemed wrong to him. When the wounds were all dressed he gave her an old-fashioned collarless shirt to wear for a nightdress and tucked her into bed. Only then did he allow himself the indulgence of thinking her pretty, seeing behind the cuts and swellings, the puffed eyelids, the tangled fair hair, a woman he might well have wished to invent.

She went to sleep almost immediately, her forehead marked with a frown.

He tiptoed noisily from the room and busied himself tidying up the kitchen in a haphazard fashion. But even while he worried over such problems as where to put a blackened saucepan his face broke continually into a grin. 'Well,' he said, 'wonders will never cease.'

When dinner came he presented her with two rainbow trout and a bowl of potatoes.

4.

It would be two days before she decided to talk and he passed these much as he would normally have, collecting the crayfish both morning and afternoon, gardening before lunch, fishing before dinner. Yet now he carried with him a new treasure, a warm white egg which he stored in some quiet dry part of his mind and as he worked his way down the rows of tomato plants, removing the small green grubs with his fingers, he smiled more often than he would have done otherwise.

When a shadow passed over the tangled garden and he looked up to admire the soft drift of a small white cloud, he did not look less long than he would have normally but there was another thing which danced around his joy, an aura of a brighter, different colour.

Yet he was, through force of habit, frugal with his emotions, and he did not dwell on the arrival of the girl. In fact the new entry into his life slipped his mind completely or was squeezed out by his concentration on the job at hand. But then, without warning, it would pop up again and then he would smile. 'Fancy that,' he'd say. Or: 'Well I never.'

The girl seemed to prefer staying in the house, sometimes reading, often sleeping with one of Dermott's neglected books clutched to her chest. The swellings were subsiding, revealing a rather dreamy face with a wide, sad mouth and slightly sleepy blue eyes. A haze of melancholy surrounded her. When she walked it was with the quiet distraction of a sleep-walker. When she sat, her slow eyes followed Dermott's progress as he moved to and fro across the room, carrying hot water from the fire to the grimy porcelain sink, washing a couple of dishes, or one knife or two forks, stewing peaches from the tree in the garden, brewing a herb tea with a slightly bitter flavour, sweeping the big flagstone floor while he spread dirt from his hob-nailed boots behind him, cleaning four bright-eyed trout, feeding the tame magpie that wandered in and out through the sunlit patch in the back door.

He whistled a lot. They were old-fashioned optimistic songs, written before she was born.

When, finally, she spoke, it was to talk about the sweeping.

'You're bringing more dirt in than you're sweeping out.'

He did not look surprised that she had spoken but he noticed the softness of her voice and hoarded it away with delight. He considered the floor, scratching his bristly head and rubbing his hand over his newly shaven chin. 'You're quite correct,' he said. He sat on the long wooden bench beneath the windows and began to take off his boots, intending to continue the job in stockinged feet.

'Here,' she said, 'give it to me.'

He gave her the broom. A woman's touch, he smiled, never having heard of women's liberation.

HE FOUND HER IN LATE SUMMER

5.

That night at dinnner she told him her story, leaning intently over the table and talking very softly.

It was beyond his experience, involving drugs, men who had abused her, manipulated her, and finally wished to kill her. He was too overwhelmed by it to really absorb it. He sat at the table absently cleaning a dirty fork with the table-cloth. 'Fancy that,' he would say. Or: 'You're better off now.' And again: 'You're better off without them, that's all.'

From the frequency of these comments she judged that he wished her to be quiet, but really they were produced by his feeling of inadequacy in the face of such a strange story. He was like a peasant faced with a foreigner who speaks with a strange accent, too overcome to recognise the language as his own.

What he did absorb was that Anna had been treated badly by the world and was, in some way, wounded because of it.

'You'll get better here,' he said, 'You've come to the right place.'

He smiled at her, a little shyly, she thought. For a brief instant she felt as safe and comfortable as she had ever been in her life and then fear and suspicion, her old friends, claimed her once more. Her skin prickled and the wind in the trees outside sounded forlorn and lonely.

She sat beside the kerosene lamp surrounded by shadows. That the light shone through her curling fair hair, that Dermott was almost unbearably happy, she was completely unaware.

6.

Weeks passed and the first chill of autumn lay along the river. Dermott slowly realised that Anna's recovery would not be as fast as he had imagined, for her lips remained sad and the sleepy eyes remained lustreless and defeated.

He brought things for her to marvel at: a stone, a dried-out frog, a beetle with a jewel-like shell, but she did not welcome the interruptions and did not try to hide her lack of interest so he stood there with the jewel in his hand feeling rather stupid.

He tried to interest her in the river, to give to her the pleasure the old inspector had given him, but she stood timidly on the bank wearing a dress she had made from an old sheet, staring anxiously at the ground around her small flat feet.

He stood in the water wearing only baggy khaki shorts and a battered pair of tennis shoes. She thought he looked like an old war photo.

'Nothing's going to bite you,' he said, 'You can stand in the water.'

'No,' she shook her head.

'I'll teach you how to catch crays.'

'No.'

'That's a silky oak.'

She didn't even look where he pointed. 'You go. I'll stay here.'

He looked up at the sky with his hands on his hips. 'If I go now I'll be away for two hours.'

'You go,' she insisted. The sheet dress made her look as sad as a little girl at bedtime.

'You'll be lonely. I'll be thinking that you're lonely,' he explained, 'so it won't be no fun. Won't you be lonely?'

She didn't say no. She said, 'You go.'

And he went, finally, taking that unsaid no with him aware that his absence was causing her pain. He was distracted and cast badly. When a swarm of caddis flies hatched over a still dark pool he did not stay to cast there but pushed on home with the catch he had: two small rainbows. He had killed them without speaking to them.

He found her trying to split firewood, frowning and breathing hard.

'You're holding the axe wrong,' he said, not unkindly.

'Well how should I hold it then?'

She stood back with her hands on her hips. He showed her how to do it, trying to ignore the anger that buzzed around her.

'That's what I was doing,' she said.

He retired to tend the garden and she thought he was angry with her for intruding into his territory. She did not know that his mother had been what they called 'a woman stockman' who was famous for her toughness and self-reliance. When she saw him watching her she thought it was with disapproval. He was keeping an anxious eye on her, worried that she was about to chop a toe off.

7.

'Come with me.'

'No, you go.'

That is how it went, how it continued to go. A little litany.

'Come, I'll teach you.'

'I'm happy here.'

'When I get back you'll be unhappy.'

Over and over, a pebble being washed to and fro in a rocky hole.

'I can't enjoy myself when you're unhappy.'

'I'm fine.'

And so on, until when he waded off downstream he carried her unhappiness with him and a foggy film lay between him and the river.

The pattern of his days altered and he in no way regretted the change. Like water taking the easiest course down a hillside, he moved towards those things which seemed most likely to minimise her pain. He helped her on projects which she deemed to be important, the most pressing of which seemed to be the long grass which grew around the back of the house. They denuded the wild vegetable garden of its dominant weed. He had never cared before and had let it grow beside the tomatoes, between the broad leaves of the pumpkin, and left it where it would shade the late lettuce.

As he worked beside her it did not occur to him that he was, in fact, less happy than he had been, that his worry about her happiness had become the dominant factor of his life, clouding his days and nagging at him in the night like a sore tooth. Yet even if it had occurred to him, the way she extended her hand to him one evening and brought him silently to her bed with a soft smile on her lips, would have seemed to him a joy more complex and delightful than any of those he had so easily abandoned.

He worked now solely to bring her happiness. And if he spent many days in shared melancholy with her there were also rewards of no small magnitude: a smile, like a silver spirit breaking the water, the warmth of her warm white body beside him each morning.

He gave himself totally to her restoration and in so doing became enslaved by her. Had he been less of an optimist he would have abandoned the project as hopeless.

And the treatment was difficult, for she was naked and vulnerable, not only to him, to the world, but to all manner of diseases which arrived, each in their turn, to lay her low. In moments of new-found bitterness he reflected that these diseases were invited in and made welcome, evidence of the world's cruelty to her, but these thoughts, alien to his nature and shocking for even being thought, were banished and put away where he could not see them.

HE FOUND HER IN LATE SUMMER

She lay in his bed pale with fever. He picked lad's love, thyme, garlic and comfrey and ministered to her with anxious concern.

'There,' he said, 'that should make you better.'

'Do you love me, Dermott?' she asked, holding his dry dusty hand in her damp one. They made a little mud between them.

He was surprised to hear the word. It had not been in his mind, and he had to think for a while about love and the different things he understood by it.

'Yes,' he said at last, 'I do.'

He felt then that he could carry her wounded soul from one end of the earth to the other. He was bursting with love.

8.

As he spent more and more time dwelling with her unhappiness he came to convince himself that he was the source of much of her pain. It was by far the most optimistic explanation, for he could do nothing to alter her past even if he had been able to understand it. So he came to develop a self-critical cast of mind, finding fault with himself for being stubborn, silent, set in his ways, preferring to do a thing the way he always had rather than the way she wished.

Eager to provide her with companionship he spent less and less time on the river, collecting the crays just once, early in the morning while she slept. In this way he lost many but this no longer seemed so important.

When she picked up a book to read in the afternoons he did likewise, hoping to learn things that he might share with her. He felt himself unlettered and ignorant. When he read he followed the lines of words with his broken-nailed finger and sometimes he caught her watching his lips moving and he felt ashamed. He discovered things to wonder at in every line and he often put his book down to consider the things he had found out. He would have liked to ask Anna many things about what he read but he imagined that she found his questions naive and irritating and did not like to be interrupted. So he passed over words he did not understand and marvelled in confused isolation at the mysteries he found within each page.

The True Nature of Vampires had been written long ago by a certain A. A. Dickson, a man having no great distinction in the world of the occult, whose only real claim to public attention had been involved with extracting twenty thousand pounds from lonely old women. Needless to say none of this was mentioned in the book.

Dermott, sitting uncomfortably on a hard wooden bench, looked like a farmer at a stock sale. He learned that vampirism does not necessarily involve the sucking of blood from the victim (although this often is the case) but rather the withdrawal of vital energy, leaving the victim listless, without drive, prey to grey periods of intense boredom.

On page ten he read, 'The case of Thomas Deason, a farmer in New Hampshire provides a classic example. In the spring of 1882 he befriended a young woman who claimed to have been beaten and abandoned by her husband. Deason, known to be of an amiable disposition, took the woman into his home as a housekeeper. Soon the groom and farm workers noticed a change in Deason: he became listless and they remarked on the "grey pallor of his skin". The groom, who was a student of such matters, immediately suspected vampirism and using rituals similar to those described in the Dion Fortune episode drove the woman from the house. It was, however, too late to save Deason who had already become a Vampire himself. He was apprehended in a tavern in 1883 and brought to trial. After his conviction and execution there was still trouble in the area and it was only after a stake was driven through the heart of his exhumed corpse in 1884 that things returned to normal in the area.'

One night, when making love, Anna bit him passionately on the neck. He leapt from her with a cry and stood shivering beside the bed in the darkness.

Suspicion and fear entered him like worms, and a slow anger began to spread through him like a poison, nurtured and encouraged each day by further doses of A. A. Dickson's musty book. His mind was filled with stories involving marble slabs, bodies that did not decompose, pistol wounds and dark figures fleeing across moonlit lawns.

His eyes took on a haunted quality and he was forever starting and jumping when she entered the room. As he moved deeper and deeper into the book his acknowledgment of his own unhappiness became unreserved. He felt that he had been tricked. He saw that Anna had taken from him his joy in the river, turned the tasks he had enjoyed into chores to be endured.

He began to withdraw from her, spending more and more time by himself on the river, his mind turning in circles, unable to think what to do. He moved into another bed and no longer slept with her. She did not ask him why. This was certain proof to him that she already knew.

Yet his listlessness, his boredom, his terrible lethargy did not decrease, but rather intensified.

When the jeep arrived to pick up the crayfish its driver was staggered to see the haunted look in Dermott's eyes and when he went back to town he told his superiors that there was some funny business with a woman down at Enoch's Point. The superiors, not having seen the look in Dermott's eyes, smiled and clucked their tongues and said to each other: 'That Dermott, the sly old bugger.'

9.
He had nightmares and cried in his sleep. He dreamed he had made a silver stake and driven it through her heart. He dreamed that she cried and begged him not to, that he wept too, but that he did it anyway driven by steel wings of fear. He shrieked aloud in his sleep and caused the subject of his dreams to lie in silent terror in her bed, staring into the blackness with wide open eyes.

He thought of running away, of leaving the river and finding a new life somewhere else, and this is almost certainly what he would have done had he not, returning from a brooding afternoon beside the river, discovered the following note: 'Dear Dermott, I am leaving because you do not like me any more and I know that I am making you unhappy. I love you. Thank you for looking after me when I was sick. I hate to see you unhappy and I know it is me that is doing it.' It was signed: 'With all the love in my heart, Anna.'

The words cut through him like a knife, slicing away the grey webs he had spun around himself. In that moment he recognised only the truth of what she wrote and he knew he had been duped, not by her, but by a book.

It was evening when he found her, sitting on the bank of a small creek some three miles up the jeep track. He said nothing, but held out his hand. They walked back to the river in darkness.

He did not doubt that she was a vampire, but he had seen something that A. A. Dickson with his marble tombs and wooden stakes had never seen: that a vampire feels pain, loneliness and love. If vampires fed on other people, he reflected, that was the nature of life: that one creature drew nourishment and strength from another.

When he took her to his bed and embraced her soft white body he was without fear, a strong animal with a heavy udder.

The Ultimate Act of Living
Eric Rolls

The pleasure is unimaginable. No matter how many times one makes love, realisation is greater than expectation. I suppose it is the same as the pain of childbirth: the experience is so almighty that it is remembered at a lower level until it is experienced again.

Whoever made the world—whether male, female or a supreme, disembodied intelligence—exceeded the capacity of gods in the design of reproduction. When it was done, Hir looked at the work and said: 'I did not plan this, or that, or that. I am proud. And somewhat uneasy.'

Derogatory words for sex have always repelled me, 'a dirty weekend', 'a naughty', 'a good fuck', 'a bit on the side', 'muff diving', so many. They express an incapacity for life. I believe that celebration is the profoundest expression of gratitude for being alive and lovemaking is the ultimate act of celebration.

The standard emblems, the penis rampant and the vulva couchant, that appear in red ochre and white clay in cave drawings thousands of years old and in white chalk on brick walls today, reveal no more than a flag reveals the people of its country. The infinity of detail is missing.

The attention paid to the penis as propagator is ridiculous. For all its flamboyance, fifteen centimetres of penis has the same number of nerve endings as fifteen millimetres of clitoris. The penis can create nothing, neither child, nor joy, nor relief, nor encouragement, without the flaring funnel of the inner lips to direct it and the pulsating channel of the vagina to receive it. The most marvellous event of orgasm is not the penis spurting but the upside-down parrot beak of the cervix dipping into the pool of semen. Havelock Ellis wrote about it, quoting a doctor who observed it with special equipment almost a hundred years ago. Now it has been filmed.

The whole of a woman's body organises this movement, her eyes, her cheeks, her breasts, her thighs, her womb, her ovaries, all the muscles of her pelvis. She throbs and her womb feeds. The first four or five dips of the cervix are quick and hungry. It takes more than it can hold and semen drips back into the pool from its sides as it tosses each beakful on its way. Then it grows less hungry and the dips become tentative and spaced seconds apart. The last, perhaps the twenty-fifth, is little more than a token gesture.

But the winning spermatozoon, the one out of hundreds of millions to fertilise the egg, might have missed most of this urgent event. Hours later it might have swum up from the vestibule of the vagina, dodging its dead compatriots, the disabled without any tail, the deformed with two tails, the fools swimming the wrong way, until it had to make its own entrance through the cervix into the uterus. Then it shouldered its way up a Fallopian tube already crammed with hopefuls until it reached the goal, where it hammered its head so vigorously against the egg, already spiked with a dozen sperm who had got halfway in, that the egg opened, received it and sealed again.

Although Elaine and I can no longer produce children, these events still take place. All that is missing is the finale, the fertilisation. It astonishes me, the amount of liquid we produce together, far more than either of us can produce alone. 'Where does it all come from? Look at the bed!' 'Not from me.' 'Nor me.'

Lovemaking is not only the meeting of temporarily solid flesh but an organisation of liquids so complicated that their formulae are still beyond human capacity. The first clear, viscous emission from the erect penis still amazes me, it is so wondrously slippery. It rolls up in beads, sometimes it flows a little. One is unaware of any muscle moving but one can feel its passage up the full length of the urethra. It seems a distillation of excitement. Its purpose is mainly antacid, the texture is a bonus.

The female fluids are less viscous and of more than one kind. One set of glands invitingly smears the vestibule with a light, antacid lubricant, the vagina sweats an alkaline fluid until it is deep enough for sperm to swim in. They are projected from the penis in a carrying fluid that holds them alive but inert. As the male and female fluids blend, stirred together a little by the withdrawing penis, the sperm come to life. Tails lash, the rush for life is on.

There are some women who have a gland—undeveloped in the majority—that squirts yet another liquid out of the urethra at the time of orgasm. I have not seen it. That is one of my immense curiosities about sex that has never been satisfied. Havelock Ellis and others have written about a South African race who perform what they call 'spray the wall'. The women teach maturing girls how to develop their pelvic muscles and how to masturbate. They station the girls a metre or so from a wall and the girls practise until they eject with enough force to hit it. And then other races practise the appalling operation of clitoridectomy so that the women experience no sexual enjoyment.

One reads often that it is rare for a woman to have an orgasm during lovemaking, that the clitoris is not positioned to receive sufficient stimulation. The head of the penis can pull on the inner lips, tightening them on the hood of the clitoris, sliding the hood along it and across it, relaxing it, teasing again. Surely the flaring glans exists for just that purpose. And after several minutes of that it is easy to shift position a little so that the head of the clitoris slides along the shaft of the penis. With each downstroke the clitoris pushes down, lifts with the upstroke. Neither of us can maintain that sensation for long. The penis spouts gratitude and the pulsating walls of the vagina grip it thankyou.

I have known two vital women with whom it seemed, it seems, normal for lovemaking to produce orgasm, my first wife Joan Stephenson, and now Elaine van Kempen. With Joan I built books and a farm and three remarkable children and led the sort of life that seemed impossible until I met her. Most women of the 1950s had domestic ideas. Joan was a pharmacist who intended to remain her own person although she bowed to convention enough to change her name. Our lives were stimulating not stultifying.

When Joan died the future seemed to be work with no compensation. Then came Elaine van Kempen, a heritage consultant and researcher of history, with four remarkable children and a determination to keep her name. Life became joy again, a different stimulation, my world wa normal.

With Elaine I am building more books and we are now remodelling a 1940s house that she found for sale in nearby town. An expert removalist brought it to our bloc of land in two pieces and joined it together with exquisit accuracy, rolling it on little caterpillar tracks. Now it is raised on steel piers and storerooms are being built under it and rooms extended on top. The carpenters are at work as I write. It is a dream of thirty years, to go fishing after a day's writing. There is an oyster lease thirty metres from our still-to-be-erected front entrance and fish in an unpolluted inlet as innocent and plentiful as those of the 1950s. When the house is finished in a couple of months, Elaine and I will make love in every room to condition it. Houses respond to attention.

One of my first jobs in the new writing room (which will still bear the old oak writing table that I have sat at for twenty-six years) will be to write a book on food and wine: of wine that tells of a March morning in the Hunter valley twenty-five years before the cork is drawn or a champagne that sings of fifteen years in French caves, and of food that acknowledges its origins like a four-year-old wether off Riverina saltbush or potatoes, white, black, purple, yellow with dirt on their skins, or of Gloucester Old Spot pigs that have fed on windfall apples.

All the family can cook, all nine of us. Cooking is not a domestic task, food is another of life's glories. Elaine and I will put in a big Zanussi commercial stove to write the book. It will sing of Italy as we work. Food and lovemaking go together. The mouth knows how to appreciate marvels. The tongue is the best instrument for stroking flesh, the lips the best instrument for massaging the delicate extensions.

In the book *Citizens* that I have just finished writing I completed the story of the Chinese and Australia. Naturally I dealt with their attitude to sex since it is as important to understanding a people as language and art. And one of their old books advises that a man should enjoy the great medicines of the three mountain peaks, a woman's saliva taken from the Red Lotus Peak, her tongue, the energy sucked from the Double Lotus Peak, her breasts, and the effusions from the Mysterious Gateway or the Lair of the White Tiger that lies below the Peak of the Purple Fungus, her *mons veneris*. The luxuriant pubic hair usually extends from the vulva in a narrow black rectangle, it does not spread into the European map of Tasmania.

They had richly imaginative names for all the sexual functions and all the parts of the body. Feminists would object to the description of the clitoris as 'the man in the boat', though they would not object to calling its hood 'the jewel box'. The clitoris is small in most Chinese women, indeed, the majority of Chinese men are strangely repelled by a big clitoris. However, the unevenly scalloped inner lips are well developed and, when they are excited, they flare into an impressive ruff known as the 'cockscomb'. That sounds like a pun in English but neither Mandarin nor Cantonese, the languages of punning, allows for a pun here. The meaning is simply 'the comb of a rooster'. The groove below the clitoris is the 'golden gully', the vestibule is 'the examination hall'. 'Jade veins' lead to the perineum.

The penis is a jade stalk and it plucks the strings of the lute, the inner lips. To make love is 'to perfect joy' or 'the ecstasy of hovering between life and death' or to experience 'clouds and rain'. The positions for making love, thirty-six in all in one of the illustrated books, bear such wonderful names as the fluttering butterfly in search of flowers, the queen bee making honey, the lost bird finding its way back to its nest in the thicket, the hungry horse galloping to the feed crib. And when the lovers are sated they lie together like 'dragons weary of battle'.

Despite their imagery the Chinese have been no more comfortable with sex than any other race. Lust is defined as a knife which hacks the bones. At times Chinese men have been seized by a ludicrous mass obsession that their penises were receding into their groins. Great fear does cause an uncomfortable shrinkage of the penis—soldiers commented on it during World War II—so the fears of a few spread quickly to hysterical hundreds. There was an outbreak in Singapore in 1967. Young men went to hospital in cars and ambulances with weights dangling from glandes, with string knotted to foreskins, even with safety pins pierced through. Grandmothers, the accustomed carers, sat beside some youths with chopsticks clamped behind exposed coronas.

An old Taoist belief held that a man absorbed vital energy from the fluids of a woman's orgasm but that he lost it if he ejaculated, so that a man who could bring several of his wives and concubines and servants to orgasm on the one night by measured thrusting—with practice he should be able to manage a thousand strokes—was assured of good health. The idea of *coitus reservatus* is still prevalent in many countries. But the advised climax to the long Chinese exercise was dangerous. As the man was about to ejaculate he had to press down on the duct between his scrotum and his anus, even clamp the thumb of his other hand over the eye of the penis, and 'the Yellow River would flow back to its source', his semen would travel through his spinal cord to his brain. The only place it could possibly go was into his bladder which meant intolerable strain on vital valves.

All the openness, much of the delight in sex in China is in the past. The puritanism of the Manchu dynasties followed by the extreme puritanism and population restraints of the Communists interfered with Chinese morals as much as the grim Victorians interfered with England's. It was over-reaction. It curbed licentiousness which had certainly become extravagant, then curbed natural lovemaking along with it. Sex became not only difficult but dirty, something to be discouraged. It had led to desperate unhappiness in both men and women, to widespread sexual incompetence.

The Gold Lotus, a great novel, accommodated sex exactly and naturally, yet few Chinese have ever had the chance to read it. In modern China none but a handful of scholars even know that the book exists. It was probably written in the sixteenth century. The author fixed its time in the twelfth century, the Sung Dynasty, but the setting is at the time of writing. He is not definitely known: novels were not regarded as literature and no records were kept of them. It is a supreme work—a big cast lead lives astonishingly corrupt, even murderous, in business and in private. It is a comedy of manners on a grand scale, probably the deepest accounting of a culture that there is. The characters portray in intimate detail their houses, food, furniture, clothes, jewellery, musical instruments, language, births, deaths, religion, the grades of society, sex.

Hsi-Men Ch'ing, a young man with a considerable estate, gives himself up to pleasure, wine and women mostly. In a poem on the first page the author warns that such a life leads to ruin.

She is beautiful, this girl. Her form, her manner promise gracious womanhood.
A double blade hangs between her thighs on which a foolish man
will spill his blood.

The sexual antics of the whole cast are treated so frankly that when Clement Egerton translated the work into English in 1939 he put big slabs of it into Latin. It is only in recent times that translations have been able to be published. Hsi-men is cruel. He whips his wives, he has servants beaten till their flesh hangs from them. He spends days at a time in bawdy houses then comes home drunk to his six scheming wives. He enters his wives and their servants by their front doors and their back doors. Some protest about rear entry but Porphyry, his mistress and the wife of his clerk, especially enjoys the approach of the flowering branch to the full moon, her buttocks. He urinated in the women's mouths when it was too cold to get out of bed. 'Do you like it?' 'It is a little bitter'. Folded in a silk handkerchief that he carries in his sleeve are a silver clasp that clamps to the base of his penis and holds it engorged, a silken cord for the same purpose, a ring of sulphur that he slides down to the silver clamp both to increase the diameter of his penis and to inflame the women as it moistens and dissolves, and a box of pills and a red powder given him by a wandering Indian monk to improve his performance. The monk gave him strict instructions that he was never to take an overdose.

If he pays them enough attention, if he gives them enough presents, the women meet him on equal footing. Here I wished to quote a passage but the translation that I was reading had so many strictures—it seemed that the reproduction of one sentence required publisher's consent and a cheque—that I turned to the 1939 edition with the slabs of Latin and got out my fifty-five-year-old school dictionary, an astonishingly comprehensive one for the time of publication. It was an interesting exercise and I was delighted to find that my translation was the better. *Caesar de Bello Gallico*, which we studied at some length at Fort Street Boys' High School, although it contained fascinating detail about his conduct of war, including taking elephants over the Pyrenees, did not arouse us with anything like this.

Golden Lotus, the fifth wife of Hsi-Men Ch'ing, 'had undressed until not a thread of silk remained on her body. She lay on her back, her scarlet sandals still on her feet, fanning herself with a white silk fan to relieve the heat.' Hsi-men 'took off his clothes, sat on a stool and stretched his toes to feel the heart of her beautiful flower. Evidence of her arousal exuded from her as the slime from a snail making its silver and sinuous way. Hsi-men took off her ornate scarlet sandals, unwound the ends of the ribbons that bound her feet and tied them to the trellis so that she looked like a golden dragon with its claw unsheathed. The gate to her womanhood was open and its watchful guard overlooked a dark red valley.'

Hsi-men was interrupted by Plum Blossom, a servant bringing wine. She ran away, Hsi-men chased her and carried her back to watch him play the game of Striking the Silver Swan with a Golden Ball. He took up an iced bowl with three plums in it, sat on a chair at a distance from Golden Lotus and cast the plums at her vulva. One stuck in it. Golden Lotus pleaded to be released. Hsi-men ignored her. He commanded Plum Blossom to fan him, pour him wine, then he went to sleep. Plum Blossom escaped again. He woke after an hour or so and remembering the now distressed Golden Lotus, engaged her so vigorously that he broke his sulphur ring. She fainted and in some alarm he untied her and called Plum Blossom and Chrysanthemum, another maid, to help her to her room.

Such abandonment had to meet a just end. After a night of prolonged lovemaking with Porphyry, Hsi-men got drunk and rode home to Golden Lotus who was randy after days of inattention. He went to bed and went to sleep. Golden Lotus lay naked beside him trying to arouse his tipsy penis. She shook him awake and asked him where his medicine was. The last four pills were in a little gold box. She took one, then she gave the others to Hsi-men in a cup of wine. It was three times the correct dose. His penis stiffened, she tightened the silk cord on its base and rode it till she had soaked five handkerchiefs with her effusions. He could get no relief. He asked her to untie the cord but his penis would not subside. She sucked it at his urgent bidding and semen squirted in quantities she could not swallow. Sudden spurts of blood followed, then a continuous flow. When his penis began to hiss cold air, Hsi-men fainted. He died within days and his evil household disintegrated until it was restored by the Moon Lady, a good woman who had been his principal wife.

A circle of wives and concubines trivialises lovemaking as nightingales' tongues trivialise food. Sex is too important and too intimate to make it a general thing just as food is too important to degrade with something that has no relevance beyond scarcity. I do not wish to eat a steak from a frozen mastodon or to find three women in our bed. Sex ought never to be tragic, it is too beautiful an experience. Animals exhibit every human facet of the relationship.

I have watched wonderfully delicate foreplay from an animal that one does not associate with gentleness at all, a very big goanna. When raiding a bird's nest, these ruthless creatures ignore the cries and wing claps of the frantic parents, they ignore the alarm calls of the young, they seize them one by one and swallow them with no more than one chomp to still them on the way down. Yet this male was chinning the spiny back of the female. They were on the trunk of a tree no more than a metre off the ground and both were so engrossed that, although they are usually cautious, they did not see me standing close and watching. His chin made scratching noises on her scales. It seemed to be part of the play as he made long, steady strokes out and in, up and down her spine. Then he began to lick her lips and under her eyes and down her side. His tongue rasped too, even on the scales around her cloaca which he circled gently. She turned a little to present it to him. Then his right penis everted and he moved up over her back, twisted and inserted it.

The penises of snakes and lizards are known by the belittling name of hemipenes, which is not fair. Reptiles have two complete penises, one for this time, one for next, and some of them have a remarkable complication of appendages on the tip. A dried tiger's penis that the Chinese once sold for medicine (unfortunately it would sometimes still be accurate to say 'sell for medicine' though it is now done secretly) is a vicious-looking instrument fitted with two-centimetre backward-sloping barbs along fifteen centimetres of the tip. It looks like a spearhead. When alive those gristly extensions that erect with the penis must be decidedly more stimulating to the tigress than a mere thin prong. The penis of a Yellow-footed Marsupial Mouse splits into two parts at the end. It is a long penis for a small creature, at least two centimetres, and the prongs on the end extend it by eight millimetres. He inserts it so deeply that these prongs reach right into the horns of the womb.

Theirs is a savage mating. The female mouse can ovulate only when under shock, so the male grabs her by the neck, throws her about, then seizes the skin above her shoulder in his teeth and mounts. He rides her for about twenty minutes and if she tries to pull away, he will tear strips of skin off. The females survive this awful treatment, the males of some species expend so much energy that they die soon after.

Male hairy flower wasps take great care of the females. The winged males approach the wingless females as they are feeding on nectar. When a male is accepted, he mates, then he carries the female off to find the larva of a Christmas beetle or other scarab on which their larvae feed. Somehow they can detect the grub a few centimetres underground. The male lowers the female to the ground, she scratches down to the grub, deposits an egg inside it, then the male carries her back to her favourite shrub. He can carry her up to 200 metres. If he has to fly that distance, he needs the rest while she is digging so that he can carry her back.

The amazing reproduction of ferns is regarded by botanists as primitive. Ferns developed millions of years before flowering plants, even more millions of years before mammals. Yet it seems to me that their reproduction is so advanced that they showed the way to mammals. Some of the leaflets on a frond develop spore capsules under them. These capsules split and fling out the spores which are about one tenth of a millimetre in diameter. The spores germinate and form fleshy, heart-shaped, flat green prothalli one to five millimetres across on which male and female sex organs develop at different sites. The female organs have an egg at the bottom of an irregular tube. On a dewy morning or a rainy day, the male organs burst and scatter active sperm over the ground. Those that land on a damp prothallus lash their long coiled tails, swim to the female organs then down the tubes to the eggs. Millions lash themselves to futile death among the forest litter.

Egrets acknowledge mating time by a change of plumage, a subtle manifestation of need. As I write, the beaks of cattle egrets have changed from yellow to red and their once white necks, breasts and backs glow with orange yellow. These migratory birds have now stationed themselves with cattle around the whole coast of Australia, following the beasts about to eat the insects that the cattle disturb while grazing. Little egrets, graceful birds with long thin black legs and black beaks, do not colour their dazzling white, but grow long delicate plumes from the back of the head, from under the lower neck and from the lower back. When the birds alight on ground or branch the plumes shiver like exquisitely delicate veils.

The huge males of the Australian Bustard standing up to 1.5 metres tall and weighing fourteen kilograms, the heaviest of flying birds, have to put on a fantastic display to attract a female. A bird takes up position on a mound where he can be seen from a distance, then he begins to stamp, to roar like a distant lion and to extend a bright red cheek pouch which stretches until it almost touches his toes. There could be four or five males on mounds several hundred metres apart. The smaller females stride about, beaks held up at an angle of forty-five degrees. They study each male at a distance, sometimes walk up for a closer inspection, then make a choice.

Many species of male frogs have inflatable pouches under the lower jaw that act as such efficient amplifiers that their calls can be heard more than a kilometre away. The males station themselves according to species where females might expect to find them, in damp grass, on the branch of a tree, on the edge of water, in reeds, they blow up their pouches which can be almost as big as their bodies, then they croak. They do nothing more, they squat in one place and croak. A female will spend several nights moving about among them, listening and deciding. When she has made up her mind, she hops to the chosen mate and presents herself, whereupon he makes an impassioned leap on to her back. Alas, the male is completely unselective. He does not notice the female at all. If one rolls a table tennis ball under him he will grasp it as eagerly. But he does take great care of the eggs as the female lays them, shepherding them with his hind legs as he squirts semen over them. The male of one species of small frog that lives in damp vegetation has pockets on his hind legs to receive the eggs. He picks them up carefully, fills his pocket and holds them there until they hatch.

I brought my books to Elaine. What else was there? They are my cheek pouch, my attractive plumage, my croak.

THE ULTIMATE ACT OF LIVING

Without my words I do not exist. Without Elaine I would exist imperfectly.

The symbol of life is not the penis, not the vulva, but a woman's breasts. I never tire of feeling them, mouthing them, watching them move. They act independently or together, erecting, collapsing. The areolae grow dark, draw in and crinkle roughly, they relax and spread out as smooth, browny-pink circles. To watch a nipple thrusting towards a baby's mouth is a marvel as old as humankind and as recent. What is the greatest image of all? The tracery of blue veins on a swollen breast.

Acknowledgements

Acknowledgements are due to the following authors, publishers and agents for permission to include the following stories:

'Upstream' © Ian Beck 1986, from *The Diver's Reluctance to Ascend*, Angus & Robertson, reproduced here with the permission of the author and Margaret Connolly Associates.

'He Found Her in Late Summer' © Peter Carey 1979, from *War Crimes*, University of Queensland Press.

'Ngomo Manza' © Tom Carment, first published in slightly different form in *Days and Nights in Africa*, Public Pictures, 1985.

'Baby Oil' © Robert Drewe 1983, from *The Bodysurfers* by permission of Pan Macmillan Australia Pty Ltd.

'Three Ways' © Gerard Lee 1993, from *Eating Dog*, University of Queensland Press.

'Ex-Wife Re-Wed' © Frank Moorhouse 1988, from *Forty-Seventeen*, Viking Books.

'Running Hot and Cold' © Chad Taylor 1995, from *The Man Who Wasn't Feeling Himself*, David Ling Publishing Ltd., NZ, with permission of the publishers and Michael Gifkins & Associates.

'His Eternal Boy' © Peter Wells 1994, from *The Duration of a Kiss*, Reed Publishing NZ, with permission of the publishers and Michael Gifkins & Associates.

'Neighbours' © Tim Winton 1985, from *Scission*, McPhee Gribble.

'Japan' © William Yang 1994, from *Fruit*, Blackwattle Press.

List of Contributors

Venero Armanno was born in Brisbane in 1959. After studying he spent ten years working in the computer industry. His first book of stories was *Jumping at the Moon* (1989) followed by the novels *The Lonely Hunter* (1993), *Romeo of the Underworld* (1994) and *My Beautiful Friend* (Random House 1995).

Ian Beck was born in Sydney in 1946. He has worked as a journalist, encyclopedia salesman, storeman and packer, clerk and builder's labourer. His first collection of stories, *The Diver's Reluctance to Ascend*, was nominated for the 1986 NSW Premier's Literary Award and the 1986 Commonwealth Literary Prize. His second collection was *Jumping the Chasm*.

John Birmingham is on the run from some mistakes he made in Queensland. He is the author of *He Died With a Felafel in His Hand*, *The Search For Savage Henry* and *How to Be a White Man*. He has written for a number of pornographic magazines including *Playboy*, *Penthouse* and *Inside Sport*. Sometimes he writes for less pornographic magazines, such as *The Independent Monthly*, *Juice* and *Rolling Stone*.

Peter Carey's books have received international acclaim and won many awards. They include *The Fat Man in History*, *War Crimes*, *Bliss*, *Illywhacker*, *Oscar and Lucinda* (which won the Booker Prize in 1989), *The Tax Inspector* and *The Unusual Life of Tristan Smith*. He presently lives in New York City.

Tom Carment was born in Sydney in 1954. As a painter, mainly of landscapes and portraits, he has been exhibiting regularly in Sydney for twenty years. His collection of writings, paintings and drawings, *Days and Nights in Africa*, was published by Public Pictures in 1985.

LIST OF CONTRIBUTORS

James Cockington grew up in Adelaide and now lives in Sydney. After a brief, unsuccessful career as a shoe designer he now works as a writer of books, films and newspaper columns. Previous books include *Mondo Weirdo* and *Mondo Bizarro*, personalised histories of the 60s and 70s, and *He Did it Her Way*, the biography of Australia's foremost drag artiste, Carlotta. His hobby is competing in demolition derbys and he has a tattoo of a cigar-smoking woodpecker on his left arm.

Matthew Condon was born in Brisbane in 1962. He has written four novels, *The Motorcycle Cafe* (1988), *Usher* (1991), *The Ancient Guild of Tycoons* (1994), and his latest, *A Night at the Pink Poodle*, which explores the life and loves of Icarus, the premier penthouse salesman on the Gold Coast.

Christopher Cyrill's first novel, *The Ganges and its Tributaries*, was published in 1993 and was shortlisted for both the NSW and Victorian Premier's Awards. In 1994 he won the Marten Bequest travelling scholarship and travelled in England, France and India. He lives in Melbourne and is working full-time on his second novel.

John Dale was born in Sydney and grew up in Tasmania. His novel *Dark Angel* was published in Australia and England in 1995. He lives in Sydney.

Julian Davies was born in Melbourne in 1954 and is the author of three novels, *Revival House* (1991), *Love Parts* (1992) and *Moments of Pleasure* (1994). He is also a potter and painter, having run his own workshop and gallery in Canberra for over ten years. He lives in the tall forests on the Great Divide near Braidwood NSW.

Robert Drewe was born in Melbourne in 1943 and grew up in Western Australia. His four novels and two books of stories have received wide praise and several prizes. *The Bodysurfers* became

LIST OF CONTRIBUTORS

a best-seller and has been adapted for film, TV, radio and the stage. He is also a playwright and screenwriter and in 1992 was awarded an Australian Creative Artists Fellowship.

Jonathan Griffiths works mainly in the theatre, directing stage translations of real life dramas. 'Whisper It' was originally performed as 'Tristram's True Story', a monologue in *A Man's Affront*. He also drives taxis and teaches job skills to the unemployed.

Mike Johnson has published four books of fiction and three of poetry. His first novel, *The Shakespeare Company Plays Lear at Babylon*, was shortlisted for the NZ Book Awards. He lives on Waiheke Island in the north of New Zealand.

Steven Lang was born and raised in Scotland. He came to Australia in 1970, meaning to pass through, but stayed. He has earned a living as a roofing contractor, cook and tour guide and had work published in literary magazines and newspapers—but his primary role over the past seventeen years has been as a father.

Gerard Lee is the author of *True Love and How to Get It*, *Pieces For a Glass Piano*, *Troppo Man*, and *Eating Dog*. He won an AFI Best Screenplay Award for the film *Sweetie* which he co-wrote with Jane Campion, and has recently written and directed his first film, *All Men are Liars*.

Damien Lovelock is lead singer with The Celibate Rifles. He played right wing with Rose Bay Rugby Union 1960–68, and is an occasional sporting commentator on ABC radio JJJ. He is the proud and frequently dumbstruck/astonished father of Luke, reinventor of the long lost E-sus 4 guitar chord, and is pleased to be able to tell people he has met the Dalai Lama.

LIST OF CONTRIBUTORS

Roger McDonald writes novels, non-fiction, essays and screenplays covering a wide range of the Australian experience. His most recent novel, *Water Man*, was shortlisted for the 1994 Miles Franklin Prize and the NSW State Literary Awards. *Shearer's Motel* won the 1993 CUB Banjo Award for non-fiction, with an adaptation being filmed for the ABC TV series *Naked*. Other novels include *1915*, *Slipstream* and *Rough Wallaby*.

Lex Marinos was born in Wagga Wagga into a family of Greek cafe owners. He graduated with an Honours BA in Drama from the University of NSW and for the past 25 years has worked in radio, film, TV and theatre as an actor and director, and was co-writer of the Kennedy/Miller mini-series *Bodyline*. He is married with 4 children, 2 dogs, 10 fishing rods and 67 flying ducks (at last count) on the lounge room wall.

Frank Moorhouse's most recent book is *Grand Days*, a novel set at the League of Nations in Geneva in the 1920s. It has been widely praised in Australia, the UK and the US, and has been published in French translation. The story in this volume is from his book *Forty-Seventeen* which is linked to *Grand Days*.

Mark Mordue was born in Newcastle in 1960. He writes for many leading Australian magazines and newspapers, and is the editor of the bi-monthly *Australian Style*. He won a Human Rights Media Award for his article 'Lust For Life', on people living with HIV/AIDS, and received the inaugural 1994 Women And The Media Award for 'Pillars Of Strength', about Aboriginal and Torres Strait Island women.

David Owen migrated to Australia in 1985 and has been living near Hobart since 1990. His publications here and overseas include five novels and two novellas, including *Bitters End* and *South Arm*.

LIST OF CONTRIBUTORS

Eric Rolls was born at Grenfell NSW in 1923 and for almost forty years farmed at Boggabri, and later Baradine, NSW. His twelve books of history, poetry, children's verse and memoir have received many awards. His books include *They All Ran Wild*, *A Million Wild Acres*, *A Celebration of the Senses*, and *Sojourners*, the first volume of the story of the Chinese in Australia. The second volume, *Citizens*, will be published in 1996. Eric was awarded the Order of Australia in 1992.

John Stapleton was born in Bangalow NSW in 1952 and brought up in Sydney. He has had stage plays produced in Adelaide and Sydney and was a freelance journalist before spending seven years as a reporter on the *Sydney Morning Herald*. He presently works for the *Australian* in Sydney.

Angus Strachan was born in Sydney in 1965. His first novel was shortlisted for the *Australian*/Vogel Award in 1982, he has published stories and articles in magazines, made two short films, and in 1995 completed a play about men and intimacy called *The Boarding House*.

Chad Taylor has written the novels *Pack of Lies* and *Heaven* and the short film *Funny Little Guy*, and his stories have appeared in a number of magazines and anthologies. His collection of stories, *The Man Who Wasn't Feeling Himself* (David Ling Publishing Ltd.) was released in New Zealand in 1995.

Clinton Walker was born in Bendigo, Victoria, in 1957. His first book, *Highway to Hell*, a biography of rock icon Bon Scott, was published in 1994 and in the UK in 1995. *Football Life* will be published in 1996, and next will be a book about stock-car racing in Australia in the 1960s. He is married with a young daughter and lives in Sydney.

Archie Weller was born in Perth in 1957. His first novel, *The Day of the Dog*, was runner-up in the 1981 inaugural *Australian*/Vogel

Award. It was published in Australia in 1982, and subsequently in the USA and Holland, and was made into the 1992 film *Blackfellas*. His book of stories, *Going Home*, appeared in 1986, and his poem 'Frankie, My Man' was joint winner of the 1988 ABC Bicentennial Poetry Award. His novel, *The Land of the Golden Clouds* will be published by Allen & Unwin in 1996.

Peter Wells lives and works in Sydney and Auckland. His first book, *Dangerous Desires*, won the 1991 New Zealand Book Award. His second book is *The Duration of a Kiss*. He also wrote and directed the film *Desperate Remedies*.

Tim Winton was born in Perth in 1960 and has an international reputation as one of Australia's finest writers. He has published six novels, two collections of stories and four books for children. His first novel, *An Open Swimmer*, won the *Australian*/Vogel Award and he has twice won the Miles Franklin Award, for *Shallows* and *Cloudstreet*. His most recent novel, *The Riders*, was published in Australia and the UK in 1994, and in the USA in 1995.

William Yang was born in North Queensland and grew up on a tobacco farm in Dimbulah. He is third generation Australian Chinese and a well known freelance photographer. His books include *Sydney Diary* and *Starting Again*. He now mainly concentrates on performance monologues, which combine writing with slide projection and are presented in theatres. His third monologue, *Sadness*, has toured Australia, New Zealand, Hong Kong and England.